DORLAND'S

Cardiology
Word Book

for Medical
Transcriptionists

DORLAND'S

Cardiology Word Book

for Medical Transcriptionists

Series Editor
SHARON B. RHODES, CMT, RHIT

Edited & Reviewed by:
Mary David, CMT

W.B. SAUNDERS COMPANY
A Harcourt Health Sciences Company

Philadelphia London New York St. Louis Sydney Toronto

W.B. Saunders Company
A Harcourt Health Sciences Company

The Curtis Center
Independence Square West
Philadelphia, Pennsylvania 19106

Dorland's Cardiology Word Book for
Medical Transcriptionists   ISBN 0-7216-9151-X

Printed in the United States of America.

Last digit is the print number: 9 8 7 6 5 4 3 2 1

I am proud to present the *Dorland's Cardiology Word Book for Medical Transcriptionists* — the first of a series of word books compiled for the professional medical transcriptionist. For one hundred years, W.B. Saunders has published the *Dorland's Illustrated Medical Dictionary*. With the advent of medical transcription, it became the dictionary of choice for medical transcriptionists.

When approached last year to help develop a new series of word books for W.B. Saunders, I have to admit the thought absolutely overwhelmed me. The *Dorland's Illustrated Medical Dictionary* was one of my first book purchases when I began my transcription career over thirty years ago. To be invited to participate in this project is an honor I could never have imagined for myself!

Transcriptionists need and will continue to need trusted up-to-date resources to help them research difficult terms quickly. In developing the *Dorland's Cardiology Word Book for Medical Transcriptionists,* I had access to the entire *Dorland's* terminology database for the book's foundation. In addition to this immense database, a context editor, Mary David, CMT, a recognized expert in the field of cardiology transcription, was selected to review the material from the database, to contribute new and unique terms, and to remove outdated and obsolete ones. With Mary's extensive research and diligent work, I believe this to be the most up-to-date word book for the field of cardiology.

In developing the cardiology word book, I wanted the size to be manageable so the book would be easy to handle, with a durable, long-lasting binding, and using a type font large enough to read while providing extensive terminology.

Anatomical plates of the heart and cardiovascular system were added as well as identification of anatomical landmarks and major veins and arteries throughout the body.

Although I have tried to produce the most thorough word book for cardiology available to medical transcriptionists, it is difficult to include every term as the field of cardiology is constantly evolving.

As you discover new terms, please feel free to share them with me for inclusion in the next edition of the *Dorland's Cardiology Word Book for Medical Transcriptionists.*

I may be reached at the following e-mail address: Sharon@TheRhodes.com.

SHARON B. RHODES, CMT, RHIT
Brentwood, Tennessee

A
A band
A fib (atrial fibrillation)
A-line (arterial line)
A-mode
A point
A wave

A2 multipurpose catheter

A_2
aortic second sound
A_2 incisural interval
A_2 to opening snap interval

AA
ascending aorta

A–A interval

A_1–A_2 interval

AAA
abdominal aortic aneurysm

AAI
atrial demand–inhibited
AAI pacemaker
AAI pacing
AAI rate–responsive mode

AAI-RR pacing

AAT
atrial demand–triggered
AAT pacemaker
AAT pacing

abacterial thrombotic endocarditis

Abbe
A. flap
A. operation

Abbokinase
A. catheter
A. Open-Cath

Abbott infusion pump

abciximab

abdominal
a. angina
a. aorta
a. aortic aneurysm (AAA)
a. aortic aneurysmectomy
a. aortic counterpulsation device
a. aortic endarterectomy
a. aortography
a. bruit
a. heart
a. jugular test
a. left ventricular assist device
a. patch electrode
a. pocket
a. vascular retractor

abdominalis
aorta a.

abdominocardiac reflex

abdomino-jugular reflux

abdominothoracic
a. arch
a. pump

ABE
acute bacterial endocarditis

Abee support

Abell-Kendall equivalent

Abelson cannula

aberrancy
acceleration-dependent a.
atrial trigeminy with a.
bradycardia-dependent a.
deceleration-dependent a.
paradoxical a.
paroxysmal atrial tachycardia with a.
postextrasystolic a.
tachycardia-dependent a.

aberrant
a. artery

aberrant *(continued)*
    a. conduction
    a. QRS complex
    a. thyroid
    a. ventricular conduction

aberrantly conducted beat

aberration
    intraventricular a.
    nonspecific T wave a.
    ventricular a.

abetalipoproteinemia
    Bassen-Kornzweig a.
    familial a.

ABG
    arterial blood gas

Abiomed
    A. biventricular support
        system
    A. BVAD 5000 biventricular
        device
    A. Cardiac device

ablater
    radiofrequency a.

ablation
    Ablatr temperature control
        device a.
    accessory conduction a.
        (ACA)
    atrioventricular junction-
        al a.
    atrioventricular nodal a.
    a. catheter
    catheter-induced a.
    chemical a.
    continuous-wave laser a.
    coronary rotational a.
    direct-current shock a.
    electrical catheter a.
    endocardial catheter a.
    fast-pathway radiofre-
        quency catheter a.
    His bundle a.
    Kent bundle a.
    laser a.
    percutaneous radiofre-
        quency catheter a.

ablation *(continued)*
    radiofrequency a.
    RF a.
    rotational a.
    slow-pathway a.
    surgical a. of pathway
        tissue a.
    transcatheter a.
    transcoronary chemical a.
    transvenous a.

ablative
    a. cardiac surgery
    a. device
    a. laser angioplasty
    a. technique

abnormal
    a. cleavage of cardiac valve
    a. left axis deviation
    a. right axis deviation

abnormality
    akinetic wall motion a.
    atrioventricular conduc-
        tion a.
    baseline ST segment a.
    brisk wall motion a.
    clotting a.
    electrical activation a.
    figure-of-8 a.
    hemodynamic a.
    immunochemical a's
    left ventricular wall mo-
        tion a.
    lusitropic a.
    nonspecific T wave a.
    perfusion a.
    persistent wall motion a.
    regional wall motion a.
    sinus node/AV conduc-
        tion a.
    snowman a.
    transient wall motion a.
    ventricular depolariza-
        tion a.
    wall motion a.

aborted systole

abouchement

ABP
   arterial blood pressure

Abrahams sign

Abrams
   A. heart reflex
   A. needle
   A.-Lucas flap heart valve

abreuography

abscess
   aortic root a.
   Brodie a.
   embolic a.
   myocardial a.
   papillary muscle a.
   periaortic a.
   ring a.

absent
   a. breath sounds
   a. pericardium
   a. pulmonary valve
   a. respiration

absolute
   a. cardiac dullness (ACD)
   a. refractory period

absorbable
   a. gelatin film
   a. gelatin sponge
   a. sutures

absorption
   fluorescent treponemal an-
      tibody a. (FTA-ABS)
   net a.

acacia
   gum a.

acanthocytosis

acarbia

acardiotrophia

acaryote

accelerated
   a. conduction
   a. hypertension

accelerated *(continued)*
   a. idioventricular rhythm
   a. idioventricular tachycar-
      dia
   a. junctional rhythm

acceleration time

accelerator
   a. globulin (AcG) blood co-
      agulation factor
   proconvertin prothrombin
      conversion a.
   serum prothrombin con-
      version a.

accelerometer
   Caltrac a.

Accent-DG balloon

accentuated antagonism

access
   A-Port vascular a.
   Low Profile Port vascular a.
   side-entry a.
   venovenous a.
   venous a.

accessory
   a. arteriovenous connec-
      tion
   a. artery
   a. atrium
   a. conduction ablation
   a. cusp
   a. obturator artery
   a. pathway
   a. saphenous vein

accident
   cardiac a.
   cardiovascular a.
   cerebrovascular a. (CVA)

accidental murmur

accretio
   a. cordis
   a. pericardii

accrochage

Accucom cardiac output monitor

Accudynamic adjustable damping

Accufix
    A. pacemaker
    A. pacemaker lead

Acculith pacemaker

Accutorr
    A. A1 blood pressure monitor
    A. bedside monitor
    A. oscillometric device

Accutracker
    A. blood pressure device
    A. II ambulatory blood pressure monitor

ACD
    absolute cardiac dullness
    arrhythmia control device
        Rex-Q ACD
        ACD resuscitator

ACE
    angiotensin-converting enzyme
        ACE balloon
        ACE fixed-wire balloon catheter
        ACE inhibitor

Ace Cloud enhancer

ace of spades sign on angiogram

aceto-orcein

acetylcholine

acetylcholinesterase
    a. deficiency

acetyl-CoA

acetylcysteine

achalasia
    esophageal a.

Achiever
    A. balloon dilatation catheter
    A. balloon dilator

achromatin

achromatinic

achromatolysis

achromin

acid
    a.-base disorder
    a.-base imbalance
    a. phosphatase

acidemia

acid-fast bacilli (AFB)

acidic fibroblast growth factor (aFGF)

acidity
    total a.

acidosis
    hypercapnic a.
    hyperchloremic a.
    lactic a.
    metabolic a.

A–C interval

aCLa
    anticardiolipin antibodies

Acland
    A. microvascular clamp
    A.-Banis arteriotomy set
    A.-Buncke counterpressor

acleistocardia

Acosta disease

Acoustascope esophageal stethoscope

acoustic
    a. imaging
    a. impedance probe
    a. microscope
    a. shadowing

acoustic *(continued)*
  a. window

acquired ventricular septal defect

acquisition
  a. gate
  gated equilibrium ventriculography, frame-mode a.
  gated equilibrium ventriculography, list-mode a.
  multiple gated a. (MUGA)
  a. time

acrocyanosis

acrohypothermy

acromelalgia

acromegalic heart disease

acromegaly

acromioclavicular

acrotic

acrotism

ACS
  Advanced Cardiovascular Systems
  Advanced Catheter Systems
    ACS Angioject
    ACS angioplasty catheter
    ACS angioplasty Y connector
    ACS balloon catheter
    ACS Concorde over-the-wire catheter system
    ACS Endura coronary dilation catheter
    ACS Enhanced Torque 8/7.5 F Taper Tip catheter
    ACS exchange guidewire
    ACS extra-support guidewire

ACS *(continued)*
    ACS floppy tip guidewire
    ACS Gyroscan
    ACS Indeflator
    ACS JL4 French catheter
    ACS LIMA guidewire
    ACS microglide wire
    ACS Mini catheter
    ACS Multi-Link coronary stent
    ACS OTW Lifestream coronary dilatation catheter
    ACS OTW Photon coronary dilatation catheter
    ACS OTW Solaris coronary dilatation catheter
    ACS percutaneous introducer set
    ACS RX Lifestream coronary dilatation catheter
    ACS SULP II balloon

ACTH
  adrenocorticotropic hormone

α-actinin

actin
  a. monomer
  a.-myosin crossbridge

actinomycetoma

actinomycosis

action
  catecholamine a.
  mechanism of a.
  a. potential
  a. potential duration

activated
  a. balloon expandable intravascular stent
  a. clotting time (ACT)
  a. graft

activated *(continued)*
a. partial thromboplastin time (aPTT)

activation
eccentric atrial a.
length-dependent a.
a. map-guided surgical resection
myofilament contractile a.
a.-sequence mapping

activator
2-chain urokinase plasminogen a. (Tcu-PA)
plasminogen a.
recombinant tissue plasminogen a. (rt-PA)
recombinant tissue-type plasminogen a.
single chain urokinase-type plasminogen a.
tissue plasminogen a. (t-PA)
tissue-type plasminogen a.
t-plasminogen a.
u-plasminogen a.
urinary plasminogen a.
urokinase-type plasminogen a. (uPA)

active
a. congestion
a. dynamic stiffness
a. fixation lead
a. hyperemia

active-site inhibited factor VIIa

activity
intrinsic sympathomimetic a.
membrane-stabilizing a.
muscle sympathetic nerve a.
myocyte metabolic a.
plasma renin a.
pulseless electrical a.
sinoaortic baroreflex a.
sympathetic a.
triggered a.

Activitrax
A. single-chamber responsive pacemaker
A. variable rate pacemaker

activity-sensing pacemaker

actocardiotocograph

actuation
direct mechanical ventricular a.

Acuson
A. cardiovascular system
A. computed sonography
A. echocardiographic equipment
A. V5M multiplane TEE transducer
A. V5M transesophageal echocardiographic monitor
A. XP-5 ultrasonoscope

acute
a. allograft rejection
a. bacterial endocarditis (ABE)
a. cardiogenic pulmonary edema
a. chest syndrome
a. compression triad
a. fibrinous pericarditis
a. infective endocarditis
a. isolated myocarditis
a. myocardial infarction
a. renal failure
a. rheumatic arthritis
a. rheumatic fever
a. severe hypotension
a. tamponade
a. ventricular assist device

ACX II balloon catheter

acyanotic
a. heart disease

acyl-CoA

acyl-CoA:cholesterol acyltransferase inhibitor

acyl-coenzyme A

acyltransferase

ADA
adenosine deaminase
ADA deficiency

Adamkiewicz artery

Adams
A. disease
A.-DeWeese device
A.-DeWeese vena caval clip
A.-DeWeese vena caval ser-
rated clip
A.-Stokes attack
A.-Stokes disease
A.-Stokes syncope
A.-Stokes syndrome

adapter
Bard-Tuohy-Borst a.
BioLase laser a.
Bodai a.
butterfly a.
catheter a.
Harris a.
Peep-Keep II a.
Protex swivel a.
Rosenblum rotating a.
Shiley pressure a.
side-arm a.
Tuohy-Borst a.

Addison
A. disease
A. maneuver
A. plane

adelomorphic

adelomorphous

adenine nucleotide translocator

adenosine
a. deaminase (ADA)
a. deaminase deficiency
a. diphosphate (ADP)
a. echocardiography
a. monophosphate

adenosine *(continued)*
a. nucleotide translocator
(ANT)
a. radionuclide perfusion
imaging
a. ^{99m}Tc sestamibi SPECT
a. thallium test
a. triphosphatase (ATPase)
a. triphosphate (ATP)
a. triphosphate disodium

adenovirus

adequate
a. blood flow
a. blood supply
a. collateral
a. hemostasis maintained

ADH
antidiuretic hormone

adherence assay

adherent pericardium

adhesin-receptor interaction

adhesins

adhesiolysis

adhesion
band of a.
chest wall a.
fibrinous a.
freeing up of a.
inflammatory a.
lysed a.
pericardial a's

adhesive
Biobrane a.
Histocryl Blue tissue a.
a. inflammation
a. pericarditis
a. phlebitis

adiastole

adiemorrhysis

adiposis
a. cardiaca

adiposis *(continued)*
   a. universalis

adipositas cordis

adiposum
   cor a.

adjunctive balloon angioplasty

admixture
   venous a.

ADP
   adenosine diphosphate

adrenal
   a. adenoma
   a. cortex
   a. gland
   a. hyperplasia
   a. hypertension
   a. medulla

adrenal medullary implant

adrenaline

adrenergic
   alpha-a.
   alpha$_1$-a. blocking agent
   a. antagonist
   beta-a.
   beta-a. stimulation
   a. drive
   a. nervous system
   a. receptor
   a. stimulant

adrenoceptor
   alpha a.
   beta a.
   a. blocker

adrenocorticotropic hormone
   (ACTH)

adrenogenital syndrome

adrenomedullary triad

adrenomedullin peptide

adrenoreceptor

ADR Ultramark 4 ultrasound

Adson
   A. aneurysm needle
   A. arterial forceps
   A. forceps
   A. hemostat
   A. hook
   A. maneuver
   A. retractor
   A. test
   A.-Coffey scalenotomy

adventitia
   aortic tunica a.
   esophageal a.

adventitial
   a. bed
   a. layer
   a. sheath

adventitious
   a. breath sounds
   a. heart sounds
   a. membrane

AEC pacemaker

AECG ambulatory ECG

AED
   automated external defibrillator

Ae–H interval

Aequitron pacemaker

aequorin

aeremia

aerendocardia

aerobic
   a. capacity
   a. exercise stress test
   a. metabolism
   a. threshold

aeroembolism

aerogenous

aerophagia

aerothorax

AES Amplatz guidewire

AFB
    acid-fast bacilli
    aortofemoral bypass
    AFB graft
    AFB needle guide

afferent
    a. arteriole
    a. artery
    a. impulse
    a. never fibers

afferentia

afflux

affluxion

AFP
    alpha-fetoprotein

AFP pacemaker

African
    A. cardiomyopathy
    A. endomyocardial fibrosis

afterdepolarization
    delayed a.
    early a.
    late a.

afterload
    cardiac a.
    a. matching
    a. mismatching
    a. reduction
    a. resistance
    ventricular a.

afterloading catheter

afterpotential

agammaglobulinemia

agar diffusion assay

agarose
    a. gel electrophoresis
    MetaPhor a.

agent
    alpha blocking a.
    antianginal a.
    antiarrhythmic a.
    antihypertensive a.
    antiplatelet a.
    bacteriostatic a.
    beta-adrenergic blocking a.
    beta blocking a.
    blood-borne infectious a.
    blood-thinning a.
    calcium channel blocking a.
    cholinergic a.
    contrast a.
    diuretic a.
    dopaminergic a.
    hypertensive a.
    hypotensive a.
    immunosuppressive a.
    inotropic a.
    nonglycoside inotropic a.
    nonsteroidal anti-inflamma-
        tory a.
    sclerosing a.
    thrombolytic a.
    vasodilator a.

age-undetermined myocardial
    infarction

agger
    a. valvae venae

agglutinating antibody

agglutination

agglutinative thrombus

agglutinin
    febrile a's

aggregation
    platelet a.

aggrephore

agonal
    a. clot
    a. rhythm
    a. thrombosis
    a. thrombus

agonist
   alpha a.
   alpha-adrenoreceptor a.
   beta a.
   beta-adrenergic a.
   calcium channel a.
   muscarinic a.

agony clot

agranulocytosis

A greater than E

A–H
   A–H conduction time
   A–H curve
   A–H interval

AH:HA ratio

Ahlquist-Durham embolism
   clamp

AI
   aortic incompetence
   aortic insufficiency
   apical impulse

AICD
   automatic implantable car-
      dioverter-defibrillator
      AICD-B pacemaker
      AICD-BR pacemaker
      Cadence AICD
      AICD device
      Guardian AICD
      AICD pacemaker
      Res-Q AICD
      AICD shocks
      Ventak P3 AICD
   automatic internal cardio-
      verter-defibrillator

AID
   automatic implantable de-
      fibrillator
      AID-B pacemaker

air
   a. embolism
   a. embolus
   a. inflatable tube

air (continued)
   a. inflatable vessel occlu-
      der
   a. hunger
   mediastinal a.

airborne transmission

air-drive artificial heart

akaryocyte

akaryota

akaryote

akinesia
   regional a.

akinesis
   apical a.

akinetic
   a. left ventricle
   a. posterior wall

Akutsu III total artificial heart

AL II guiding catheter

alanine aminotransferase

Albertini treatment

Albini nodules

Albright syndrome

albumin
   a.-coated vascular graft

albuminized woven Dacron
   tube graft

albuminuria

Alcatel pacemaker

Alcock catheter plug

alcoholic
   a. cardiomyopathy
   a. malnutrition
   a. myocardiopathy

Alcon
   A. Closure System
   A. Digital B 2000 ultra-
      sound

aldehyde-tanned bovine carotid
   artery graft

aldesleukin

aldosterone
   a. antagonist
   a. depression

aldosteronism

aldosteronoma

Aldrete needle

Alexander
   A. rib raspatory
   A. rib stripper
   A.-Farabeuf costal perios-
      teotome
   A.-Farabeuf rib rasp

alexandrite laser

Alfred M. Large vena cava
   clamp

algiovascular

alglucerase

algorithm
   Levenberg-Marquardt a.

algovascular

aliasing
   a. artifact
   image a.

alinidine

aliquot

Alivi aggregometer

alkaline
   a. phosphatase

alkaloid
   ergot a.

alkalosis
   altitude a.
   metabolic a.
   respiratory a.

alkaptonuria

Allain method

allantoic
   a. circulation
   a. vein

allele
   mutant a.

Allen test

Allen Brown
   A. B. criteria
   A. B. prosthesis
   A. B. shunt

allergen-induced mediator release

alligator pacing cable

Allis
   A. clamp
   A. forceps
   A. hemostat
   A. periosteal elevator
   A. thoracic forceps

Allison retractor

Alliston procedure

allogeneic
   a. graft
   a. transplant

allograft
   bovine a.
   cardiac a.
   cryopreserved heart val-
      ve a.
   cryopreserved human aor-
      tic a.
   CryoVein saphenous vein a.
   a. reaction
   a. survival
   a. vasculopathy

allometric

alloplasmatic

allorhythmia

allorhythmic

all or none law

allosome
  paired a.

allosteric modification of enzyme

Allport-Babcock searcher

Aloka
  A. color Doppler
  A. color Doppler system for
    blood flow mapping
  A. echocardiograph ma-
    chine
  A. ultrasound

alpha
  a.-1 adrenergic blocker
  a.-1 adrenergic blocking
    agent
  a.-1 antitrypsin (AAT)
  a.-1 antitrypsin deficiency
  a. agonist
  a. blocker
  a. blocking agent
  a. lipoprotein
  a. receptor
  a.-2 macroglobulin
  a.-1 proteinase inhibitor

alpha-adrenergic
  a.-a. blocker
  a.-a. blocking agent
  a.-a. stimulation

alpha-adrenoreceptor
  a.-a. agonist
  a.-a. blocker

alpha-fetoprotein (AFP)

AlphaNine
  A. clotting agent

Alport syndrome

alteplase
  recombinant a.

alteration
  ST a's

alternans
  auscultatory a.
  cardiac a.
  concordant a.
  electrical a.
  mechanical a.
  pulsus a.
  QRS a.
  ST segment a.
  total a.

alternating
  a. bidirectional tachycardia
  a. pulse

alternation
  cardiac a.
  concordant a.
  cycle length a.
  discordant a.
  electrical a. of the heart
  mechanical a.

Alvarez
  A. prosthesis
  A.-Rodriguez cardiac cathe-
    ter

alveolar
  a. capillary membrane
  a. hypoventilation
  a. proteinosis
  a.-septal amyloidosis

Alzate catheter

amazon thorax

Ambrose plaque type

Ambu
  A. bag
  A. CardioPump

ambulatory
  a. ECG
  a. electrocardiographic
    monitoring
  a. electrocardiography
  a. Holter monitoring

AMC needle

Amcath catheter

ameba
    a. verrucosa

amebic
    a. pericarditis

amebocyte

ameboid cell

ameboma

ameiosis

American
    A. Bentley cardiopulmonary bypass system
    A. Heart Association (AHA)
    A. Heart Association classification of stenosis
    A. Heart Association diet
    A. Optical CardioCare pacemaker
    A. Optical R-inhibited pacemaker
    A. vascular stapler

AMI
    acute myocardial infarction
    anterior myocardial infarction

amine
    sympathomimetic a.

amino acid

aminocaproic acid

aminoethyl ethanolamine

aminoglycoside

aminoguanidine

aminophylline

aminosalicylic acid

aminoterminal propeptide

aminotransferase

amitosis

amitotic

AML
    anterior mitral leaflet

A-mode
    A-m. echocardiography
    A-m. Echo-tracking device

amphiaster

amphicentric

amphikaryon

amphipathic helix

amphipyrenin

amphitene

amphoric
    a. echo
    a. murmur
    a. rales
    a. respiration

amphoriloquy

Amplatz
    A. angiography needle
    A. aortography catheter
    A. cardiac catheter
    A. catheter
    A. coronary catheter
    A. dilator
    A. femoral catheter
    A. guide
    A. Hi-Flo torque-control catheter
    A. left I, II catheter
    A. right coronary catheter
    A. right I, II catheter
    A. Super Stiff guide wire
    A. technique
    A. torque wire
    A. tube guide
    A. II curve

Amplex guide wire

amplitude
    aortic a.
    apical interventricular septal a.
    atrial pulse a.

amplitude *(continued)*
    C to A mitral valve a.
    C to E a.
    cardiac signal a.
    contractile a.
    D to E a.
    diminished wave a.
    a. of ECG wave
    a. image
    a. linearity
    low a.
    mid-interventricular sep-
        tal a.
    posterior left ventricular
        wall a.
    pulse a.
    P wave a.
    a. of QRS complex
    R wave a.
    septal a.
    valve opening a.
    ventricular pulse a.
    wall a.
    wave a.

ampulla *pl.* ampullae
    Bryant a.
    a. of Thoma

ampullary aneurysm

Amtech-Killeen pacemaker

amylase
    serum a.

amyloid
    a. A protein
    a. heart disease

amyloidosis
    alveolar-septal a.
    cardiac a.
    familial a.
    heredofamilial a.
    mediastinal a.
    nodular pulmonary a.
    parenchymal a.
    primary systemic a.
    pseudotumoral mediastin-
        al a.
    senile a.

amyloidosis *(continued)*
    systemic a.

amyocardia

amyotrophic chorea

ANA
    antinuclear antibody

anabolic steroid

anacrotic
    a. limb of carotid arterial
        pulse
    a. notch of carotid arterial
        pulse

anacrotism

anadicrotic
    a. pulse

anadicrotism

anadicrotus
    pulsus a.

anaerobe

anaerobic
    a. bacteria
    a. decomposition
    a. gram-negative rods
    a. infection

anaerobiosis

analgesic
    patient-controlled a. (PCA)
    a. requirements

analysis *pl.* analyses
    backscatter a.
    beat-to-beat a.
    centerline method of wall
        motion a.
    Doppler spectral a.
    Doppler waveform a.
    fast Fourier spectral a.
    Fourier series a.
    frequency-domain a.
    multilinear regression a.
    phase image a.
    pressure-volume a.
    probability a.

analysis *(continued)*
    quantitative coronary an-
      giographic a.
    regression a.
    sensitivity a.
    spectral a.
    wall motion a.

anaphase
    flabby a.

anaphylaxis

anaphylactic
    a. antibody
    a. crisis
    a. reaction
    a. shock

anaphylactoid
    a. purpura
    a. reaction

anaplerosis

anaplerotic sequence

anapnea

anapneic

anapnotherapy

anasarca

anastomose

anastomosis *pl.* anastomoses
    aortic a.
    aorticopulmonary a.
    arterial a.
    a. arteriolovenularis
    a. arteriovenosa
    a. of ascending aorta to
      pulmonary artery
    Baffe a.
    bidirectional cavopulmon-
      ary a.
    Blalock-Taussig a.
    cavopulmonary a.
    a. clamp
    cobra-head a.
    a. forceps
    conjoined a.
    Clado a.

anastomosis *(continued)*
    Cooley intrapericardial a.
    Cooley modification of Wa-
      terston a.
    crucial a.
    cruciate a.
    distal a.
    elliptical a.
    end-to-end a.
    end-to-side a.
    Fontan atriopulmonary a.
    Glenn a.
    heterocladic a.
    homocladic a.
    internal mammary artery to
      coronary artery a.
    Kugel a.
    left pulmonary artery to de-
      scending aorta a.
    Nakayama a.
    portacaval a.
    portosystemic a.
    postcostal a.
    Potts a.
    Potts aortic-pulmonary ar-
      tery a.
    Potts-Smith side-to-side a.
    precapillary a.
    right atrium to pulmonary
      artery a.
    right pulmonary artery to
      ascending aorta a.
    right subclavian to pulmo-
      nary artery a.
    a. of Riolan
    side-to-side a.
    stirrup a.
    Sucquet-Hoyer a.
    superior vena cava to dis-
      tal right pulmonary ar-
      tery a.
    superior vena cava to pul-
      monary a.
    tensionless a.
    terminoterminal a.
    Waterston extrapericardi-
      al a.

anastomotic

anastral

anatomic
    a. assessment
    a. block

anatomy
    distorted a.
    left-dominant coronary a.
    native coronary a.
    right-dominant coronary a.

anatricrotic

anatricrotism

anchor
    Harpoon suture a.

ANCOR imaging system

Ancure system treatment device

Andersen
    A. syndrome
    A. triad

Anderson
    A. procedure
    A. test
    A.-Keys method

Andral decubitus

Andrews
    A. retractor
    A. suction tip

Andrews Pynchon tube

Androsov vascular stapler

anechoic

Anel
    A. method
    A. operation

anemia
    aplastic a.
    chronic hemolytic a.
    Cooley a.
    hemolytic a.
    Mediterranean a.
    megaloblastic a.

anemia *(continued)*
    microangiopathic a.
    sickle cell a.
    splenic a.

anemic
    a. hypoxia
    a. murmur

anemometry

anergy

anesthesia
    Bier block a.
    crash induction of a.
    MacIntosh blade a.

anesthetic

aneurysm
    abdominal a.
    abdominal aortic a. (AAA)
    ampullary a.
    aortic a.
    aortic arch a.
    aortoiliac a.
    aortic sinusal a.
    apical a.
    arterial a.
    arteriosclerotic a.
    arteriovenous a.
    arteriovenous pulmonary a.
    atherosclerotic a.
    atrial septal a.
    axial a.
    axillary a.
    bacterial a.
    Bérard a.
    berry a.
    brain a.
    cavernous-carotid a.
    cardiac a.
    cerebral a.
    Charcot-Bouchard a.
    cirsoid a.
    compound a.
    congenital aortic a.
    congenital cerebral a.
    consecutive a.
    coronary a.
    Crawford technique for a.

aneurysm *(continued)*
   Crisp a.
   cylindroid a.
   cystogenic a.
   DeBakey technique for a.
   descending thoracic a.
   dissecting a.
   dolichoectatic a's
   ectatic a.
   embolic a.
   embolomycotic a.
   endogenous a.
   erosive a.
   exogenous a.
   false a.
   fusiform a.
   hernial a.
   infected a.
   infrarenal abdominal aortic a.
   innominate a.
   interventricular septum a.
   intracranial a.
   Kommerell diverticulum a.
   lateral a.
   left ventricular a.
   luetic a.
   mesh-wrapping of aortic a.
   miliary a.
   mitral valve a.
   mixed a.
   mural a.
   mycotic a.
   orbital a.
   Park a.
   phantom a.
   popliteal a.
   Potts a.
   racemose a.
   Rasmussen a.
   renal a.
   Richet a.
   Rodriguez a.
   ruptured aortic a.
   sacciform a.
   saccular a.
   sacculated a.
   serpentine a.

aneurysm *(continued)*
   Shekelton a.
   sinus of Valsalva a.
   spindle-shaped a.
   spurious a.
   suprasellar a.
   syphilitic a.
   thoracic a.
   thoracoabdominal aortic a.
   traction a.
   traumatic aortic a.
   true a.
   tubular a.
   varicose a.
   venous a.
   ventricular a.
   verminous a.
   windsock a.
   wrapping of abdominal aortic a.

aneurysmal
   a. bone cyst
   a. bruit
   a. bulging
   a. dilatation
   a. hematoma
   a. murmur
   a. phthisis
   a. thrill
   a. wall

aneurysmatic
   a. bone cyst
   a. bruit
   a. bulging
   a. dilatation
   a. hematoma
   a. murmur
   a. phthisis
   a. thrill
   a. wall

aneurysmectomy

aneurysmography

aneurysmogram

aneurysmoplasty
   Matas a.

aneurysmorrhaphy

aneurysmotomy

AneuRx stent graft system

ANF
   atrial natriuretic factor

AngeLase combined mapping-
   laser probe

Angelchik antireflux prosthesis

Angell-Shiley bioprosthetic
   valve

Angell-Shiley xenograft prosthetic valve

angel's trumpet

Ange-Med Sentinel ICD device

Anger scintillation camera

Angestat hemostasis introducer

Angetear tearaway introducer

angialgia

angiasthenia

angiectasis

angiectatic

angiectomy

angiectopia

angiemphraxis

angiitis
   allergic granulomatous a.
   Churg-Strauss a.
   hypersensitivity a.
   leukocytoclastic a.
   necrotizing a.
   nonnecrotizing a.

angina
   abdominal a.
   accelerated a.
   anxiety a.
   atypical a.
   bandlike a.
   benign croupous a.
   Bretonneau a.

angina (continued)
   chronic stable a.
   classic a.
   clinical a.
   cold-induced a.
   a. cordis
   coronary spastic a.
   crescendo a.
   crescendo-decrescendo a.
   a. crouposa
   a. cruris
   a. decubitus
   a. dyspeptica
   effort a.
   ergonovine maleate provo-
      cation a.
   esophageal a.
   exercise-induced a.
   exertional a.
   false a.
   first-effort a.
   focal a.
   a. gangrenosa
   a.-guided therapy
   Heberden a.
   hippocratic a.
   hypercyanotic a.
   hysteric a.
   intractable a.
   a. inversa
   ischemic rest a.
   lacunar a.
   a. laryngea
   Ludwig a.
   a. membranacea
   microvascular a.
   mixed a.
   neutropenic a.
   new onset a.
   nocturnal a.
   nonexertional a.
   a. nosocomii
   a. notha
   office a.
   pacing-induced a.
   a. pectoris
   a. pectoris decubitus
   a. pectoris electrica

angina *(continued)*
   a. pectoris sine dolore
   a. pectoris vasomotoria
   a. phlegmonosa
   Plaut a.
   Plaut-Vincent a.
   postinfarction a.
   postprandial a.
   preinfarction a.
   Prinzmetal a.
   progressive a.
   pseudomembranous a.
   rate-dependent a.
   rebound a.
   reflex a.
   refractory a.
   rest a.
   a. rheumatica
   a. scarlatinosa
   Schultz a.
   sexual a.
   silent a.
   a. simplex
   smoking-induced a.
   a. spuria
   stable a.
   streptococcus a.
   sudden onset of a.
   toilet-seat a.
   a. tonsillaris
   a. trachealis
   treadmill-induced a.
   typical a.
   a. ulcerosa
   unstable a.
   variable threshold a.
   variant a.
   variant a. pectoris
   vasomotor a.
   vasospastic a.
   vasotonic a.
   Vincent a.
   walk-through a.
   white-coat a.
anginal
   a. equivalent
   a. perceptual threshold
anginiform

anginoid

anginophobia

anginosa
   syncope a.

anginosis

anginous

angioataxia

angioblast

angioblastic

angioblastoma

angiocardiogram

angiocardiography
   equilibrium radionuclide a.
   first-pass radionuclide a.
   gated equilibrium radionu-
     clide a.
   radionuclide a.
   transseptal a.

angiocardiokinetic

angiocardiopathy

angiocarditis

Angiocath PRN catheter

angiocatheter
   Brockenbrough a.
   Corlon a.
   Deseret a.
   Eppendorf a.
   Mikro-tip a.

angiocentric

angiocheiloscope

angioclast

Angio-Conray

Angiocor
   A. prosthetic valve
   A. rotational thrombolizer

angiodermatitis
   disseminated pruritic a.

angiodiascopy

angiodiathermy

angiodynia

angiodysplasia
a. of colon
gastrointestinal a.

angiodysplastic
a. lesions

angiodystrophia

angiodystrophy

angioectatic

angioedema

Angioflow high-flow catheter

angiogenesis

angiogenic

Angiografin

angiogram
biplane orthogonal a.
Brown-Dodge a.
cardiac a.
cineangiogram
coronary a.
digital subtraction a.
ECG-synchronized digital
subtraction a.
equilibrium radionuclide a.
first-pass nuclide rest and
exercise a.
first-pass radionuclide a.
fluorescein a.
gated blood pool a.
gated nuclear a.
left ventricular cineangiogram
inferior mesenteric a.
pulmonary artery wedge a.
radioisotope a.
selective coronary cineangiogram
sitting-up view a.
superior mesenteric a.

angiogram (continued)
transvenous digital sub-
traction a.
wedge a.

angiograph
3DFT magnetic resonan-
ce a.

angiographic
a. assessment
a. catheter
a. contrast
a. instrumentation

angiographically occult intracranial vascular malformation

angiography
aortography a.
balloon-occlusion pulmon-
ary a.
biplane orthogonal a.
carotid a.
cerebral a.
color power a.
coronary a.
digital subtraction a. (DSA)
digitized subtraction a.
equilibrium radionuclide a.
fluorescein a.
gated blood-pool a.
gated radionuclide a.
indocyanine green a.
internal mammary artery
graft a.
intraoperative digital subtraction a.
intraoperative vascular a.
intravenous digital subtraction a.
left aortic a.
left atrial a.
left coronary artery a.
left ventricular a.
magnetic resonance a.
mesenteric a.
multigated a.
noncardiac a.
nonselective coronary a.
peripheral a.

angiography *(continued)*
pulmonary wedge a.
quantitative coronary a.
radionuclide a.
renal a.
renovascular a.
rest and exercise gated nuclear a.
rest radionuclide a.
right coronary artery a.
saphenous vein bypass graft a.
selective a.
subtraction a.
supra-aortic a.
surveillance a.
synchrotron-based transvenous a.
thermal a.
ultrasound a.
vascular a.
ventricular a.
wedge pulmonary a.

Angioject
ACS A.

angiohemophilia

angiohyalinosis

angiohypertonia

angiohypotonia

angioinvasive

Angio-Jet rapid thrombectomy system

angioid

angiokeratoma
a. corporis diffusum

angiokinesis

angiokinetic

Angio-Kit catheter

angioleiomyoma

angiolipoma

angiolith

angiologia

angiology

angioma
cherry a.
spider a.
a. venosum racemosum

angiomatosis
bacillary a.

Angiomedics catheter

angiomegaly

angiometer

angiomyocardiac

angionecrosis

angioneoplasm

angioneurography

angioneuropathic

angioneuropathy

angioneurosis

angioneurotic edema

angioneurotomy

angionoma

Angiopac

angioparalysis

angioparesis

angiopigtail catheter

angioplasia

angiopathy

angioplasty
ablative laser a.
adjunctive balloon a.
balloon catheter a.
balloon coarctation a.
balloon coronary a.
balloon laser a.
bootstrap two-vessel a.
complementary balloon a.

angioplasty *(continued)*
coronary artery a.
culprit lesion a.
Dotter-Judkins percutaneous transluminal a.
excimer laser coronary a. (ELCA)
facilitated a.
Grüntzig balloon catheter a.
high-risk a.
Ho:YAG laser a.
Kensey rotation atherectomy extrusion a.
kissing balloon a.
laser a.
laser-balloon a.
laser thermal a.
multilesion a.
one-vessel a.
Osypka rotational a.
patch-graft a.
percutaneous balloon a.
percutaneous laser a.
percutaneous transluminal coronary a.
peripheral laser a.
rescue a.
salvage balloon a.
stand-alone balloon a.
supported a.
Tactilaze a.
thermal/perfusion balloon a.
thulium:YAG laser a.
tibioperoneal vessel a.
transluminal coronary a.
vibrational a.
angioplasty-related vessel occlusion
angiopneumography
angiopoiesis
angiopoietic
angiopressure
angioreticuloma
angiorrhaphy

angiosarcoma
angioscintigraphy
angiosclerosis
angiosclerotic gangrene
angioscope
Imagecath rapid exchange a.
Masy a.
Mitsubishi a.
Olympus a.
angioscopy
fiberoptic a.
percutaneous transluminal a.
Angio-Seal hemostatic puncture closure device
Angioskop-D
angiospasm
angiospastic
Angiosol
angiostenosis
angiosteosis
angiosthenia
angiostomy
angiotelectasis
angiotensin (ACE)
a.-converting enzyme
a.-converting enzyme inhibitor
a.-I converting enzyme
a.-II receptor blockade
a.-II receptor blocker
renin a.
angiotensinase
angiotensinogen
a. gene
angiotomy
angiotonia

angiotonic

angiotrophic

angitis

angle
　blunted costophrenic a.
　cardiodiaphragmatic a.
　cardiohepatic a.
　cardiophrenic a.
　costophrenic a.
　costovertebral a. (CVA)
　Ebstein a.
　flip a.
　intercept a.
　Louis a.
　Ludwig a.
　nail-to-nail bed a.
　phase a.
　phrenopericardial a.
　Pirogoff a.
　a. port pump
　QRS–T a.
　sternoclavicular a.
　venous a.
　xiphoid a.

angled
　a. ball-end electrode
　a. balloon catheter
　a. DeBakey clamp
　a. peripheral vascular
　　clamp
　a. vein retractor

angle-tip
　a.-t. electrode
　a.-t. guide wire

angor
　a. animi
　a. pectoris

angulated multipurpose catheter

angulation
　RAO a.

angulus
　a. venosus

angusta
　aorta a.

Anichkow myocyte

animi
　angor a.

A–N interval

anion
　a. exchange resin
　a. gap
　superoxide a.

anisokaryosis

anisopiesis

anisorrhythmia

anisosphygmia

anisotropic conduction

anisotropy

anisoylated plasminogen strep-
　tokinase activator complex

anistreplase

Ankeney sternal retractor

ankle
　a.-arm index
　a.-brachial blood pressure
　　ratio
　a.-brachial index
　a. edema
　a. exercise

anlagen

annihilation photon

annular
　a. abscess
　a. array transducer
　a. calcification
　a. constriction
　a. dehiscence
　a. dilatation
　a. disruption
　a. phased array system
　a. plication

annular *(continued)*
a. thrombus
annuloaortic ectasia
annulocuspid hinge
annuloplasty
Carpentier a.
DeVega tricuspid valve a.
Gerbode a.
Kay a.
prosthetic ring a.
septal a.
tricuspid valve a.
Wooler-type a.
annulus *pl.* annuli
aortic a.
atrioventricular annuli
calcified a.
annuli fibrosi cordis
a. fibrosus
friable a.
mitral a.
mitral valve a.
a. of nuclear pore
a. ovalis
pulmonary valve a.
septal tricuspid a.
tricuspid valve a.
Vieussens a.
anodal
a. closure
a. closure contraction
a. opening contraction
anode
transvenous a.
anomalous
a. atrioventricular excitation
a. bronchus
a. complex
a. conduction
a. first rib thoracic syndrome
a. left main coronary artery
a. mitral arcade
a. origin

anomalous *(continued)*
a. origin of the left coronary artery from the pulmonary artery
a. pulmonary vein
a. pulmonary venous connection
a. pulmonary venous drainage
a. pulmonary venous return
a. rectification
a. retroesophageal right subclavian artery
anomaly
aortic arch a.
atrioventricular connection a.
congenital cardiac a.
conotruncal congenital a.
conotruncal a.
coronary artery a.
Ebstein a.
Freund a.
pulmonary valve a.
pulmonary venous connection a.
pulmonary venous return a.
Shone a.
Taussig-Bing a.
Uhl a.
ventricular inflow a.
viscerobronchial cardiovascular a.
anoxemia test
anoxia
myocardial a.
stagnant a.
ANP
atrial natriuretic polypeptide
AN region
Anrep
A. effect

Anrep *(continued)*
    A. phenomenon

ansa cervicalis

ansamycin

antagonism
    accentuated a.
    salt a.

antagonist
    adrenergic a.
    aldosterone a.
    beta a.
    beta-1 a.
    beta-2 a.
    calcium a's
    calcium channel a.
    dihydropyridine calcium a.
    thromboxane receptor a.
    vitamin K a.

antecedent
    plasma thromboplastin a.

antecubital
    a. approach
    a. fossa
    a. space

antegrade
    a. aortogram
    a. approach
    a. block cycle length
    a. conduction
    a. double balloon/double
      wire technique
    a. fashion
    a. flow
    a. internodal pathway
    a. refractory period

antegrade/retrograde cardioplegia technique

antemortem
    a. clot
    a. thrombus

antephase

anterior
    a. anodal patch electrode

anterior *(continued)*
    a. approach
    a. axillary line
    a. chamber
    a. descending coronary artery
    a. inferior communicating artery
    a. internodal pathway
    a. leaflet
    a. mitral leaflet (AML)
    a. motion of posterior mitral valve leaflet
    a. myocardial infarction (AMI)
    a. oblique projection
    a. papillary muscle
    a. sandwich patch technique
    a. table
    a. view on thallium imaging
    a. wall
    a. wall dyskinesis
    a. wall myocardial infarction

anteriorly directed jet

anteroapical
    a. dyskinesis

anterograde
    a. block
    a. conduction
    a. flow
    a. transseptal technique

anteroinferior myocardial infarction

anterolateral
    a. myocardial infarction

anteromesial hypokinesis

anteroposterior
    a. paddles
    a. projection
    a. thoracic diameter

anteroseptal
    a. myocardial infarction

antesystole

anthraconecrosis

anthracosilicosis

anthracosis

anthracycline-induced cardiomyopathy

anthracycline toxicity

Anthron
A. heparinized antithrom-
bogenic catheter
A. II catheter

anthropometric evaluation

antiadhesin antibody

antiadrenergic
a. agent

antialdosterone therapy

anti-aliasing technique

antianginal
a. agent
a. drug
a. treatment

antiarrhythmic
a. agent
a. drug
a. drug classification (Ia, Ib,
Ic, II, III, IV)

antiatherogenic

antiatherosclerotic

antibacterial

antibasement membrane

antibiotic
antipseudomonas a.
azalide class of a's
macrolide a's
perioperative a.
preoperative a.
prophylactic a.

antibody
agglutinating a.

antibody *(continued)*
anaphylactic a.
antiadhesin a.
anticardiolipin a's (aCLa)
anti-DNA a.
antidystrophin a.
antiglomerular basement
membrane a's
anti-La a's
antimyosin monoclonal a.
antineutrophil cytoplasmic
a's
antinuclear a. (ANA)
antiphospholipid a.
antireceptor a.
anti-Ro SS-A a's
anti-Sm a.
anti-SSA/Ro a's
anti-SSB/La a's
B cell a.
CD18 a's
cross-reactive a.
digitalis-specific a.
direct fluorescent a.
7E3 glycoprotein IIb/IIIa
platelet a.
7E3 monoclonal Fab a.
fibrin-specific a.
fluorescent antimembra-
ne a. (FAMA)
indium-111 antimyosin a.
monoclonal antimyosin a.
monoclonal a. 3G4
myosin-specific a.
OKT3 a.
platelet a.
polyclonal anticardiac
myosin a.
Rh a.
sheep antidigoxin Fab a.
streptococcal a.
streptokinase a.
teichoic acid a.
thyroid a.
tissue-specific a's
treponemal a.
TR-R9 antithrombin recep-
tor polyclonal a.

antibody *(continued)*
  Y2B8 a.

antibradycardia

anticardiolipin antibody (aCLa)

anticholinergic

anticipated systole

anticoagulant
  lupus a.
  oral a.
  a. therapy

anticoagulation
  long-term a.

anti-deoxyribonuclease

antidiuretic hormone (ADH)

antidromic
  a. circus-movement tachy-
    cardia
  a. tachycardia

antidysrhythmic

anti-elastase

antiembolism stockings

antiendotoxin therapy

antifibrillatory

antifibrin antibody imaging

antifilarial

antifungal

antigen
  Australia a.
  carcinoembryonic a. (CEA)
  Epstein-Barr nuclear a.
  human leukocyte a. (HLA)
  human lymphocyte a.
    (HLA)
  inhalant a.
  KI a.
  O a.
  p24 a.
  PLA-I platelet a.
  proliferating cell nuclear a.

antigenicity

anti-G suite

antiheart antibody titer

antihemophilic
  a. factor
  a. factor (human)
  a. factor (recombinant)

antihistamine

antihyperlipidemic

antihypertensive

antihypotensive

anti-inflammatory

anti-inhibitor coagulant complex

antilymphocyte serum

antimicrobial
  a. catheter cuff
  a. therapy

antimitotic

antimony
  a. compound
  a. toxicity

antimyosin
  a. antibody imaging
  a. infarct-avid scintigraphy
  a. monoclonal antibody
    with Fab fragment

antinuclear
  a. antibody (ANA)

antioxidative

antiphospholipid
  a. antibody
  a. syndrome

antiplasmin

antiplatelet
  a. agent
  a. therapy

antipodal

antipode

antiport

Anti-Sept bactericidal scrub solution

antishock garment

antisialagogue

antistasin

antistreptokinase

antistreptolysin O (ASO)

antistreptozyme

antitachycardia
a. pacemaker (ATP)
a. pacing

antitemplate

antithrombin
a. III (AT-III)

antithromboplastin

antithrombotic

antithymocyte

antitrypsin
α-1 a.
alpha-1 a. (AAT)
M-type alpha 1-a.
plasma alpha 1-a. (pAAT)
recombinant alpha-1 a.
(rAAT)

antitubulin

antler sign

antrectomy

antrum *pl.* antra
cardiac a.

Antyllus method

anuclear

anucleated

anuloplasty (*variant of* annuloplasty)

anulus (*variant of* annulus)

anxiolytic

aorta *pl.* aortae
abdominal a.
a. abdominalis
a. angusta
arch of a.
arcus aortae
a. ascendens
ascending a.
bifurcation of a.
biventricular origin of a.
buckled a.
buckling of a.
button of a.
calcified a.
a. chlorotica
coarctation of a.
a. descendens
descending a.
dextropositioned a.
dissecting a.
dissection of a.
double-barrelled a.
dynamic a.
infrarenal abdominal a.
kinked a.
a.-left atrium ratio
medionecrosis of a.
overriding a.
palpable a.
paravisceral a.
porcelain a.
preductal coarctation of a.
primitive a.
pseudocoarctation of a.
recoaractation of a.
retroesophageal a.
sacrococcygeal a.
straddling a.
terminal a.
a. thoracalis
thoracic a.
a. thoracica
thoracoabdominal a.
throbbing a.
ventral a.

aortal

aortalgia

aortarctia

aortartia

aortectasia, aortectasis

aortectomy

aortic
  a. anastomosis
  a. aneurysm
  a. aneurysmal disease
  a. aneurysm clamp
  a. annulus
  a. arch
  a. arch arteriogram
  a. arch cannula
  a. arch interruption
  a. arch syndrome
  a. arteritis syndrome
  a. assist balloon introducer
  a. atresia
  a. balloon pump
  a. bifurcation
  a. blood pressure AoBP
  a. bulb
  a. catheter
  a. clamp
  a. closure sound
  a. coarctation
  a. commissure
  a. compliance
  a. crossclamp
  a. crossclamp time
  a. cuff
  a. cusp
  a. cusp separation
  a. diameter
  a. dicrotic notch pressure
  a. dissection (type A, type B)
  a. dwarfism
  a. embolism
  a. envelope
  a. facies
  a. hiatus
  a. homograft
  a. impedance
  a. incompetence

aortic (continued)
  a. insufficiency (AI)
  a. intramural hematoma
  a. isthmus
  a. jet velocity
  a. knob
  a. knuckle
  left atrial to a. (La:A)
  a.-left ventricular tunnel murmur
  a.-mitral combined disease murmur
  a. nipple
  a. notch
  a. obstruction
  a. occluder
  a. occlusion clamp
  a. opening
  a. orifice
  a. override
  a. perfusion cannula
  a. plexus
  a. pressure gradient
  a. prosthesis
  a. pullback
  a. pullback pressure
  a. pulmonary window
  a. reflex
  a. regurgitation (AR)
  a. regurgitation murmur
  a. ring
  a. root
  a. root dimension
  a. root perfusion needle
  a. root ratio
  a. runoff
  a. rupture
  a. sac
  a. sclerosis
  a. second sound (A_2)
  a. septal defect
  a. sinotubular junction
  a. sinus
  a. spindle
  a. stenosis (AS)
  a. stenosis jet
  a. stenosis murmur
  a. sulcus

aortic *(continued)*
   a. suprarenal artery
   a. thrill
   a. thromboembolic disease
   a. thrombosis
   a. triangle
   a. tube graft
   a. tunica adventitia
   a. tunica intima
   a. tunica media
   a. valve
   a. valve area
   a. valve brush
   a. valve disease
   a. valve endocarditis
   a. valve gradient
   a. valve leaflet
   a. valve prosthesis
   a. valve regurgitation
   a. valve replacement (AVR)
   a. valve resistance
   a. valve restenosis
   a. valve retractor
   a. valve rongeur
   a. valve vegetation
   a. valve velocity profile
   a. valvotomy
   a. valvular insufficiency
   a. valvulitis
   a. valvuloplasty
   a. valvulotomy
   a. vasa vasorum
   a. vent needle
   a. window

aorticopulmonary
   a. anastomosis
   a. septal defect
   a. shunt
   a. window

aorticorenal

aorticus

aortism

aortismus abdominalis

aortitis
   arthritis-associated a.

aortitis *(continued)*
   Döhle-Heller a.
   giant cell a.
   luetic a.
   nummular a.
   rheumatic a.
   syphilitic a.
   a. syphilitica obliterans
   Takayasu a.

aortoarteritis

aortobifemoral
   a. bypass
   a. graft

aortocaval

aortocarotid bypass

aortoclasia

aortocoronary
   a. bypass
   a. bypass graft
   a. snake graft
   a. vein bypass

aortocoronary-saphenous vein
   bypass

aortofemoral
   a. arterial runoff
   a. arteriography
   a. artery shunt
   a. bypass graft
   a. prosthesis

aortogram
   abdominal a.
   arch a.
   contrast a.
   digital subtraction supra-
      valvular a.
   flush a.
   a. with distal runoff
   retrograde a.
   retrograde femoral a.
   retrograde transaxillary a.
   supravalvular a.
   thoracic a.
   transbrachial arch a.
   translumbar a.

aortography
    abdominal a.
    a. angiography
    antegrade a.
    arch a.
    ascending a.
    atherosclerotic a.
    biplane a.
    caudally angled balloon occlusion a.
    digital subtraction supravalvular a.
    flush a.
    laid-back balloon occlusion a.
    mycotic a.
    retrograde a.
    selective a.
    single-plane a.
    sinus of Valsalva a.
    thoracic arch a.
    transbrachial a.
    translumbar a.
    traumatic a.
    true vs. false aneurysm a.

aortoiliac
    a. aneurysm
    a. bypass graft
    a. endarterectomy
    a. obstructive disease
    a. occlusive disease
    a. thrombosis

aortoiliofemoral
    a. bypass
    a. circuit
    a. endarterectomy

aortolith

aortomalacia

aorto-ostial lesion

aortopathy

aortoplasty
    patch-graft a.

aortoptosia, aortoptosis

aortopulmonary
    a. collateral
    a. fenestration
    a. shunt
    a. tunnel
    a. window

aortorenal bypass

aortorrhaphy

aortosclerosis

aortostenosis

aorto-subclavian-carotid-axilloaxillary bypass

aortotomy
    curvilinear a.

aortovelography
    transcutaneous a.
    transvenous a.

aortoventriculoplasty

apallic syndrome

apathetic hyperthyroidism

APB
    atrial premature beat
    auricular premature beat

APC
    atrial premature contraction

Apert syndrome

aperture
    transducer a.

apex *pl.* apices
    a. beat
    cardiac a.
    a. cordis
    a. of heart
    a. impulse
    left ventricular a.
    a. murmur
    right ventricular a.
    uptilted cardiac a.

apex *(continued)*
    ventricular a.
apexcardiogram
    upstsroke pattern on a.
apexcardiography
apheresis
aphonic pectoriloquy
apical
    a. bronchus
    a. aneurysm
    a. five-chamber view echo-
        cardiogram
    a. four-chamber view
    a. hypoperfusion on thal-
        lium scan
    a. impulse
    a. interventricular septal
        amplitude
    a. left ventricular puncture
    a. lordotic roentgenogram
    a. mid-diastolic heart mur-
        mur
    a. murmur
    a. scarring
    a. systolic heart murmur
    a. two-chamber view
apicoseptal aneurysmectomy
Apo
    A. A-1 deficiency
    A. A-1 LDL-cholesterol su-
        bfraction
    A. A-2 LDL-cholesterol su-
        bfraction
    A. E3 isoform
    A. E test
Apogee CX 100 Interspec ultra-
    sound machine
apolipoprotein
    a. A-I
    a. B
    a. C-II
    a. D
    a. E
aponeurosis

aponeurotic
apoplectic
apoplexy
    abdominal a.
    adrenal a.
    asthenic a.
    capillary a.
    ingravescent a.
apoprotein
    a. A
    a. B
    a. C
    a. D
    a. E
apoptosis
apoptotic cell death
A-Port vascular access
aposome
apparatus
    anastomosis a.
    central a.
    chromidial a.
    Golgi a.
    Jaquet a.
    Nakayama anastomosis a.
    spindle a.
    vasomotor a.
appendage
    atrial a.
    auricular a.
    left atrial a.
    right atrial a.
    truncated atrial a.
appendectomy
    auricular a.
appendix
    auricular a.
applanation tonometry
applesauce sign
apposition
    mitral-septal a.

apposition *(continued)*
    stent a.

approach
    antegrade a.
    anterior a.
    brachial artery a.
    central a.
    cephalic a.
    external jugular a.
    femoral a.
    groin a.
    internal jugular a.
    Lortat-Jacob a.
    percutaneous a.
    percutaneous transfemoral a.
    posterior a.
    retrograde femoral a.
    subcostal a.
    transdiaphragmatic a.
    transradial a.
    transxiphoid a.
    trap-door a.

aprotinin

approximation
    Friedewald a.
    loose a.

approximator
    Ablaza-Morse rib a.
    Bailey rib a.
    Leksell sternal a.
    Lemmon rib a.
    Lemmon sternal a.
    microanastomosis a.
    Nunez sternal a.
    Pilling Wolvek sternal a.
    pivot microanastomosis a.
    rib a.
    sternal a.
    Wolvek sternal a.

aPTT
    activated partial thromboplastin time

apyrene

AR
    aortic regurgitation

AR-1 diagnostic guiding catheter

AR-2 diagnostic guiding catheter

arachidonate metabolism

arachidonic acid
    a. a. metabolites

Araki-Sako technique

araldehyde-tanned bovine carotid artery graft

araneus
    nevus a.

Arani double-loop guiding catheter

Arantii
    ductus A.

Arantius
    bodies of A.
    A. body
    canal of A.
    A. nodule

arborization
    a. block

Arbrook Hemovac

arcade
    anomalous mitral a.
    arterial a's
    a. collateral
    Flint a.
    septal a.

arch
    abdominothoracic a.
    a. of aorta
    aortic a.
    aortic a., cervical
    aortic a., double
    a. aortography
    a. arteriography
    axillary a.
    azygos vein a.
    bifid aortic a.
    carotid a.

arch *(continued)*
    a. and carotid arteriography
    carpal a., anterior
    carpal a., dorsal
    carpal a., palmar
    carpal a., posterior
    cervical aortic a.
    circumflex aortic a.
    congenital interrupted aortic a.
    digital venous a's
    dorsal venous a. of foot
    double aortic a.
    FemoStop femoral artery compression a.
    hypoplastic a.
    jugular venous a.
    Langer axillary a.
    palmar arterial a., deep
    palmar arterial a., superficial
    palmar venous a., deep
    palmar venous a., superficial
    palpebral a., inferior
    palpebral a., superior
    plantar a., deep
    plantar arterial a.
    plantar venous a.
    pharyngeal a.
    pulmonary a.
    right aortic a.
    tarsal a's
    transverse aortic a.
    Treitz a.
    volar venous a., deep
    volar venous a., superficial
    Zimmerman a.

archamphiaster

arching of mitral valve leaflet

Arco
    A. atomic pacemaker
    A. lithium pacemaker

Arcomax
    A. FMA cardiac angiography system

arcus
    a. plantaris
    a. venosi digitales
    a. volaris profundus
    a. volaris superficialis
    a. volaris venosus profundus
    a. volaris venosus superficialis

area
    aortic valve a.
    arrhythmogenic a.
    Bamberger a.
    body surface a.
    a. of superficial cardiac dullness
    cross-sectional a.
    echo-spared a.
    effective balloon dilated a.
    end-diastolic a.
    Erb a.
    Krönig a.
    a.-length method for ejection fraction
    midsternal a.
    mitral valve a.
    pulmonary valve a.
    pulmonic a.
    regurgitant jet a.
    secondary aortic a.
    subxiphoid a.
    tricuspid valve a.
    truncoconal a.
    valve orifice a.
    watershed a.

ArF excimer laser

arginine vasopressin

argon
    a. beam coagulator
    a. ion laser
    a.-krypton laser
    a. laser
    a. laser photocoagulator cautery
    a.-pumped dye laser

argon *(continued)*
  a.-pumped tunable dye laser
  a. needle
  a. vessel dilator

Argyle
  A. arterial catheter
  A. catheter
  A. Sentinel Seal chest tube
  A.-Turkel safety thoracentesis system
  A.-Turkel thoracentesis

Argyll Robertson pupils

Arloing-Courmont test

arm
  a.-ankle indices
  a. ergometry treadmill
  a. exercise stress test
  a.-leg gradient

armored heart

Army-Navy retractor

array
  convex linear a.
  multi-element linear a.
  PRx Endotak-Sub-Q a.
  sock a.
  symmetrical phased a.

arrest
  asystolic a.
  bradyarrhythmic a.
  cardiac a.
  cardioplegic a.
  cardiopulmonary a.
  cardiorespiratory a.
  circulatory a.
  cold cardioplegia a.
  cold ischemic a.
  deep hypothermic circulatory a.
  heart a.
  hypothermic fibrillating a.
  intermittent sinus a.
  respiratory a.
  sinoatrial a.
  sinus a.

arrest *(continued)*
  total circulatory a.
  transient sinus a.

Arrhigi
  point of A.

arrhythmia
  atrial a.
  atrioventricular junctional a.
  AV nodal Wenckebach a.
  baseline a.
  cardiac a.
  chronic a.
  a. circuit
  compound a.
  continuous a.
  a. control device (ACD)
  exercise-aggravated a.
  exercise-induced a.
  a. focus
  high-density ventricular a.
  hypokalemia-induced a.
  inducible a.
  inotropic a.
  juvenile a.
  lethal a.
  Lown a.
  malignant ventricular a.
  Mönckeberg a.
  nodal a.
  nonphasic a.
  nonrespiratory sinus a.
  paroxysmal supraventricular a.
  pause-dependent a.
  perpetual a.
  phasic sinus a.
  postperfusion a.
  reentrant a.
  reperfusion a.
  respiratory a.
  respiratory sinus a.
  Singh-Vaughn-Williams classification of a's
  sinus a.
  spontaneous a.
  stress-related a.
  supraventricular a.

arrhythmia *(continued)*
tachybrady a.
vagus a.
ventricular a.

Arrhythmia Net arrhythmia monitor

arrhythmic

arrhythmogenesis

arrhythmogenic
a. area of ventricle
a. right ventricular disease
a. right ventricular dysplasia
a. substrate
a. ventricular activity

arrhythmogenicity

arrhythmokinesis

Arrow
A. balloon wedge catheter
A. Flex intra-aortic balloon catheter
A. Hi-flow infusion set
A. QuadPolar electrode catheter
A. pulmonary artery catheter
A. sheath
A. TwinCath multilumen peripheral catheter
A.-Berman angiographic balloon
A.-Berman balloon angioplasty catheter
A.-Clarke thoracentesis device
A.-Fischell EVAN needle
A.-Howes multilumen catheter
A.-Howes quad-lumen catheter

artegraft

artemisin

arteralgia

arterectomy

arteria *pl.* arteriae
a. acetabuli
a. adrenalis media
a. anastomotica auricularis magna
a. aorta
arteriae arciformes renis
a. ascendens ileocolica
a. auditiva interna
arteriae auriculares anteriores
arteriae bronchiales
a. buccinatoria
a. bulbi urethrae
a. cecalis anterior
a. cecalis posterior
a. centralis brevis
a. centralis longa
a. cerebelli inferior anterior
a. cerebelli inferior posterior
a. cerebelli superior
a. cervicalis superficialis
arteriae cervicovaginales
a. circumflexa anterior humeri
a. circumflexa humeri posterior
a. circumflexa posterior humeri
a. comitans nervi sciatici
a. coronaria [cordis] dextra
a. coronaria dextra
a. coronaria [cordis] sinistra
a. coronaria sinistra
a. deferentialis
a. descendens genicularis
arteriae digitales volares communes
arteriae digitales volares propriae
a. frontalis
a. gastroepiploica dextra
a. gastroepiploica sinistra
a. genus inferior lateralis
a. genus inferior medialis
a. genus media

arteria *(continued)*
- a. genus superior lateralis
- a. genus superior medialis
- a. glutealis inferior
- a. glutealis superior
- a. gyri angularis
- a. haemorrhoidalis inferior
- a. haemorrhoidalis media
- a. haemorrhoidalis superior
- a. hepatica
- a. hypogastrica
- arteriae ileae
- arteriae ilei
- a. innominata
- a. interossea dorsalis
- a. interossea volaris
- arteriae intestinales
- arteriae labiales anteriores vulvae
- arteriae labiales posteriores vulvae
- a. lusoria
- a. mammaria interna
- a. maxillaris externa
- a. maxillaris interna
- a. mediana
- arteriae mediastinales anteriores
- a. meningea anterior
- a. mentalis
- arteriae metacarpeae dorsales
- arteriae metacarpeae palmares
- arteriae metatarseae dorsales
- arteriae metatarseae plantares
- a. nasi externa
- a. paracentralis
- arteriae parietooccipitales
- a. perinei
- a. peronea
- a. precunealis
- a. pulmonalis
- a. recurrens

arteria *(continued)*
- arteriae recurrentes ulnares
- a. scapularis descendens
- a. scapularis dorsalis
- arteriae scrotales anteriores
- arteriae scrotales posteriores
- a. spermatica externa
- a. spinalis posterior
- arteriae sternocleidomastoideae
- a. temporalis posterior
- arteriae thalamostriatae anterolaterales
- arteriae thalamostriatae anteromediales
- a. thoracica suprema
- arteriae thymicae
- a. transversa scapulae
- arteriae metacarpeae volares
- a. nutriens tibialis

arterial
- a. anastomosis
- a. aneurysm
- a. bleeding
- a. blood flow
- a. blood gas (ABG)
- a. blood pressure (ABP)
- a. calcification
- a. cannula
- a. carbon dioxide pressure
- a. circle of Willis
- a. cone
- a. coupling
- a. cutdown
- a. decortication
- a. dicrotic notch pressure
- a. dissection
- a. embolectomy catheter
- a. embolism
- a. entry site
- a. filter
- a. graft
- a. groove
- a. hyperemia

arterial *(continued)*
  a. hypertension
  a. hypotension
  a. hypoxemia
  a. impedance
  a. insufficiency
  a. line (A-line)
  a. line pressure bag
  a. line transducer
  a. mean
  a. mean line
  a. media
  a. murmur
  a. needle
  a. occlusive disease
  a. oscillator endarterec-
    tomy instrument
  a. oxygen saturation
  a. pressure
  a. pulse
  a. remodeling
  a. runoff
  a. saturation
  a. sclerosis
  a. sheath
  a. spasm
  a. spider
  a. stick
  a. switch operation
  a. switch procedure
  a. thrill
  a. thrombosis
  a. vein of Soemmering
  a. wave
  a. wedge

arterialization

arteriarctia

arteriasis

arteriectasia

arteriectasis

arteriectomy

arteriectopia

arterioatony

arteriocapillary
  a. sclerosis

arteriodilating

arteriofibrosia

arteriogenesis

arteriogram
  aorta and runoff a.
  arch a.
  biplane quantitative coron-
    ary a.
  brachial a.
  femoral a.
  runoff a.
  subclavian a.

arteriograph

arteriographic
  a. regression

arteriography
  aortofemoral a.
  arch a.
  biplane pelvic a.
  biplane quantitative coron-
    ary a.
  carotid a.
  catheter a.
  cine a.
  coronary a.
  digital subtraction a.
  femoral a.
  Judkins technique for co-
    ronary a.
  left coronary cine a.
  percutaneous femoral a.
  pulmonary artery a.
  quantitative a.
  renal a.
  selective a.
  Sones selective coronary a.

arteriohepatic dysplasia syndrome

arteriolar
  a. hyalinosis
  a. narrowing
  a. resistance
  a. sclerosis

arteriole
  afferent a.
  efferent a.
  ellipsoid a's
  Isaacs-Ludwig a.
  macular a., inferior
  macular a., superior
  medial a. of retina
  nasal a. of retina, inferior
  nasal a. of retina, superior
  precapillary a.
  sheathed a's
  temporal a. of retina, infe-
    rior
  temporal a. of retina, supe-
    rior

arteriolith

arteriolitis
  necrotizing a.

arteriology

arteriolonecrosis

arteriolopathy

arteriolosclerosis
  hyaline a.
  hyperplastic a.

arteriolosclerotic

arteriolovenular bridge

arteriomalacia

arteriometer

arteriomotor

arteriomyomatosis

arterionecrosis
  hyaline a.

arteriopalmus

arteriopathy
  hypertensive a.
  plexogenic pulmonary a.
  thrombotic pulmonary a.

arteriophlebotomy

arterioplania

arterioplasty

arteriopressor

arteriorenal

arteriorrhagia

arteriorrhaphy

arteriorrhexis

arteriosclerosis
  cerebral a.
  coronary a.
  decrudescent a.
  diffuse a.
  hyaline a.
  hypertensive a.
  infantile a.
  intimal a.
  medial a.
  Mönckeberg a.
  nodose a.
  nodular a.
  a. obliterans
  peripheral a.
  presenile a.
  senile a.

arteriosclerotic
  a. cardiovascular disease
    (ASCVD)
  a. heart disease (ASHD)
  a. peripheral vascular dis-
    ease
  a. vascular disease (ASVD)

arteriospasm

arteriospastic

arteriostenosis

arteriosteogenesis

arteriostosis

arteriostrepsis

arteriosus
  conus a.
  ductus a.
  patent ductus a. (PDA)
  persistent ductus a.

arteriosus *(continued)*
  persistent truncus a.
  pseudotruncus a.
  reversed ductus a.
  truncus a.
arteriotomy
  brachial a.
arteriotony
arteriovenous (AV, A-V)
  a. anastomosis
  a. aneurysm
  a. communication
  a. crossing changes
  a. fistula
  a. malformation (AVM)
  a. nicking
  a. oxygen difference
  a. pulmonary aneurysm
  a. shunt
arterioversion
arteritis *pl.* arteritides
  aortic arch a.
  brachiocephalic a.
  a. brachiocephalica
  coronary a.
  cranial a.
  a. deformans
  fibrinoid a.
  giant cell a.
  granulomatous a.
  Horton a.
  a. hyperplastica
  infantile a.
  infectious a.
  localized visceral a.
  mesenteric a.
  necrotizing a.
  a. nodosa
  a. obliterans
  rheumatic a.
  rheumatoid a.
  syphilitic a.
  Takayasu a.
  temporal a.
  tuberculous a.
  a. umbilicalis
  a. verrucosa

artery
  aberrant coronary a.
  accessory a.
  accompanying a. of ischiadic nerve
  accompanying a. of median nerve
  acetabular a.
  acromiothoracic a.
  a's of Adamkiewicz
  adipose a's of kidney
  adrenal a., middle
  afferent a. of glomerulus
  alveolar a's, anterior superior
  alveolar a., inferior
  alveolar a., posterior superior
  anastomotic atrial a.
  angular a.
  a. of angular gyrus
  appendicular a.
  arcuate a's of kidney
  arcuate a. of foot
  atrial anastomotic a.
  atrioventricular nodal a.
  auditory a., internal
  auricular a's, anterior
  auricular a., deep
  auricular a., left
  auricular a., posterior
  auricular a., right
  axillary a.
  azygos a's of vagina
  basilar a.
  beading of a's
  brachial a.
  brachial a., deep
  brachial a., superficial
  brachiocephalic a.
  bronchial a's
  bronchial a's, anterior
  buccal a.
  buccinator a.
  a. of bulb of penis
  bulbourethral a.
  a. of bulb of vestibule
  capsular a., inferior

artery *(continued)*
    capsular a., middle
    caroticotympanic a's
    carotid a., common
    carotid a., external
    carotid a., internal
    caudal a.
    cecal a., anterior
    cecal a., posterior
    central a's, anterolateral
    central a's, anteromedial,
      of anterior cerebral a.
    central a's, anteromedial,
      of anterior communica-
      ting a.
    central a's of spleen
    central a's, posterolateral
    central a's, posteromedial,
      of posterior cerebral a.
    central a's, posteromedial,
      of posterior communica-
      ting a.
    central a., long
    central a. of retina
    central a., short
    a. of central sulcus
    cerebellar a., anterior infe-
      rior
    cerebellar a., posterior infe-
      rior
    cerebellar a., superior
    cerebral a's
    cerebral a., anterior
    cerebral a., middle
    cerebral a., posterior
    a. of cerebral hemorrhage
    a's of cerebrum
    cervical a., ascending
    cervical a., deep
    cervical a., deep descend-
      ing
    cervical a., superficial
    cervical a., transverse
    cervicovaginal a's
    choroid a., anterior
    choroidal a., anterior
    ciliary a's, anterior

artery *(continued)*
    ciliary a's, long
    ciliary a's, long posterior
    ciliary a's, short
    ciliary a's, short posterior
    circumflex a.
    circumflex a., internal deep
    circumflex a. of scapula
    circumflex femoral a., lat-
      eral
    circumflex femoral a., me-
      dial
    circumflex humeral a., ante-
      rior
    circumflex humeral a., pos-
      terior
    circumflex iliac a., deep
    circumflex iliac a., superfi-
      cial
    coccygeal a.
    cochlear a.
    colic a., accessory superior
    colic a., inferior right
    colic a., left
    colic a., middle
    colic a., right
    collateral a., inferior ulnar
    collateral a., middle
    collateral a., radial
    collateral a., superior ulnar
    communicating a., anterior
    communicating a., anterior
      inferior (AICA)
    communicating a., poste-
      rior
    conal a.
    conducting a's
    conjunctival a's, anterior
    conjunctival a's, posterior
    conus a., left
    conus a., right
    conus a., third
    copper-wire a's
    corkscrew a's
    coronary a., left (LCA)
    coronary a., left anterior
      descending (LAD)

artery *(continued)*

coronary a., left anterior
descending, diagonal
branch
coronary a., left circumflex
(LCX)
coronary a. of stomach, left
coronary a., posterior descending (PDA)
coronary a., right
cremasteric a.
cricothyroid a.
cystic a.
deep a. of clitoris
deep a. of penis
deferential a.
deltoid a.
dental a's, anterior
dental a., inferior
dental a., posterior
diaphragmatic a's, superior
diaphragmatic a.
digital a's, collateral
digital a's, common palmar
digital a's, common plantar
digital a's, common volar
digital a's of foot, common
digital a's of foot, dorsal
digital a's of hand, dorsal
digital a's, proper palmar
digital a's, proper plantar
digital a's, proper volar
distributing a's
dorsal a. of clitoris
dorsal a. of foot
dorsal a. of nose
dorsal a. of penis
dorsal a. of tongue
a. of ductus deferens
efferent a. of glomerulus
elastic a's
end a.
epigastric a., inferior
epigastric a., superficial
epigastric a., superior
episcleral a's
esophageal a's, inferior
esophageal a.

artery *(continued)*

ethmoidal a., anterior
ethmoidal a., posterior
facial a.
facial a., transverse
fallopian a.
femoral a.
femoral a., common
femoral a., deep
femoral a., superficial
fibular a.
frontal a.
frontobasal a., lateral
frontobasal a., medial
funicular a.
gastric a's, short
gastric a., left
gastric a., left inferior
gastric a., posterior
gastric a., right
gastric a., right inferior
gastro-omental a., left
gastro-omental a., right
gastroduodenal a.
gastroepiploic a., left
gastroepiploic a., right
genicular a., descending
genicular a., lateral inferior
genicular a., lateral superior
genicular a., medial inferior
genicular a., medial superior
genicular a., middle
gluteal a., inferior
gluteal a., superior
gonadal a's
helicine a's
hemorrhoidal a., inferior
hemorrhoidal a., middle
hemorrhoidal a., superior
hepatic a., common
hepatic a., proper
hyaloid a.
a's of hybrid type
hypogastric a.
hypophysial a., inferior
hypophysial a., superior

artery *(continued)*
    ileal a's
    ileocolic a.
    ileocolic a., ascending
    a's of ileum
    iliac a., anterior
    iliac a., common
    iliac a., external
    iliac a., internal
    iliac a., small
    iliolumbar a.
    infracostal a.
    infraorbital a.
    inguinal a's
    innominate a.
    insular a's
    intercostal a's, anterior
    intercostal a's, posterior
    intercostal a., first posterior
    intercostal a., highest
    intercostal a., second posterior
    intercostal a., superior
    interlobar a's of kidney
    interlobular a's of kidney
    interlobular a's of liver
    intermediate atrial a., left
    intermediate atrial a., right
    intermetacarpal a's, palmar
    interosseous a., anterior
    interosseous a., common
    interosseous a., dorsal
    interosseous a., posterior
    interosseous a., recurrent
    interosseous a., volar
    interventricular a., anterior
    interventricular septal a's, anterior
    interventricular septal a's, posterior
    intestinal a's
    jejunal a's
    labial a's of vulva, anterior
    labial a's of vulva, posterior
    labial a., inferior
    labial a., superior

artery *(continued)*
    a. of labyrinth
    labyrinthine a.
    lacrimal a.
    laryngeal a., inferior
    laryngeal a., superior
    lateral inferior a. of knee
    lateral superior a. of knee
    lenticulostriate a.
    lingual a.
    lingual a., deep
    lingular a.
    lingular a., inferior
    lingular a., superior
    lobar a's of left lung, superior
    lobar a's of left lung, inferior
    lobar a's of right lung, superior
    lobar a's of right lung, inferior
    lobar a. of right lung, middle
    a's of lower limb
    lumbar a's
    lumbar a's, fifth
    lumbar a's, lowest
    malleolar a., lateral anterior
    malleolar a., lateral posterior
    malleolar a., medial anterior
    mammary a., external
    mammary a., internal
    mammary a., left internal (LIMA)
    mandibular a.
    marginal a., left
    marginal a. of colon
    marginal a. of Drummond
    marginal a., right
    masseteric a.
    mastoid a.
    maxillary a.
    maxillary a., external
    maxillary a., internal

artery *(continued)*
   medial a. of foot, superficial
   medial inferior a. of knee
   medial superior a. of knee
   median a.
   mediastinal a's, anterior
   mediastinal a's, posterior
   medullary a.
   meningeal a., accessory
   meningeal a., anterior
   meningeal a., middle
   meningeal a., posterior
   mental a.
   mesencephalic a's
   mesenteric a., inferior
   mesenteric a., superior
   metacarpal a's, dorsal
   metacarpal a's, palmar
   metacarpal a's, ulnar
   metacarpal a's, volar
   metacarpal a., deep volar
   metatarsal a's, dorsal
   metatarsal a's, plantar
   a's of mixed type
   a's of Mueller
   muscular a's
   musculophrenic a.
   mylohyoid a.
   myomastoid a.
   nasal a's, lateral posterior
   nasal a., dorsal
   nasal a., external
   nasopalatine a.
   Neubauer's a.
   nodal a.
   nutrient a's of femur
   nutrient a's of humerus
   nutrient a.
   nutrient a. of fibula
   nutrient a. of tibia
   obturator a.
   obturator a., accessory
   occipital a.
   occipital a., lateral
   occipital a., middle
   ophthalmic a.
   ovarian a.

artery *(continued)*
   palatine a's, lesser
   palatine a., ascending
   palatine a., descending
   palatine a., greater
   palpebral a's, lateral
   palpebral a's, medial
   pancreatic a., dorsal
   pancreatic a., great
   pancreatic a., inferior
   pancreaticoduodenal a's, inferior
   pancreaticoduodenal a., anterior superior
   pancreaticoduodenal a., posterior superior
   paracentral a.
   paramedian a's
   parietal a's, anterior and posterior
   pelvic a., posterior
   perforating a's
   pericallosal a.
   pericardiac a's, posterior
   pericardiacophrenic a.
   perineal a.
   peroneal a.
   peroneal a., perforating
   pharyngeal a., ascending
   phrenic a., great
   phrenic a., inferior
   phrenic a., superior
   plantar a., deep
   plantar a., external
   plantar a., lateral
   plantar a., medial
   pontine a's
   popliteal a.
   a. of postcentral sulcus
   a. of precentral sulcus
   precuneal a.
   prepancreatic a.
   principal a. of thumb
   pterygoid a's
   a. of pterygoid canal
   pubic a.
   pudendal a., deep external
   pudendal a., internal

artery *(continued)*
- pudendal a., superficial external
- pulmonary a.
- pulmonary a., left (LPA)
- pulmonary a., right
- a. of the pulp
- pyloric a.
- quadriceps a. of femur
- radial a.
- radial a., collateral
- radial a. of index finger
- radial a. of index finger, volar
- radiate a's of kidney
- ranine a.
- rectal a., inferior
- rectal a., middle
- rectal a., superior
- recurrent a.
- recurrent a., anterior tibial
- recurrent a., posterior tibial
- recurrent a., radial
- recurrent a., ulnar
- renal a.
- retrocostal a.
- retroduodenal a's
- a. of round ligament of uterus
- sacral a's, lateral
- sacral a., median
- sacrococcygeal a.
- scapular a., descending
- scapular a., dorsal
- scapular a., transverse
- sciatic a.
- a. to sciatic nerve
- scrotal a's, anterior
- scrotal a's, posterior
- segmental a., inferior lingular
- segmental a., lingular
- segmental a. of kidney, anterior superior
- segmental a. of kidney, anterior inferior

artery *(continued)*
- segmental a. of kidney, inferior
- segmental a. of kidney, posterior
- segmental a. of kidney, superior
- segmental a. of left lung, lateral basal
- segmental a. of left lung, superior
- segmental a. of left lung, apical
- segmental a. of left lung, medial basal
- segmental a. of left lung, posterior basal
- segmental a. of left lung, anterior descending
- segmental a. of left lung, posterior
- segmental a. of left lung, anterior ascending
- segmental a. of left lung, anterior basal
- segmental a. of left lung, posterior ascending
- segmental a. of left lung, anterior
- segmental a. of left lung, posterior descending
- segmental a. of liver, anterior
- segmental a. of liver, lateral
- segmental a. of liver, medial
- segmental a. of liver, posterior
- segmental a. of right lung, posterior descending
- segmental a. of right lung, apical
- segmental a. of right lung, lateral
- segmental a. of right lung, anterior ascending
- segmental a. of right lung, anterior basal

artery *(continued)*

  segmental a. of right lung, anterior descending
  segmental a. of right lung, posterior basal
  segmental a. of right lung, lateral basal
  segmental a. of right lung, medial
  segmental a. of right lung, medial basal
  segmental a. of right lung, posterior ascending
  segmental a. of right lung, posterior
  segmental a. of right lung, superior
  segmental a. of right lung, anterior
  segmental a., superior lingular
  segmental a. to inferior lobe of right lung, superior
  septal a's, anterior
  septal a's, posterior
  sheathed a's
  sigmoid a's
  sinoatrial nodal a.
  sinuatrial nodal a.
  sinus node a.
  spermatic a., external
  spermatic a., internal
  sphenopalatine a.
  spinal a's
  spinal a., anterior
  spinal a., posterior
  splenic a.
  sternal a's, posterior
  sternocleidomastoid a's
  sternocleidomastoid a., superior
  striate a's
  striate a's, lateral
  striate a's, medial
  stylomastoid a.
  subclavian a.
  subcostal a.

artery *(continued)*

  sublingual a.
  submental a.
  subscapular a.
  superior a. of cerebellum
  supraduodenal a.
  suprahyoid a.
  supraorbital a.
  suprarenal a's, superior
  suprarenal a., aortic
  suprarenal a., inferior
  suprarenal a., middle
  suprascapular a.
  supratrochlear a.
  sural a's
  sylvian a.
  tarsal a's, medial
  tarsal a., lateral
  temporal a's, deep
  temporal a., anterior
  temporal a., anterior deep
  temporal a., intermediate
  temporal a., middle
  temporal a., posterior
  temporal a., posterior deep
  temporal a., superficial
  terminal a.
  testicular a.
  thalamostriate a's, anterolateral
  thalamostriate a's, anteromedial
  thoracic a., highest
  thoracic a., internal
  thoracic a., lateral
  thoracic a., superior
  thoracicoacromial a.
  thoracoacromial a.
  thoracodorsal a.
  thymic a's
  thyroid a., inferior
  thyroid a., lowest
  thyroid a. of Cruveilhier, inferior
  thyroid a., superior
  tibial a., anterior
  tibial a., posterior
  tonsillar a.

artery *(continued)*
    transverse a. of face
    transverse a. of neck
    transverse cervical a.
    tubo-ovarian a.
    tympanic a., anterior
    tympanic a., inferior
    tympanic a., posterior
    tympanic a., superior
    ulnar a.
    ulnar collateral a., inferior
    ulnar collateral a., superior
    umbilical a.
    a's of upper limb
    urethral a.
    uterine a.
    uterine a., aortic
    vaginal a.
    venous a's
    vermiform a.
    vertebral a.
    vesical a's, superior
    vesical a., inferior
    vestibular a's
    vidian a.
    a. of Zinn
    zygomatico-orbital a.

arthritis-associated aortitis

arthropod venom

Arthus-type reaction

articulation

artifact
    aliasing a.
    baseline a.
    beam width a.
    catheter impact a.
    catheter whip a.
    coin a.
    cupping a.
    end-pressure a.
    flow a.
    pacemaker a.
    pacing a.
    reverberation a.
    side lobe a.
    T a.
    view-aliasing a.

artifact *(continued)*
    wrap-around ghosting a.
    zebra a.

artifactual bradycardia

artificial
    a. blood
    a. cardiac valve
    a. heart (LPA)
    a. pacemaker
    a. pneumothorax
    a. ventilation

Arvidsson dimension-length method

Arzco
    A. model 7 cardiac stimulator
    A. pacemaker
    A. TAPSUL pill electrode

AS
    aortic stenosis

ASC
    ASC Alpha balloon
    ASC Monorel catheter
    ASC RX perfusion balloon catheter

A-scan echography

ascariasis

ascendens
    aorta a.

ascending
    a. aorta (AA)
    a. aorta-to-pulmonary artery shunt
    a. aortic pressure
    a. aortography
    a. loop of Henle

Ascension Bird

Aschner
    A. phenomenon
    A. reflex
    A. sign
    A.-Dagnini reflex

Aschoff
    A. body
    A. cell
    A. nodules
    A.-Tawara node

ascites
    a. praecox

ascorbate dilution curve

ascorbic acid

ASCVD
    arteriosclerotic cardiovas-
        cular disease
    atherosclerotic cardiovas-
        cular disease

ASD
    atrial septal defect

asequence

ASH
    asymmetrical septal hyper-
        trophy

ASHD
    arteriosclerotic heart dis-
        ease

Asherman chest seal

Asherson syndrome

Ashley phenomenon

Ashman
    A. beat
    A. phenomenon

Ask-Upmark
    A.-U. kidney
    A.-U. syndrome

ASO
    antistreptolysin O
    ASO titer test

aspartate aminotransferase
    (AST)

asphygmia

Asserachrom
    A. D-DI ELISA assay

Asserachrom *(continued)*
    A. t-PA immunologic assay

assessment
    anatomic a.
    angiographic a.
    cardiovascular a.
    echocardiographic a.
    functional a.
    hemodynamic a.
    invasive a.
    jugular bulb catheter place-
        ment a.
    noninvasive a.
    transposition a.

assisted circulation

AST
    aspartate aminotransferase

asteroid

asthenia
    neurocirculatory a.
    vasoregulatory a.

asthenic apoplexy

asthenicus
    thorax a.

asthma
    cardiac a.
    Elsner a.
    Heberden a.
    Rostan a.

Astra
    A. profile
    A. T4, T6 pacemaker

astral

Astrand
    A. bicycle exercise stress
        test
    A. treadmill

Astrand-Rhyming protocol

astrocele

astrocinetic

astrocoele

astrocyte

astrokinetic

astrosphere

astrophorous

Astropulse cuff

astrostatic

Astro-Trace Universal adapter
clip

Astrup blood gas value

ASTZ
    antistreptozyme

Asuka PTA over-the-wire catheter

ASVD
    arteriosclerotic vascular
        disease

asymmetric
    a. septal hypertrophy
        (ASH)

asymptomatic
    a. cardiac ischemia
    a. carotid atherosclerosis
        plaque
    a. complex ectopy

asynchronism

asynchronous
    a. pacing
    a. pulse generator

asynchrony
    a. index

asyneresis

asynergy
    infarct-localized a.
    left ventricular a.
    regional a.
    segmental a.

asystole
    atrial a.
    Beau a.

asystole (continued)
    ventricular a.

asystolia

asystolic
    a. arrest

AT
    atrial tachycardia
        MemoryTace AT

Atakr system

A-T antiembolism stockings

ataxia
    a. cordis
    Friedreich a.
    hereditary a.
    spinocerebellar a.

ataxic
    a. aphasia
    a. gait

atelocardia

atherectomy
    Auth a.
    a. catheter
    coronary a.
    coronary angioplasty ver-
        sus excisional a.
    coronary rotational a.
    a. cutter
    a. device
    directional coronary a.
    high-speed rotational a.
    a. index
    Kinsey a.
    percutaneous coronary ro-
        tational a.
    retrograde a.
    rotational a.
    Simpson a. catheter
    transluminal a.
    transluminal extraction a.

atheroablation laser

AtheroCath
    Simpson Coronary A. cath-
        eter

AtheroCath *(continued)*
    Simpson Coronary A. system
    Simpson peripheral A.
    A. spinning blade catheter

atheroembolism

atheroembolus *pl.* atheroemboli

atherogenesis
    monoclonal theory of a.
    response-to-injury hypothesis of a.

atherogenic

atherogenicity index

atherolytic reperfusion guide wire

atheroma

atheromatosis

atheromatous
    a. debris
    a. embolism
    a. plaque

atheronecrosis

atherosclerosis
    cardiac allograft a.
    coronary artery a.
    de novo a.
    encrustation theory of a.
    intimal a.
    lipogenic theory of a.
    a. obliterans
    premature a.

atherosclerotic
    a. aneurysm
    a. aortic disease
    a. aortography
    a. cardiovascular disease (ASCVD)
    a. carotid artery disease
    a. coronary artery disease
    a. narrowing
    a. plaque

atherosis

atherothrombosis

atherothrombotic

atherotome

athlete's heart

athletic heart

AT-III
    antithrombin III

Atkinson tube stent

Atlas
    A. LP PTCA balloon dilatation catheter
    A. ULP balloon dilatation catheter

Atlee clamp

ATL Ultramark Y echocardiographic device

atmospheres of pressure

atmotherapy

ATnativ

ATP
    adenosine triphosphate
        ATP hydrolysis
    antitachycardia pacemaker

ATPase
    adenosine triphosphatase
        myofibrillar ATPase
        SR calcium ATPase

ATRAC-II double-balloon catheter

ATRAC multipurpose balloon catheter

atracurium

Atra-grip clamp

Atraloc needle

Atrauclip hemostatic clip

atraumatic needle

atresia
   aortic a.
   mitral a.
   pulmonary a.
   tricuspid a.
   ventricular a.

atrial
   a. activation mapping
   a. activation time
   a. anomalous bands
   a. appendage
   a. arrhythmia
   a. asynchronous pace-
      maker
   a. asystole
   a.-axis discontinuity
   a. baffle operation
   a. balloon septostomy
   a. bigeminy
   a. bolus dynamic computer
      tomography
   a. capture
   a. capture beat
   a. capture threshold
   a. chaotic tachycardia
   a. cuff
   a. defibrillation threshold
   a. demand-inhibited (AAI)
   a. demand-inhibited pace-
      maker
   a. demand-triggered (AAT)
   a. demand-triggered pace-
      maker
   a. diastole
   a. diastolic gallop
   a. dissociation
   a. echo
   a. ectopic beat
   a. ectopic tachycardia
      (AET)
   a. ectopy
   a. effective refractory pe-
      riod
   a. ejection force
   a. escape interval
   a. extrastimulus method
   a. extrasystole

atrial (continued)
   a. fibrillation (AF)
   a. fibrillation-flutter
   a. fibrillation with rapid
      ventricular response
   a. filling pressure
   a. flutter
   a. fusion beat
   a. infarction
   a. kick
   a. lead impedance
   a. liver pulse
   a. myocardial cell
   a. myocardial infarction
   a. myxoma
   a. natriuretic factor (ANF)
   a. natriuretic polypeptide
      (ANP)
   a. non-sensing
   a. notch
   a. ostium primum defect
   a. overdrive pacing
   a.-paced cycle length
   a. pacing
   a. pacing stress test
   a. pacing study
   a. pacing wire
   a. paroxysmal tachycardia
   a. premature beat
   a. premature complexes
   a. premature contraction
      (APC)
   a. premature depolariza-
      tion
   a. pulse amplitude
   a. pulse width
   a. reentry tachycardia
   a. repolarization wave
   a. rhythm
   a. ring
   a. sensing configuration
   a. sensitivity
   a. septal aneurysm
   a. septal defect (ASD)
   a. septal defect single disk
      closure device
   a. septal defect umbrella
   a. septectomy
   a. septostomy

atrial *(continued)*
    a. septum
    a. shear
    a. sound
    a. standstill
    a. stasis index
    a. synchronous pulse generator
    a. synchronous ventricular inhibited pacemaker
    a. synchrony
    a. systole
    a. tachycardia (AT)
    a. thrombus
    a. tracking pacemaker
    a. train pacing
    a. transport function
    a. triggered pulse generator
    a. triggered ventricular-inhibited pacemaker
    a. valve
    a. vector loop
    a. venous pulse
    a. ventricular nodal reentry tachycardia
    a. ventricular reciprocating tachycardia
    a. ventricular shunt
    a. VOO pacemaker
    a.-well technique

atrialized
    a. chamber
    a. ventricle

Atricor Cordis pacemaker

atriocarotid interval

atriocommissuropexy

atriocyte

atriodextrofascicular tract

atriodigital dysplasia

atriofascicular tract

atriography

atrio-His
    a.-H. pathway
    a.-H. tract

atriohisian, atrio-Hisian
    a. bypass tract
    a. fiber
    a. interval
    a. tract

atriomegaly

atrionector

atrionodal bypass tract

atriopeptin

atriopressor reflex

atriopulmonary shunt

atrioseptal
    a. defect
    a. sign

atrioseptopexy

atrioseptoplasty

atriosystolic murmur

atriotome

atriotomy

atrioventricular (AV, A-V)
    a. block
    a. bundle
    a. canal
    a. canal cushion
    a. canal defect
    a. conduction
    a. conduction abnormality
    a. conduction defect
    a. conduction system
    a. conduction tissue
    a. connection anomaly
    a. delay interval
    a. discordance
    a. dissociation
    a. extrasystole
    a. flow rumbling murmur
    a. furrow
    a. gradient
    a. groove
    a. interval

atrioventricular *(continued)*
    a. junction
    a. junctional ablation
    a. junctional arrhythmia
    a. junctional bigeminy
    a. junctional escape beat
    a. junctional escape complex
    a. junctional extrasystole
    a. junctional heart block
    a. junctional pacemaker
    a. junctional reciprocating tachycardia
    a. junctional rhythm
    a. junctional tachycardia
    a. junction motion
    a. malformation (AVM)
    a. nodal artery
    a. nodal bigeminy
    a. nodal conduction
    a. nodal disease
    a. nodal extrasystole
    a. nodal reentrant tachycardia
    a. nodal reentry
    a. nodal rhythm
    a. nodal tachycardia
    a. nodal Wenckebach arrhythmia
    a. node
    a. node artery
    a. node pathways
    a. node Wenckebach periodicity
    a. orifice
    a. reciprocating tachycardia
    a. refractory period
    a. ring
    a. septal defect
    a. sequential pacemaker
    a. situs concordance
    a. sulcus
    a. synchronous pacemaker
    a. synchrony
    a. time
    a. valve
    a. valve insufficiency

atrioventricular *(continued)*
    a. valve replacement
    a. Wenckebach block

atrioventricularis
    a. communis
    crus dextrum fasciculi a.
    crus sinistrum fasciculi a.
    nodus a.

atrioventriculostomy

Atri-pace I bipolar flared pacing catheter

Atrium Blood Recovery System

atrium *pl.* atria
    accessory a.
    common a.
    congenital single a.
    a. cordis
    a. dextrum
    a. of heart
    high right a.
    left a. (LA)
    low septal a.
    a. of lungs
    a. pulmonale
    pulmonary a.
    right a. (RA)
    single a.
    a. sinistrum
    stunned a.

atrophic
    a. cardiomyopathy
    a. thrombosis

atrophy
    brown a.
    cardiac a.
    cyanotic a. of liver
    Erb a.
    multiple system a.
    olivopontocerebellar a.
    red a.
    spinal muscular a.

Atrostim phrenic nerve stimulator

attack
    Adams-Stokes a.

attack *(continued)*
    heart a.
    transient ischemic a. (TIA)
    vagal a.
    vasovagal a.

attenuation
    heterogeneous a.

attenuator

attrition murmur

atypical
    a. atrioventricular nodal re-entrant tachycardia
    a. chest pain
    a. mycobacterial colonization
    a. tamponade
    a. verrucous endocarditis

auditory
    a. alternans
    a. fremitus

Auenbrugger sign

Aufrecht sign

Aufricht elevator

auger wire

augmentation therapy

augmentor

auricle
    left a. of heart
    right a. of heart

auricula
    atrial a.
    a. atrialis
    a. atrii dextri
    a. atrii sinistri
    a. cordis
    a. dextra cordis
    a. sinistra cordis

auricular
    a. appendage
    a. appendectomy
    a. complex
    a. extrasystole

auricular *(continued)*
    a. fibrillation
    a. flutter
    a. premature beat
    a. rate
    a. standstill
    a. systole
    a. tachycardia

auriculopressor reflex

auriculoventricular
    a. extrasystole
    a. groove
    a. interval

Aurora
    A. dual-chamber pacemaker
    A. pulse generator

aurothiomalate

Ausculoscope

auscultation
    cardiac a.
    Korányi a.
    percussion and a. (P&A)

auscultatory
    a. alternans
    a. gap
    a. sign
    a. sound

Austin Flint
    A. F. murmur
    A. F. phenomenon
    A. F. respiration
    A. F. rumble

Australia antigen

Australian Q fever

Austrian syndrome

autacoid

Auth
    A. atherectomy
    A. atherectomy catheter

Autima II dual-chamber pacemaker

autoanalyzer

autobiotic

Autoclix

autoclot

autocrine

autodecremental pacing

autodigestion of connective tissue

autogamous

autogamy

autogenic graft

autogenous
a. vein

autograft

autohypnosis

autoimmune disorder

autoinfusion

autologous
a. blood
a. clot
a. fat graft
a. pericardial patch
a. transfusion
a. vein graft

autolysosome

automatic
a. atrial tachycardia (AAT)
a. beat
a. boundary detection
a. ectopic tachycardia
a. exposure system
a. external defibrillator (AED)
a. implantable cardioverter-defibrillator (AICD)
a. implantable defibrillator (AID)
a. internal cardioverter-defibrillator (AICD)

automatic (continued)
a. internal defibrillator
a. intracardiac defibrillator
a. mode switching
a. oscillometric blood pressure monitor
a. pacemaker
a. ventricular contraction

automaticity
enhanced a.
pacemaker a.
sinus nodal a.
triggered a.

automixis

autonomic
a. dysreflexia
a. hyperreflexia
a. modulation
a. nervous system
a. sensory innervation

autoperfusion balloon catheter

autophagia

autophagolysosome

autophagosome

autophagy

Autoplex Factor VIII inhibitor bypass product

autoradiography

autoregulation
heterometric a.
homeometric a.

autosome

Autostat ligating and hemostatic clip

Auto Suture Surgiclip

autosynthesis

autotemnous

autotomy

autotoxic cyanosis

Autotransfuser
  Biosurge Synchronous A.

autotransfusion system

autotransplantation

Autotrans system

auxocardia

AV
  arteriovenous
  atrioventricular
    AV Gore-Tex fistula
    AV Miniclinic

AVAD
  acute ventricular assist device

Avanti introducer

avascular
  a. necrosis

avascularization

Avenue insertion tool

average
  a. mean pressure
  a. pulse magnitude

averaging
  digital a.
  signal a.

aVF lead

aVL lead

aVR lead

aviators' disease

Avitene topical hemostatic material

Avius sequential pacemaker

AVM
  arteriovenous malformation
  atrioventricular malformation

AV O$_2$ difference
  pulmonary AV O$_2$ difference
  systemic AV O$_2$ difference

AV-Paceport thermodilution catheter

AVR
  aortic valve replacement

avulsion

awl
  Rochester a.
  Wangensteen a.

axial
  a. computed tomography
  a. control
  a. plane

axillary
  a. arch
  a. artery
  a. block
  a. lymph nodes
  a. triangle
  a. vein

axilloaxillary bypass

axillobifemoral

axillofemoral

axillopopliteal

Axiom
  A. DG balloon angioplasty catheter
  A. double sump pump
  A. thoracic trocar

Axios 04 pacemaker

axis pl. axes
  arterial a.
  clockwise rotation of electrical a.
  celiac a.
  cell a.
  costocervical arterial a.
  a. deviation

axis *(continued)*
    a. of EKG lead
    electrical a. of heart
    a. of heart
    hypophyseal-pituitary ad-
        renal a.
    instantaneous electrical a.
    J point electrical a.
    junctional a.
    left a.
    long a.
    mean electrical a.
    mean QRS a.
    normal electrical a.
    P wave a.
    QRS a.
    right a.
    rightward a.
    a. shift
    short a.
    Strong unbridling of celiac
        artery a.
    superior QRS a.
    thoracic a.
    twisting on the electrical a.
    variable a.
    X a.

axis *(continued)*
    Y a.

axoneme

Ayers
    A. cardiovascular needle
        holder
    A. sphygmomanometer
    A. T-piece

Ayerza
    A. disease
    A. syndrome

azalide
    a. class of antibiotics

azotemia
    extrarenal a.
    postrenal a.
    prerenal a.
    renal a.

azygography

azygoportal interruption

azygos
    a. arch
    a. vein

B
  B bump
  B bump on echocardi-
    ogram
  B cell
  B cell antibody
  B cell lymphoma
B1
  B1 cell
B4
  leukotriene B4 (LTB4)
b
  b knuckle
Babcock
  B. operation
  B. thoracic tissue-holding
    forceps
Babinski
  downgoing B.
  B. reflex
  B. syndrome
  upgoing B.
baby
  blue b.
babygram x-ray
Baccelli sign
Bachmann
  B. bundle
  internodal tract of B.
  B. pathway
  pathway of B.
bacillary
  b. angiomatosis
  b. embolism
  b. phthisis
bacillus *pl.* bacilli
  acid-fast b. (AFB)
  enteric gram-negative b.
  gram-negative b.
  gram-positive b.
  Klebs-Löffler b.
  Löffler b.
  Warthin-Starry–staining b.

back-bleeding
backflow from arterial line
backflush
background subtraction technique
backscatter
  b. analysis
  two-dimensional integra-
    ted b.
backward heart failure
BACTEC
  BACTEC radiometry
  BACTEC system
bacteremia
bacteremic
bacteria (*pl. of* bacterium)
bacteria-free stage of bacterial
  endocarditis
bacterial
  b. endocarditis (BE)
  b. infection
  b. myocarditis
  b. pericarditis
  b. vegetation
bactericidal titer
bacterioid
bacteriophage
bacterium *pl.* bacteria
  facultative bacteria
BAE
  bronchial artery emboliza-
    tion
Baffe anastomosis
baffle
  fabric b.
  b. fenestration
  Gore-Tex b.
  intra-atrial b.

baffle *(continued)*
 b. leak
 Mustard atrial b.
 pericardial b.
 Senning intra-atrial b.
 Senning type of intra-
  atrial b.

bag
 Ambu b.
 Douglas b.
 eXtract specimen b.
 Hope b.
 Lifesaver disposable resus-
  citator b.
 manual resuscitation b.
 rebreathing b.
 Sones hemostatic b.
 SureGrip breathing b.
 Voorhees b.

bagassosis

bagged (ventilated)

baggy heart

bagpipe sign

bag-valve-mask

Bahnson
 B. aortic aneurysm clamp
 B. aortic cannula
 B. appendage clamp
 B. sternal retractor

Bailey
 B. aortic clamp
 B. aortic valve-cutting for-
  ceps
 B. aortic valve rongeur
 B. catheter
 B. clamp
 B. rib approximator
 B. rib contractor
 B. rib spreader
 B.-Gibbon rib contractor
 B.-Glover-O'Neill commis-
  surotomy knife
 B.-Glover-O'Neill valvulo-
  tome
 B.-Morse mitral knife

bailout
 b. autoperfusion balloon
  catheter
 b. catheter
 b. stent
 b. valvuloplasty

Baim
 B. pacing catheter
 B.-Turi cardiac device
 B.-Turi monitoring catheter
 B.-Turi pacing catheter

Bainbridge
 B. anastomosis clamp
 B. hemostatic forceps
 B. effect
 B. reflex
 B. vessel clamp

Bair Hugger
 B. H. patient warming blan-
  ket
 B. H. warmer

Bakes
 B. dilator
 B. probe

Bakst
 B. cardiac scissors
 B. valvulotome

balance
 sympathovagal b.

Balectrode
 B. pacing catheter
 B. pacing probe

Balke
 B. exercise stress test
 B. treadmill protocol
 B.-Ware test
 B.-Ware treadmill protocol

Ball
 B. reusable electrode

ball
 b.-cage prosthesis
 b.-cage valve
 b.-and-cage prosthetic
  valve

ball *(continued)*
  b.-and-cage valve prosthe-
    sis
  b. electrode
  fungus b.
  b. heart valve
  b.-occluder valve
  b. poppet of prosthetic
    valve
  b. thrombus
  b. valve
  b. valve prosthesis
  b. valve thrombus
  b. variance
  b. wedge
  b.-wedge catheter

ballerina-foot pattern

ballet
  cardiac b.

ballistocardiogram

ballistocardiograph

ballistocardiography

balloon
  Accent-DG b.
  ACE b.
  ACS Alpha b.
  ACS SULP II b.
  ACS TX 2000 b.
  ACX b.
  b. angioplasty
  b. angioplasty catheter
  b. aortic valvotomy
  b. aortic valvuloplasty
  b. atrial septostomy
  b. atrial septotomy
  Arrow Berman angiogra-
    phic b.
  b. atrial septostomy
  AVCO aortic b.
  Bandit b.
  Baxter Intrepid b.
  bifoil b.
  Blue Max high-pressure b.
  Brandt cytology b.
  cardiac b. pump
  b. catheter
  b. catheter angioplasty

balloon *(continued)*
  b.-centered argon laser
  b. coarctation angioplasty
  b. coronary angioplasty
  counterpulsation b.
  b. counterpulsation
  Cribier-Letac aortic valvu-
    loplasty b.
  Datascope intra-aortic b.
  Datascope intra-aortic b.
    pump
  b. dilation
  dilatation b.
  Distaflex b.
  b. embolectomy catheter
  Endura b. catheter
  Epistat double b.
  b.-expandable flexible coil
    stent
  b.-expandable intravascular
    stent
  Express b.
  Extractor three-lumen re-
    trieval b.
  Falcon b.
  b.-flotation pacing catheter
  Hadow b.
  Hartzler Micro II angioplas-
    ty b.
  Helix b.
  Hunter-Sessions b.
  b.-imaging catheter
  b. inflation
  Inoue self-guiding b.
  Integra II b.
  intra-aortic b.
  intra-aortic b. assist device
  intra-aortic b. counterpul-
    sation
  intra-aortic b. pump
  14K b.
  Kay b.
  kissing b.
  Kontron b.
  b. laser angioplasty
  latex b.
  LPS b.
  Mansfield b.
  Micross SL b.

balloon *(continued)*
    b. mitral commissurotomy
    b. mitral valvotomy
    b. mitral valvuloplasty
    Monorail Speedy b.
    NC Bandit b. (non-compli-
      ant)
    NoProfile b.
    b. occlusion
    b.-occlusion pulmonary an-
      giography
    b. occlusive intravascular
      lysis enhanced recanaliza-
      tion
    Olbert b.
    Omega-NV b.
    Omniflex b.
    Omni SST b.
    Orion b.
    Owens b.
    Percor DL-II (dual-lumen)
      intra-aortic b.
    Percor-Stat intra-aortic b.
    PET b.
    Piccolino b.
    pillow-shaped b.
    POC b.
    polyethylene terephthala-
      te b.
    polyolefin copolymer b.
    polyvinyl chloride b.
    Prime b.
    b. pulmonary valvotomy
    b. pulmonary valvuloplasty
    b. pump
    QuickFurl SL b.
    radiofrequency hot b.
    b. rupture
    Schneider-Shiley b.
    septostomy b. catheter
    Shadow b.
    b.-shaped heart
    Short Speedy b.
    b. shunt
    Simpson PET b. atherec-
      tomy device
    sizing b.
    Slalom b.
    Slider b.

balloon *(continued)*
    Slinky b.
    Solo b.
    Spears laser b.
    Stack autoperfusion b.
    Stretch b.
    b. tamponade
    Ten b.
    thermodilution b.
    thigh b.
    Thruflex b.
    b.-tipped angiographic
      catheter
    b.-tipped catheter
    b.-tipped flow-directed
      catheter
    b.-tipped thermodilution
      catheter
    trefoil b.
    trefoil Schneider b.
    b. tricuspid valvotomy
    b. tuboplasty
    Tyshak b.
    b. valvuloplasty
    valvuloplasty b. catheter
    waisting of b.
    windowed b.

ballooning mitral cusp syn-
    drome

Balloon-on-a-Wire

Baltaxe view

Baltherm catheter

Bamberger
    B. area
    B. bulbar pulse
    B. sign
    B.-Marie disease

band
    atelectatic b.
    atrial anomalous b's
    atrioventricular b.
    contraction b.
    CPK-BB b's
    CPK-MB b.
    CPK-MM b.
    His b.
    I b.

band *(continued)*
    moderator b.
    myocardial b. (MB)
    Parham b's
    parietal b.
    pulmonary artery b.
    b. of Reil
    b. saw effect
    Vesseloops rubber b.
    Z b.

bandage
    Esmarch's b.
    Tricodur Epi compression
        support b.
    Tricodur Omos compres-
        sion support b.
    Tricodur Talus compres-
        sion support b.

banding
    Muller b.
    pulmonary artery (PA) b.
    b. of pulmonary artery
    Trusler rule for pulmonary
        artery b.

Bandit
    B. PTCA catheter
    NC B. catheter
    POC B. catheter

bandlike angina

bandpass filter

bandwidth

bangungut syndrome

bank
    tissue b.

Bannister disease

Bannwarth syndrome

BAR
    beta-adrenergic receptor

Barbara Walters shot (20/20
    view of LAD)

barbed
    b. epicardial pacing lead
    b. hook

barbiturate

barb-tip lead

Bard
    B. arterial cannula
    B. balloon-directed pacing
        catheter
    B. cardiopulmonary sup-
        port pump
    B. cardiopulmonary sup-
        port system
    B. clamshell septal occlu-
        der
    B. clamshell septal um-
        brella
    B. electrode
    B. electrophysiology cathe-
        ter
    B. guiding catheter
    B. nonsteerable bipolar
        electrode
    B. PDA umbrella
    B. percutaneous cardiopul-
        monary support system
    B. probe
    B. PTFE graft
    B. sign
    B. soft double-pigtail stent
    B. TransAct intra-aortic bal-
        loon pump
    B.-Parker blade
    B.-Parker knife
    B.-Parker scalpel

Bardco catheter

Bardenheurer ligation

Bardic
    B. cannula
    B. cutdown catheter
    B. vein catheter

barium
    b. enema
    b.-impregnated poppet
    b. swallow

Barlow syndrome

Barnard
    B. mitral valve prosthesis

Barnard *(continued)*
    B. operation

barometer-maker's disease

barometric pressure

baroceptor

baroreceptor
    cardiac b.
    carotid b.
    perturbed carotid b.
    b. reflex
    b. sensitization

baroreflex
    carotid b.
    sinoatrial b.

barotrauma
    pulmonary b.

Barraya forceps

barrel
    b.-chested
    b.-hooping compression
    b.-shaped chest
    b.-shaped thorax

Barrett esophagus

barrier
    blood-air b.
    blood-brain b.
    blood-retina b.
    placental b.

Barron pump

Barsony-Polgar syndrome

Barth syndrome

Bartonella
    B. elizabethae
    B. bacilliformis
    B. vinsonii

Bartter syndrome

basal
    b. cell carcinoma
    b. diastolic murmurs
    b. metabolic rate (BMR)
    b.-septal hypertrophy

base
    b. of heart
    whole blood buffer b.

baseline
    b. arrhythmia
    b. artifact
    b. echocardiography
    b. EKG
    b. of EKG
    b. rhythm
    b. ST segment abnormality
    b. standing blood pressure
    b. standing pulse rate
    b. variability
    b. variability of fetal heart
      rate
    wandering b.

basement membrane

baseplate
    winged b.

basic (BCLS)
    b. cardiac life support
    b. cycle length
    b. drive cycle length
    b. fibroblast growth factor
    b. life support (BLS)
    b. rate

basicaryoplastin

basichromatin

basichromiole

basicytoparaplastin

basilic vein

basiparachromatin

basiparaplastin

basis
    b. cordis
    b. pulmonis

Basix pacemaker

basket
    Medi-Tech multipurpose b.
    pericardial b.

basophil

Bassen-Kornzweig abetalipoproteinemia

Batch least-squares method

bath
film-fixer b.
film wash b.
fixer b.
Haake water b.
Nauheim b.
wash b.

bathycardia

batrachotoxin

Batson plexus

battery
Celsa b.
external pacemaker b.
lithium b.
nickel-cadmium b.
b. voltage

battery-assisted heart assist device

Battey-avium complex

bat wing shadow on x-ray

Bauer syndrome

Baumès symptom

BAV
balloon aortic valvotomy
balloon aortic valvulo-
plasty
bicommissural aortic valve

Baxter
B. angioplasty catheter
B. Flo-Gard 8200 volumetric
infusion pump
B. Intrepid balloon
B. mechanical valve
B. mechanical valve pros-
thesis

Bayes theorem

Bayliss theory

Bayle granulations

Baylor
B. autologous transfusion
system
B. cardiovascular sump
tube
B. rapid autologous trans-
fusion (BRAT)
B. sump
B. total artificial heart

Baypress

Bazett
B. corrected QT interval
B. formula

Bazin disease

BBB
bundle-branch block

BBBB
bilateral bundle-branch
block

BCA
balloon catheter angio-
plasty
bidirectional cavopulmon-
ary anastomosis

BCD Plus cardioplegic unit

BCO_2
Cardiac Stimulator B.

BE
bacterial endocarditis

bead
Digoxin RIA B.

beading
arteriolar b.
b. of arteries

Beall
B. circumflex artery scis-
sors
B. disk valve prosthesis
B. mitral valve

Beall *(continued)*
    B. mitral valve prosthesis
    B. prosthetic valve
    B. scissors
    B.-Surgitool ball-cage pros-
        thetic valve
    B.-Surgitool disk prosthetic
        valve

beam
    b. splitter
    b. width artifact

Beardsley aortic dilator

beat
    aberrantly conducted b.
    apex b.
    Ashman b.
    asynchronous b.
    atrial capture b.
    atrial ectopic b.
    atrial escape b.
    atrial fusion b.
    atrial premature b.
    atrioventricular (AV) junc-
        tional escape b.
    atrioventricular (AV) junc-
        tional premature b.
    auricular premature b.
    automatic b.
    b.-to-b. analysis
    b.-to-b. variability
    b.-to-b. variability of fetal
        heart
    capture b's
    ciliary b.
    combination b.
    coupled b's
    dependent b.
    Dressler b.
    dropped b.
    echo b.
    ectopic b.
    ectopic ventricular b.
    entrained b.
    escape b.
    escaped b.
    extrasystolic b.
    fascicular b.
    forced b.

beat *(continued)*
    fusion b.
    heart b.
    interference b.
    interpolated b.
    interpolated ventricular
        premature b.
    junctional escape b.
    junctional premature b.
    Lown class 4a ventricular
        ectopic b's
    Lown class 4b ventricular
        ectopic b's
    malignant b.
    missed b.
    mixed b.
    nodal b.
    paired b's
    parasystolic b.
    b's per minute (bpm)
    postectopic b.
    postextrasystolic b.
    premature b.
    premature atrial b.
    premature auricular b.
    premature junctional b.
    premature ventricular b.
    pseudofusion b.
    reciprocal b.
    reentrant b.
    retrograde b.
    salvo of b's
    sinus b.
    skipped b.
    summation b.
    sustained ventricular
        apex b.
    unifocal ventricular ecto-
        pic b.
    ventricular ectopic b.
    ventricular escape b.
    ventricular fusion b.
    ventricular premature b.

beating at a fixed rate

Beatty-Bright friction sound

Beau
    B. asystole
    B. disease

Beau *(continued)*
    B. lines
    B. syndrome
Beaver
    B. blade
    B. knife
    B.-DeBakey blade
Beck
    B. cardiopericardiopexy
    B. clamp
    B. Depression Inventory
    B. epicardial poudrage
    B. I, II operation
    B. miniature aortic clamp
    B. rasp
    B. triad
    B. vascular clamp
    B.-Potts aortic and pul-
        monic clamp
Becker
    B. accelerator cannula
    B. disease
Béclard hernia
becquerel (Bq)
Becton Dickinson (B-D)
    B. D. guidewire
    B. D. Teflon-sheathed nee-
        dle
bed
    adventitial b.
    b. blocks
    capillary b.
    cyanosis of nail b's
    myocardial b.
    nail b.
    perfusion b.
    pulmonary b.
    Sanders b.
    Stress Echo b.
    vascular b.
    venous capacitance b.
Bedge antireflux mattress
beef-lung heparin
beep-o-gram

beer
    b. and cobalt syndrome
    b. heart
    b.-drinker's cardiomyopa-
        thy
Beer-Lambert principle
bee venom
behavior
    contractile b.
    type A b.
    type B b.
behavioral
    b. factor
    b. therapy
Behçet
    B. disease
    B. syndrome
Béhier-Hardy sign
bejel syphilis
Bellavar medical support stock-
    ings
bellows
    chest b.
    b. murmur
    b. sound
Belzer
    B. apparatus
    B. solution
bends
Benedict retractor
Bengash needle
Bengolea forceps
benign
    b. croupous angina
    b. early repolarization
    b. intracranial hyperten-
        sion
benigna
    endocarditis b.

benignum
empyema b.

Benjamin-Havas fiberoptic light clip

Bentall
B. cardiovascular prosthesis
inclusion technique of B.
B. inclusion technique
B. operation
B. procedure

Bentley
B. Duraflo II
B. oxygenator
B. transducer

Bentson
B. exchange straight guidewire
B. floppy-tip guidewire
B. guidewire
B.-Hanafee-Wilson catheter

beractant

Bérard aneurysm

Berenstein occlusion balloon catheter

Berger operation

Bergmeister papilla

beriberi
atrophic b.
cerebral b.
dry b.
b. heart
infantile b.
paralytic b.
wet b.

beriberic

Berkovits-Castellanos hexapolar electrode

Berlin
B. nosology

Berlin (continued)
B. TAH

Berman
B. angiographic catheter
B. aortic clamp
B. balloon flotation catheter
B. cardiac catheter
B. vascular clamp

Bernheim syndrome

Berning and Steensgaard-Hansen score

Bernoulli
B. equation
B. theorem

Bernstein test

Berry sternal needle holder

berry
b. aneurysm

berylliosis

beryllium disease

beta
$b._1$-adrenergic receptor
$b._2$-adrenergic receptor
b. adrenoceptor
b. adrenoceptor stimulation
b. agonist
b. antagonist
$b._1$-antagonist
$b._2$-antagonist
b. blockade
b. blocker
b. blocker therapy
b. blocking agent
b. lactamase
b. lipoprotein
b. lipoprotein fraction
b. ray
b. receptor
b. thromboglobulin

beta-adrenergic
b.-a. agonist
b.-a. blocker

beta-adrenergic *(continued)*
  b.-a. blocking agent
  b.-a. receptor
  b.-a. stimulation

beta-adrenoreceptor
  b.-a. agonist
  b.-a. blocker
  b.-a. blocking agent

beta-beta homodimer

Beta-Cath system

Betacel-Biotronik pacemaker

Betachron E-R

Betadine Helafoam solution

beta-endorphin

betaine diet

beta-lactam

beta-lactamase
  CAZ b.-l.
  b.-l. inhibitor

beta-myosin heavy-chain gene

beta-thromboglobulin
  plasma b.-t.

bethanidine

Bethune
  B. rib shears
  B.-Coryllos rib shears

Bettman-Fovash thoracotome

Beuren syndrome

bevel

beveled
  b. thin-walled needle
  b. vein

beveling

Bezalip

Bezold-Jarisch reflex

bFGF
  basic fibroblast growth factor

B–H interval

Bianchi
  B. nodules
  B. valve

biatrial
  b. enlargement
  b. myxoma

biatriatum
  cor pseudotriloculare b.

bibasally

bibasilar
  b. atelectasis
  b. coarse crackles
  b. crackles

bicameral

BiCAP
  Bipolar Circumactive Probe
  B unit
    BiCAP unit

bicarbonate
  sodium b.

bicarbonaturia

Bicarbon Sorin valve

bicardiogram

bicaval
  b. cannulation

Biceps bipolar coagulator

Bicer-val prosthetic valve

Bichat tunic

Bickel ring

bicommissural aortic valve
  (BAV)

Bicor catheter

bicuspid
  b. aortic valve

bicuspidization

bicycle
  Aerobicycle

bicycle *(continued)*
    Aerodyne b.
    Collins b.
    b. dynamometer
    b. echocardiography
    b. ergometer
    b. ergometer exercise
      stress test
    b. ergometry
    b. exercise test
    Siemens-Albis b.
    Tredex b.
    Tredex powered b.

bidimensional

bidirectional
    b. cavopulmonary anasto-
      mosis
    b. four-pole Butterworth
      high-pass digital filter
    b. shunt
    b. shunt calculation
    b. superior cavopulmonary
      anastomosis
    b. ventricular tachycardia

Bier block anesthesia

Biermer sign

bifascicular
    b. heart block

biferious pulse *(variant of* bisferious)

bifid P waves

bifocal demand DVI pacemaker

bifoil
    b. balloon
    b. balloon catheter

bifurcated
    b. J-shaped tined atrial
      pacing and defibrillation
      lead
    b. vein graft for vascular
      reconstruction

bifurcation
    b. of aorta
    aortic b.

bifurcation *(continued)*
    carotid b.
    coronary b.
    iliac b.
    b. lesion
    b. of pulmonary trunk

bigemina

bigeminal
    b. bisferious pulse
    b. pulse
    b. rhythm

bigeminus
    pulsus b.

bigeminy
    atrial b.
    atrioventricular junction-
      al b.
    atrioventricular nodal b.
    b. bisferious pulse
    escape-capture b.
    junctional b.
    nodal b.
    reciprocal b.
    rule of b.
    ventricular b.

bilateral
    b. adrenal hyperplasia
    b. acid binding resin
    b. acid sequestrant
    b. bundle-branch block
      (BBBB)
    b. internal mammary artery
      (reconstruction)

bilayer

bileaflet tilting-disk prosthetic
  valve

Bili mask

Billingham criteria

billowing
    cusp b.
    b. mitral leaflet
    b. mitral valve syndrome

bilobate

biloculare
    cor b.

bimanual precordial palpation

binding
    guanine nucleotide modula-
        table b.

Bing
    B. stylet
    B.-Taussig heart procedure

Binswanger disease

binuclear

binucleate

binucleation

binucleolate

bioabsorbable
    b. closure device

bioassay

bioavailability

Biobrane adhesive

Biobrane/HF graft material

Biocef

Biocell RTV implant

Bioclate

Bioclot protein S assay

biocompatibility

Biocon impedance plethysmog-
    raphy cardiac output monitor

Biocor prosthetic valve

biodegradable
    b. stent
    b. surgical tack

Biodex System

bioelectric
    b. current
    b. potential

bioelectricity

biofeedback

Biofilter cardiovascular hemo-
    concentrator

biofragmentable anastomotic
    ring

biograft
    B. bovine heterograft mate-
        rial
    Dakin b.
    Dardik B.
    B. graft
    Meadox Dardik B.

bioimpedance
    b. electrocardiograph
    thoracic electrical b.

biological
    b. fitness
    b. half-life
    b. response modifiers

Bio-Medicus
    B.-M. arterial catheter
    B.-M. pump

biomembrane

Biomer (segmented polyureth-
    rane)

Bionit
    B. vascular graft
    B. vascular prosthesis

biophysical profile (BPP)

bioplasm

bioplasmic

Bioplus dispersive electrode

BioPolyMeric
    B. femoropopliteal bypass
        graft
    B. vascular graft

bioprosthesis
    Carpentier-Edwards Peri-
        mount RSR pericardial b.
    Freestyle aortic root b.

bioprosthesis *(continued)*
 Hancock M.O. II porcine b.
 Mosaic cardiac b.
 pericarbon b.
 Perimount RSR pericardial b.
 PhotoFix alpha pericardial b.
 porcine b.
 SJM X-Cell cardiac b.
 Toronto SPV b.

bioprosthetic
 b. heart valve
 b. prosthetic valve

biopsy
 bite b.
 brush b.
 catheter-guided b.
 cytological b.
 endomyocardial b.
 endoscopic b.
 excisional b.
 fine-needle aspiration b.
 b. forceps
 mediastinal lymph node b.
 percutaneous needle b.
 pericardial b.
 punch b.
 scalene fat pad b.
 supraclavicular lymph node b.
 ventricular b.
 wedge b.

bioptic sampling

bioptome
 Bycep PC Jr b.
 Caves b.
 Caves-Schultz b.
 Cordis b.
 Cordis Bi-Pal b.
 JAWZ b.
 Kawai b.
 King b.
 Konno b.
 Mansfield b.
 Olympus b.
 Scholten endomyocardial b.

bioptome *(continued)*
 Stanford b.
 Stanford-Caves b.

Bio-Pump

Biorate pacemaker

bioresorbable implant

Bio-sentry telemetry

Biosound
 B. 2000 II ultrasound unit
 B. Phase 2 ultrasound unit
 B. Surgiscan echocardiograph
 B. wide-angle monoplane ultrasound scanner

Biostent

Biostil blood transfusion set

Biosurge Synchronous Autotransfuser

BioTac
 B. biopsy cannula
 B. ECG electrode

Biotrack coagulation monitor

Biotronik
 B. lead connector
 B. demand pacemaker

Bio-Vascular prosthetic valve

biphasic
 b. action potential
 b. complex on EKG
 b. P wave
 b. shock
 b. stridor

biplanar tomography

biplane
 b. aortography
 b. fluoroscopy
 b. formula
 b. imaging
 b. orthogonal angiography
 b. pelvic arteriography
 b. pelvic oblique study

biplane *(continued)*
   b. quantitative coronary arteriography
   b. ventriculography

bipolar
   b. catheter
   b. coagulating forceps
   b. generator
   b. hemostasis probe
   b. limb leads
   b. myocardial electrode
   b. pacemaker
   b. pacing electrode catheter
   b. temporary pacemaker catheter

Bipolar Circumactive Probe B unit (BiCAP)

BiPort hemostasis introducer sheath kit

bird's eye catheter

bird's nest
   b. n. lesion
   b. n. vena cava filter

birefringence

Birtcher defibrillator

bisferiens
   pulsus b.

bisferient

bisferious
   b. pulse

Bishop sphygmoscope

bishop's hat

bishop's nod

Bisping electrode

bistoury
   b. blade
   Jackson b.

bite biopsy

biterminal electrode

Bitpad digitizer

BIVAD centrifugal left and right ventricular assist device

bivalent

bivalve

biventricular
   b. assist device (BVAD)
   Thoratec b. assist device
   b. endomyocardial fibrosis
   b. hypertrophy
   b. support

Björk
   B. method of Fontan procedure
   B.-Shiley aortic valve prosthesis
   B.-Shiley convexoconcave 60-degree valve prosthesis
   B.-Shiley floating disk prosthesis
   B.-Shiley graft
   B.-Shiley heart valve holder
   B.-Shiley heart valve sizer
   B.-Shiley mitral valve
   B.-Shiley Monostrut valve
   B.-Shiley prosthesis
   B.-Shiley prosthetic valve
   B.-Shiley valve

b knuckle

Blackfan-Diamond syndrome

blade
   arthroscopic banana b.
   AtheroCath spinning b. catheter
   b. atrial septostomy
   Bard-Parker b.
   Beaver b.
   Beaver-DeBakey b.
   bistoury b.
   Collin radiopaque sternal b.
   b. control wire holder
   Cooley-Pontius sternal b.

blade *(continued)*
    DeBakey b.
    electrosurgical b.
    knife b.
    Lite B.
    SCA-EX ShortCutter catheter with rotating b's
    b. septostomy catheter
    sternal retractor b.

blade and balloon atrial septostomy

Blake exercise stress test

Blalock
    B. anastomosis
    B. clamp
    B. pulmonic stenosis clamp
    B. shunt
    B.-Hanlon atrial septectomy
    B.-Hanlon operation
    B.-Niedner pulmonic stenosis clamp
    B.-Taussig anastomosis
    B.-Taussig operation
    B.-Taussig procedure
    B.-Taussig shunt

blanche
    tache b.

blanch test

bland
    b. edema
    b. embolism

Bland
    B.-Altman method
    B.-Garland-White syndrome

blanket
    Bair-Hugger patient warming b.
    circulating water b.
    cooling b.
    Gaymar water-circulating b.
    hypothermia b.

blast
    b. chest

blastomycosis

blastin

blastogenesis

blastogenetic

blastogenic

bleed
    arterial b.
    intracerebral b.
    low-pressure b.
    sentinel b.

bleeding
    arterial b.
    back-b.
    b. diathesis
    b. time

blender
    Bird low-flow b.
    Virtis b.

blind
    b. coronary dimple

bloater
    blue b.

bloc
    en b.
    heart-lung b.

Bloch equation

Block
    B. cardiac device
    B. right coronary guiding catheter

block
    acquired symptomatic AV b.
    alveolar-capillary b.
    anatomic b.
    anterior fascicular b.
    anterograde b.
    arborization b.
    arteriovenous b.
    atrioventricular (AV) b.
    atrioventricular junctional heart b.
    2:1 AV b.

block *(continued)*
  AV Wenckebach b.
  axillary b.
  bed b's
  bifascicular b.
  bifascicular bundle-
    branch b.
  bifascicular heart b.
  bilateral bundle-branch b.
  bundle-branch b.
  complete AV b.
  complete heart b.
  conduction b.
  congenital heart b.
  congenital complete
    heart b.
  congenital symptomatic
    AV b.
  b. cycle length
  divisional heart b.
  entrance b.
  exit b.
  familial heart b.
  fascicular b.
  fascicular heart b.
  first-degree AV b.
  first-degree heart b.
  fixed third-degree AV b.
  focal b.
  functional b.
  heart b.
  3:1 heart b.
  3:2 heart b.
  heparin b.
  high-degree AV b.
  high-grade atrioventricu-
    lar b.
  His bundle heart b.
  incomplete atrioventricu-
    lar b.
  incomplete heart b.
  incomplete left bundle-
    branch b.
  incomplete right bundle-
    branch b.
  inflammatory heart b.
  infra-His b., infrahisian b.
  intermittent third-degree
    AV b.

block *(continued)*
  interventricular b.
  intra-atrial b.
  intra-His b., intrahisian b.
  intranodal b.
  intraventricular b.
  intraventricular conduc-
    tion b.
  ipsilateral bundle branch b.
  left anterior fascicular b.
  left bundle-branch b.
  left posterior fascicular b.
  Luciani-Wenckebach atriov-
    entricular b.
  Mobitz I second-degree
    AV b.
  Mobitz II second-degree
    AV b.
  Mobitz type I atrioventricu-
    lar b.
  Mobitz type II atrioventri-
    cular b.
  Mobitz type I b. on Wenck-
    ebach heart
  paraffin b.
  paroxysmal AV b.
  partial heart b.
  peri-infarction b.
  posterior fascicular b.
  protective b.
  pseudo-AV b.
  retrograde b.
  right bundle-branch b.
  second-degree AV b.
  second-degree heart b.
  shock b's
  sinoatrial b.
  sinoatrial exit b.
  sinoauricular b.
  sinus b.
  sinus exit b.
  sinus node exit b.
  subjunctional heart b.
  suprahisian b.
  third-degree atrioventricu-
    lar b.
  third-degree heart b.
  transient AV b.
  transient heart b.

block *(continued)*
    trifascicular b.
    unifascicular b.
    unidirectional b.
    vagal b.
    ventricular b.
    ventriculoatrial (VA) b.
    voltage-dependent b.
    Wenckebach b.
    Wenckebach atrioventricular b.
    Wenckebach AV b.
    Wenckebach periodicity b.
    Wilson b.

blockade
    alpha-adrenergic b.
    angiotensin-II receptor b.
    beta b., β-b.
    stellate ganglion b.

blocked
    b. APC (atrial premature contraction)
    b. heart artery
    b. pleurisy

blocker
    adrenoceptor b.
    alpha-adrenergic b.
    alpha-adrenoceptor b.
    alpha-adrenoreceptor b.
    angiotensin-II receptor b.
    beta b.
    beta-adrenergic b.
    beta-adrenoceptor b.
    beta-adrenoreceptor b.
    calcium channel b.
    calcium entry b.
    ganglionic b.
    renin-angiotensin b.
    slow channel b.

blocking
    b. vagal afferent fibers
    b. vagal efferent fibers

blood
    b.-air barrier
    arterial b.
    artificial b.
    autologous b.

blood *(continued)*
    b.-brain barrier
    b. cardioplegia
    clot of b.
    b. clot
    b. clot lysis
    cord b.
    b. coagulation factor (I–XIII)
    b. coagulation time
    b. count
    b. culture
    defibrinated b.
    deoxygenated b.
    b. dyscrasia
    b. expander
    b. flow
    b. flow on Doppler echocardiogram
    b. flow measurement
    b.-flow probe
    Fluosol artificial b.
    frank b.
    b. gas
    b. gases on oxygen
    b. gases on room air
    heparinized b.
    laky b.
    mixed venous b.
    b. murmur
    occult b.
    b. oxygen
    b. oxygen level
    oxygen saturation of the hemoglobin of arterial b.
    oxygenated b.
    b. patch injection
    peripheral b.
    b. perfusion
    b. perfusion monitor
    b. platelet thrombus
    b. plate thrombus
    b. pool
    b.-pool imaging
    b.-pool radionuclide scan
    b. pressure
    b. pressure cuff
    b. products
    b. pump

blood *(continued)*
    b. replacement
    b. sampling instrument
    shear rate of b.
    shunted b.
    sludged b.
    peripheral b. smear
    b. staining
    b. thinning agents
    tonometered whole b.
    b. transfusion
    unoxygenated b.
    b. urea nitrogen (BUN)
    venous b.
    b. vessel bridges
    b. vessel supporter
    b. viscosity
    b. volume
    b. volume distribution
    b. volume studies
    b. warmer
    b. warmer cuff
    whole b.
    b. workup

bloodless
    b. field
    b. fluid
    b. phlebotomy

bloodletting

blood pressure–lowering effect

bloodstream

Bloodwell vascular forceps

bloody
    b. tap

Bloom
    B. DTU 201 external stimu-
    lator
    B. programmable stimula-
    tor
    B. syndrome

blooming effect

blot
    b. test
    Western b.

blow
    diastolic b.

blow-by
    b.-b. oxygen

blowing
    b. murmur
    b. wound

blubbery diastolic murmur

Blue FlexTip catheter

Blue Max high-pressure balloon

Blue Max triple-lumen catheter

blue
    b. baby
    b. bloater
    b. disease
    b. finger syndrome
    methylene b.
    b. phlebitis
    b. toe syndrome ("trash
    foot")
    b. velvet syndrome

Blum arterial scissors

Blumenau test

Blumenthal lesion

blunt
    b. eversion
    b. eversion carotid endar-
    terectomy
    b. injury
    b. and sharp dissection
    b. trauma

blunted costophrenic angle

bluntly dissected

blush
    capillary b.
    myocardial b.
    b. phenomenon
    tumor b.

BMI
    body mass index

B-mode
   B-m. echocardiography
   B-m. ultrasonography
   B-m. ultrasound

BMP-2
   bone morphogenetic pro-
      tein type 2

boat-shaped heart

Bochdalek hernia

Bock ganglion

Bodai adapter

body
   aortic b's
   Arantius b's
   b's of Arantius
   Arnold b.
   asbestos b's
   asbestosis b's
   Aschoff b's
   aspiration of foreign b.
   asteroid b.
   Auer b.
   Babès-Ernst b's
   Bracht-Wächter b's
   Cabot ring b's
   carotid b.
   cell b.
   central b.
   central fibrous b.
   central fibrous b. of heart
   coccygeal b.
   carotid b.
   creola b's
   Döhle inclusion b's
   b. fat
   ferruginous b's
   fibrous b.
   foreign b.
   Gamna-Gandy b's
   gelatin compression b.
   glomus b.
   Golgi b.
   Gordon elementary b.
   Heinz b.
   intermediate b. of Flem-
      ming

body *(continued)*
   jugulotympanic b.
   LCL b's
   Luschka's b.
   Masson b's
   Medlar b's
   metachromatic b's
   multilamellar b.
   multivesicular b.
   Negri b's
   para-aortic b's
   paranuclear b.
   b. plethysmograph
   b. position
   psammoma b's
   residual b.
   b. surface area (BSA)
   b. surface Laplacian map-
      ping
   thoracic vertebral b.
   tympanic b.
   vagal b.
   Weibel-Palade b's
   Zuckerkandl b's

Boeck
   B. disease
   B. sarcoidosis

Boerema hernia repair

Boerhaave
   B. syndrome
   B. tear

Boettcher
   B. arterial forceps
   B. pulmonary artery clamp
   B. pulmonary artery for-
      ceps

Bogalusa criteria

boggy edema

Bohr
   B. formula
   B. isopleth method

BOILER
   balloon occlusive intravas-
      cular lysis enhanced re-
      canalization

bois
   bruit de b.

bolometer

bolster
   Teflon felt b.

bolt
   Camino microventricular b.

Boltzmann distribution

bolus
   b. injection
   b. intravenous injection
   b. of medication

Bonchek
   B.-Shiley cardiac jacket
   B.-Shiley vein distention
      system

bond
   soldered b.

bone
   b. demineralization
   fibrous dysplasia of b.
   b. marrow aplasia
   b. marrow aspiration
   b. marrow embolism
   b. marrow tap
   b. marrow transplant
   b. morphogenetic protein
      type 2 (BMP-2)
   Paget disease of b.
   b. wax

Bonferroni
   B. correction
   B. test

bony heart

Bonzel Monorail balloon catheter

Bookwalter retractor

booming
   b. diastolic rumble
   b. rumble

booster heart

boot
   Bunny b.
   compression b.
   Cryo/Cuff pressure b.
   gelatin compression b.
   IPC b's
   PNS Unna b.
   sheepskin b.
   Unna b.
   Unna paste b.

boot-shaped heart

bootstrap
   b. dilation
   b. two-vessel angioplasty
   b. two-vessel technique

border
   brush b.
   cardiac b.
   b. of cardiac dullness
   inferior b. of heart
   lower sternal b.
   b. of oval fossa
   right b. of heart
   sternal b.
   striated b.
   upper sternal b.

borderline
   b. cardiomegaly
   b. EKG
   b. hypertension
   b. left ventricular fullness
   b. right ventricular fullness

Bordet-Gengou test

Borg
   B. numerical scale
   B. scale
   B. scale of treadmill exer-
      tion
   B. treadmill exertion scale

Born aggregometry

Bornholm disease

borreliosis
   Lyme b.

Borst side-arm introducer set

Bosch ERG 500 ergometer

Bosher commissurotomy knife

BosPac cardiopulmonary bypass system

Bostock
    B. catarrh
    B. disease

Botallo duct

bottle
    Castaneda b.
    b. sound

bottle-neck stenosis

bougie
    Celestin b.
    EndoLumina illuminated b.

Bouillaud
    B. disease
    B. sign
    B. syndrome
    B. tinkle

bounding pulse

bouquet of vessels

Bourassa catheter

Boutin thoracoscope

bouts of tachycardia

Bouveret
    B. disease
    B. syndrome

Bovie
    B. coagulation cautery
    B. electrocautery
    B. ultrasound aspirator

bovied

bovine
    b. allograft
    b. biodegradable collagen
    b. collagen plug device
    b. heart
    b. heart valve

bovine *(continued)*
    b. heterograft
    b. lavage extract surfactant
    pegademase b.
    b. pericardial bioprosthesis
    b. pericardial heart valve
        xenograft
    b. pericardial valve
    b. pericardium strips

bovinum
    cor b.

Bowditch
    B. law
    B. phenomenon
    B. staircase effect

bowing of mitral valve leaflet

box
    digital constant-current pa-
        cing b.
    Elecath switch b.

Boyce sign

Boyd
    B. perforating vein
    B. point

Bozzolo sign

BP
    blood pressure

BPD
    bronchopulmonary dyspla-
        sia

bpm
    beats per minute

BQ-123

brachial
    b.-ankle index
    b. arteriogram
    b. arteriotomy
    b. artery
    b. artery approach
    b. artery cutdown
    b. artery thrombosis
    b. bypass
    b. catheter

brachial *(continued)*
    b. dance
    b. plexus
    b. pulse
    b. syndrome
    b. vein

brachioaxillary bridge graft fistula

brachiocephalic
    b. arteritis
    b. artery
    b. ischemia
    b. system
    b. trunk
    b. vein
    b. vessel angioplasty

brachiogram

brachiosubclavian bridge graft fistula

Bracht
    B.-Wächter bodies
    B.-Wächter lesion

brachycardia

Bradbury-Eggleston syndrome

bradied down

Bradilan

Bradshaw-O'Neill aorta clamp

bradyarrhythmia
    digitalis-induced b.

bradyarrhythmic arrest

bradycardia
    atrial b.
    artifactual b.
    baseline b.
    Branham's b.
    cardiomuscular b.
    central b.
    clinostatic b.
    essential b.
    fetal b.
    idiopathic b.
    idioventricular b.
    intermittent junctional b.

bradycardia *(continued)*
    junctional b.
    nodal b.
    postinfectious b.
    postinfective b.
    postoperative b.
    pulseless b.
    sinoatrial b.
    sinus b.
    vagal b.
    ventricular b.

bradycardiac

bradycardia-dependent aberrancy

bradycardia-tachycardia syndrome

bradycardic

bradycrotic

bradydiastole

bradydiastolia

bradydysrhythmia

bradykinin

bradyrhythmia

bradysphygmia

bradytachycardia
    b. syndrome

bradytachydysrhythmia
    b. syndrome

brady-tachy syndrome

braidlike lesion

brain
    b. aneurysm
    b. death
    b.-heart infusion
    b. infarct
    b. murmur
    b. natriuretic peptide
    b. wave

branch
    acute marginal b.

branch *(continued)*
    AV b. block
    AV groove b.
    bifurcating b.
    bundle b.
    diagonal b.
    first diagonal b.
    first major diagonal b.
    first septal perforator b.
    inferior wall b.
    left b. of atrioventricular
      bundle
    left bundle b.
    b. lesion
    marginal b.
    obtuse marginal b. (OMB)
    posterior descending b.
    pulmonary b. stenosis
    ramus b.
    b. retinal vein occlusion
    right b. of atrioventricular
      bundle
    right bundle b.
    septal b.
    septal perforating b.
    side b.
    ventricular b.
    b. vessel occlusion
    b. vessel pruning

branched chain alpha ketoacid
  dehydrogenase

branching
    mirror-image brachioce-
      phalic b.

Brandt cytology balloon

Branham
    B. bradycardia
    B. sign

Brasdor method

brash
    water b.

BRAT
    Baylor rapid autologous
      transfusion
    BRAT system

Brauer
    B. cardiolysis
    B. operation

Braun-Stadler sternal shears

Braunwald
    B. classification (I–IIIB)
    B. heart valve
    B. prosthesis
    B. sign
    B.-Cutter ball prosthetic
      valve
    B.-Cutter ball valve pros-
      thesis

brawny edema

bread-and-butter pericardium

bread-and-butter textbook sign

bread knife valvulotome

breakaway splice

breast
    b. pang
    thrush b.

Brechenmacher
    B. fiber
    B. tract

Brecher and Cronkite technique

bregmocardiac reflex

Brehmer treatment

Bremer AirFlo Vest

Brenner carotid bypass shunt

Brescia-Cimino AV (arteriovenous) fistula

Bretonneau angina

Bretschneider-HTK cardioplegic
  solution

Brett syndrome

bridge
    arteriolovenular b.
    cell b's

bridge *(continued)*
>cytoplasmic b.
>muscle b.
>myocardial b.
>protoplasmic b.
>Wheatstone b.

bridging
>muscular b.
>myocardial b.

Bright
>B. disease
>B. murmur

bright echo

brightness modulation

Brill-Zinsser disease

Brisbane method

Broadbent inverted sign

Brock
>B. auricular clamp
>B. cardiac dilator
>B. clamp
>B. commissurotomy knife
>B. infundibular punch
>B. infundibulectomy
>B. knife
>B. mitral valve knife
>B. operation
>B. probe
>B. procedure
>B. pulmonary valve knife
>B. valvulotome
>B. valvulotomy

Brockenbrough
>B. angiocatheter
>B. cardiac device
>B. catheter
>B. commissurotomy
>B. curved needle
>B. curved-tip occluder
>B. effect
>B. mapping catheter
>B. modified bipolar catheter
>B. sign

Brockenbrough *(continued)*
>B. transseptal catheter
>B. transseptal commissurotomy
>B.-Braunwald sign

Broders index ((grades 1–4))

Brodie
>B. abscess
>B.-Trendelenburg tourniquet test

Brompton
>B. cocktail
>B. solution

Brom repair

broth
>b. test
>Todd-Hewitt b.

Broviac atrial catheter

brown
>b. atrophy
>b. edema

Brown-Adson forceps

Brown-Dodge method

Brozek formula

Bruce
>B. bundle
>B. exercise stress test
>B. protocol, modified
>B. protocol, standard
>B. tract
>B. treadmill exercise protocol

brucellosis

Brugada syndrome

Brughleman needle

bruissement

bruit
>abdominal b.
>aneurysmal b.
>asymptomatic b.
>AV fistula with good b.

bruit *(continued)*
    audible b.
    carotid b.
    b. d'airain
    b. de bois
    b. de canon
    b. de choc
    b. de clapotement
    b. de claquement
    b. de craquement
    b. de cuir neuf
    b. de diable
    b. de drapeau
    b. de fêlé
    b. de froissement
    b. de frolement
    b. de frottement
    b. de galop
    b. de grelot
    b. de Leudet
    b. de la roué de moulin
    b. de lime
    b. de moulin
    b. de parchemin
    b. de piaulement
    b. de pot fêlé
    b. de rape
    b. de rappel
    b. de Roger
    b. de scie
    b. de scie ou de rape
    b. de soufflet
    b. de tabourka
    b. de tambour
    b. de triolet
    epigastric b.
    false b.
    flank b.
    Leudet b.
    musical b.
    palpable b.
    renal artery b.
    Roger b.
    seagull b.
    skodique b.
    subclavian b.
    supraclavicular b.
    systolic b.
    thyroid b.

bruit *(continued)*
    Traube b.
    Verstraeten b.

brunescent

Brunner rib shears

Brunschwig artery forceps

Brush electrocardiographic
    score

brush
    b. biopsy
    Edwards-Carpentier aortic
      valve b.
    Mill-Rose Protected Speci-
      men microbiology b.
    protected b.

Brushfield spot

Bryant
    B. ampulla
    B. mitral hook

BSA ejection fraction

B-scan
    B-s. frame

BTF-37 arterial blood filter

bucardia

Buchbinder
    B. catheter
    B. Omniflex catheter
    B. Thruflex over-the-wire
      catheter

buckled aorta

buckling
    b. of aorta
    chordal b.
    midsystolic b.
    midsystolic b. of mitral
      valve

bud
    vascular b.

Budd-Chiari syndrome

budding

Buerger
 B. disease
 B.-Allen exercise
 B.-Grütz disease

Buerhenne steerable catheter

buffer
 Krebs-Henseleit b.

buffered aspirin

buffy coat smear

bulb
 b. of aorta
 aortic b.
 carotid b.
 b. of jugular vein, inferior
 b. of jugular vein, superior
 thrombosis of jugular b.

bulbar pulse

bulbospiral

bulboventricular
 b. fold
 b. foramen
 b. groove
 b. loop
 b. sulcus
 b. tube

bulbus
 b. aortae
 b. arteriosus
 b. caroticus
 b. cordis
 b. venae jugularis
 b. venae jugularis inferior
 b. venae jugularis superior

bulge
 precordial b.

bulging
 infarct b.

bulldog clamp

bullet-tip catheter

bull's-eye
 b. plot
 b. polar coordinate map-
  ping

bump
 B b.
 ductus b.

BUN
 blood urea nitrogen

bundle
 atrioventricular b.
 AV b.
 Bachmann b.
 b.-branch block (BBB)
 b.-branch fibrosis
 b.-branch reentrant tachycardia
 b.-branch reentry
 Bruce b.
 commissural b.
 common b.
 Helie b.
 His b.
 image b.
 James b.
 Keith b.
 Keith sinoatrial b.
 Kent b.
 Kent-His b.
 Mahaim b.
 main b.
 myocardial fiber b.
 neurovascular b.
 sinoatrial b.
 b. of His
 b. of Stanley Kent
 Thorel b.
 vascular b.

bur
 atherectomy b.
 b.-bearing catheter
 diamond-coated b.

burden
 ischemic b.

Burdick
 B. EKG machine
 B. electrocardiogram

Burford
 B. retractor
 B. rib retractor

Burford *(continued)*
  B. rib spreader
  B.-Finochietto rib spreader
  B.-Lebsche sternal knife

Burger
  B. scalene triangle
  B. technique for scapulo-
    thoracic disarticulation
  B. triangle

Bürger-Grütz disease

Burghart symptom

Burns
  space of B.

Burow
  B. quantitative method
  B. solution
  B. vein

bursa
  Calori b.

burst
  b. of arrhythmia
  b. atrial pacing
  b. pacemaker
  b. of pacing
  paroxysmal b.
  respiratory b.
  b. shock
  spider b.
  b. of ventricular ectopy
  b. of ventricular tachycar-
    dia

Buschke
  B. disease
  scleredema of B.

Buselmeier shunt

butterfly
  b. needle
  b. shadow on x-ray
  silicone b.

Butterworth bidirectional filter

buttock claudication

button
  b. of aorta
  cell b.
  DiaTAP vascular access b.
  b. electrode
  Perspex b.
  skin b.
  b. technique

buttoned device

buttonhole
  b. deformity
  b. incision
  mitral b.
  b. mitral stenosis

buttress
  Teflon pledget suture b.

BV-2 needle

BvgAS regulon

BvgS protein

BVS
  biventricular support
  BVS pump

BW755C
  cyclooxygenase-lipoxygen-
    ase blocking agent
  BW755C

Bycep
  B. biopsy forceps
  B. PC Jr bioptome

bypass
  aorta to first obtuse mar-
    ginal branch b.
  aorta to LAD b.
  aorta to marginal branch b.
  aorta to posterior descen-
    ding b.
  aortic-femoral b.
  aortobifemoral b.
  aortobi-iliac b.
  aortocarotid b.
  aortocoronary b.
  aortocoronary-saphenous
    vein b.

bypass *(continued)*
    aortoiliofemoral b.
    aortofemoral b.
    aortofemoral b., thoracic
    aortoiliac b.
    aortoiliofemoral b.
    aortorenal b.
    aortosubclavian b.
    aorto-subclavian-carotid-ax-
      illoaxillary b.
    atrial-femoral artery b.
    axillary b.
    axillary-axillary b.
    axilloaxillary b.
    axillobifemoral b.
    axillofemoral b.
    axillopopliteal b.
    brachial b.
    cardiopulmonary b.
    carotid-axillary b.
    carotid-carotid b.
    carotid-subclavian b.
    b. circuit
    coronary b.
    coronary artery b.
    coronary artery b. graft
      (CABG)
    cross femoral-femoral
      graft b.
    crossover b.
    descending thoracic aorto-
      femoral-femoral b.
    extra-anatomic b.
    extracranial/intracranial
      (EC/IC) b.
    fem-fem b.
    femoral crossover b.
    femoral-femoral b.
    femoral-popliteal b.
    femoral-tibial b.
    femoral-tibial-peroneal b.
    femoral to tibial b.
    femoral vein-femoral ar-
      tery b.
    femoroaxillary b.
    femorodistal b.
    femorofemoral b.
    femorofemoral crossover b.
    femorofemoropopliteal b.

bypass *(continued)*
    femoropopliteal b.
    femoropopliteal saphenous
      vein b.
    femorotibial b.
    fem-pop b.
    b. graft
    b. graft catheter
    b. graft catheterization
    b. graft visualization
    heart-lung b.
    hepatorenal b.
    iliofemoral b.
    iliopopliteal b.
    infracubital b.
    infrainguinal b.
    inframalleolar b.
    infrapopliteal b.
    in situ b.
    internal mammary artery b.
    ipsilateral nonreversed
      greater saphenous vein b.
    left atrium to distal arterial
      aortic b.
    left heart b.
    Litwak left atrial-aortic b.
    b. machine
    obturator b.
    obturator foramen b.
    partial b.
    partial cardiopulmonary b.
    percutaneous cardiopul-
      monary b.
    percutaneous femoral-fem-
      oral cardiopulmonary b.
    percutaneous left heart b.
    pulsatile cardiopulmon-
      ary b.
    renal artery–reverse sa-
      phenous vein b.
    reversed b.
    right heart b.
    saphenous vein b.
    subclavian-carotid b.
    subclavian-subclavian b.
    superior mesenteric ar-
      tery b.
    b. surgery
    temporary aortic shunt b.

bypass *(continued)*
    b. time
    total cardiopulmonary b.
    b. tract

bypassable

by-product
    eosinophil b's

Byrel
    B. SX pacemaker
    B. SX/Versatrax pacemaker

C
 C to E amplitude
 C point of cardiac apex
  pulse

c
 c wave
 c wave of jugular venous
  pulse
 c wave pressure on right
  atrial catheterization

CA
 cardiac arrest
 coronary artery

C-A amplitude of mitral valve

CABG
 coronary artery bypass
  graft

cable
 alligator pacing c.
 OxyLead interconnect c.

Cabot-Locke murmur

Cabral coronary reconstruction

cachectic
 c. endocarditis

cachexia
 cardiac c.
 thyroid c.

CAD
 coronary artery disease

CADD-Plus intravenous infusion
 pump

Cadence
 C. AICD
 C. biphasic ICD
 C. implantable cardiover-
  ter-defibrillator
 C. tiered therapy defibrilla-
  tor system
 C. TVL nonthoracotomy
  lead

Cadet V-115 implantable cardioverter-defibrillator

cadmiosis

cadmium (Cd)
 c. fumes

café-au-lait spot

café coronary

cage
 c. catheter device
 chest c.
 rib c.
 thoracic c.
 titanium c.

caged-ball
 c.-b. valve
 c.-b. valve prosthesis

CAGEIN
 catheter-guided endo-
  scopic intubation

caisson disease

calcicardiogram

calcicosilicosis

calcicosis

calcific
 c. debris
 c. mitral stenosis
 c. nodular aortic stenosis
 c. pericarditis

calcification
 annular c.
 arterial c.
 coronary c.
 dystrophic c.
 linear c.
 mitral annular c.
 Mönckeberg c.
 napkin-ring c.
 pericardial c.
 subannular c.
 valve c.

88

calcification *(continued)*
    valvular c.

calcified
    c. aortic valve
    c. lesion
    c. mitral leaflet
    c. nodule
    c. pericardium
    c. plaque
    c. thrombus
    c. valvular leaflets

calcineurin

calcinosis

calciphylaxis

calcitonin gene–related peptide

calcium
    c. antagonist
    c. channel
    c. channel agonist
    c. channel antagonist
    c. channel blocker
    c. channel blocking agent
    c. chloride
    c. deposit
    c. entry blocker
    fenoprofen c.
    c. gluceptate
    c. gluconate
    c. ion
    c. ionophore A23187
    mitral annular c.
    myoplasmic c.
    nadroparin c.
    c. oxalate
    c. oxalate deposition
    c. paradox
    c. product
    c. rigor
    c. score
    c. sign
    c. transient

calcofluor stain

calculation
    bidirectional shunt c.

calculosa
    pericarditis c.

calculus *pl.* calculi
    cardiac c.

caldesmon

calf
    c. claudication

calibration

calibrator
    Fogarty c.

Califf score

California disease

calipers
    digital c.
    Lange c.
    Mipron digital computer-assisted c.
    Tenzel c.

callosa
    pericarditis c.

Calman
    C. carotid artery clamp
    C. ring clamp

calmodulin

Calori bursa

Calot triangle

calpain

Caltrac accelerometer

Caluso PEG tube

Cambridge
    C. defibrillator
    C. electrocardiograph
    C. jelly electrode

camera
    Anger scintillation c.
    cine c.
    gamma scintillation c.
    multicrystal gamma c.

camera *(continued)*
    multiwire gamma c.
    scintillation c.
    Siemens Orbiter gamma c.
    single-crystal gamma c.
    Sopha Medical gamma c.
    video c.

cameral fistula

Cameron-Haight elevator

Camino
    C. intracranial catheter
    C. mitroventricular bolt
    C. mitroventricular bolt
      catheter

Campbell de Morgan spots

Camp-Sigvaris stockings

CAMP test

camsylate
    trimethaphan c.

canal
    c. of Arantius
    arterial c.
    atrioventricular c.
    carotid c.
    common atrioventricular c.
    complex atrioventricular c.
    c. of Cuvier
    femoral c.
    His c.
    Holmgren-Golgi c's
    Hunter c.
    intercellular c's
    interfacial c's
    intracytoplasmic c's
    c's of Lambert
    partial atrioventricular c.
    perivascular c.
    persistent common atriov-
      entricular c.
    pulmoaortic c.
    Sucquet-Hoyer c.
    Theile c.
    Van Hoorne c.
    ventricular c.
    Verneuil c.

canalization

candidiasis
    endocardial c.

Cannon
    C. a wave
    C. endarterectomy loop
    C. formula
    C. theory

cannon
    c. sound

cannonball
    c. pulse

cannula
    Abelson c.
    aortic arch c.
    aortic perfusion c.
    arterial c.
    atrial c.
    Bard arterial c.
    Bardic c.
    Becker accelerator c.
    cardiovascular c.
    Churchill cardiac suction c.
    Chimochowski cardiac c.
    Cobe small vessel c.
    Cope needle introducer c.
    coronary artery c.
    coronary perfusion c.
    femoral artery c.
    Flexicath silicone subclavi-
      an c.
    Floyd loop c.
    Fluoro Tip c.
    Gregg c.
    Grüntzig femoral stiffen-
      ing c.
    high-flow c.
    infusion c.
    intra-arterial c.
    left ventricular apex c.
    Litwak c.
    Mayo c.
    metallic tip c.
    Morris c.
    outlet c.
    perfusion c.

cannula *(continued)*
  Polystan perfusion c.
  Portnoy ventricular c.
  Research Medical straight
    multiple-holed aortic c.
  Rockey c.
  saphenous vein c.
  Sarns aortic arch c.
  Sarns soft-flow aortic c.
  Sarns two-stage c.
  Sarns venous drainage c.
  Silastic coronary artery c.
  Soresi c.
  2-stage c.
  Tibbs arterial c.
  vein graft c.
  vena cava c.
  Venflon c.
  venous c.
  Wallace Flexihub central
    venous pressure c.
  washout c.
  Webster infusion c.

cannulate

cannulated

cannulation
  bicaval c.
  ostial c.

canon
  bruit de c.

canrenoate potassium

cantering rhythm

Cantlie line

Cantrell pentalogy

capacitance
  c. vessel

capacitor forming time

capacity
  aerobic c.
  diffusing c.
  diffusion c.
  exercise c.
  metabolic vasodilatory c.
  work c.

Capetown
  C. aortic prosthetic valve
  C. aortic valve prosthesis

capillarectasia

capillariomotor

capillarioscopy

capillaritis

capillaropathy

capillaroscopy

capillary
  c. apoplexy
  arterial c.
  c. bed
  c. blush
  compensatory c. filling
  continuous c's
  erythrocytic c's
  fenestrated c's
  Meigs c's
  c. refill
  sheathed c's
  sinusoidal c.
  venous c.

Capintex
  C. nuclear VEST monitor
  C. VEST system

Capiox-E bypass system oxygenator

Capiscint

Caplan syndrome

Capnocheck

capnograph

capnography

capped lead

caprisans
  pulsus c.

caprizant

capsule
  Glisson c.

capsule *(continued)*
　　c. of heart

CapSure cardiac pacing lead

capture
　　atrial c.
　　c. beats
　　c. complex
　　failure to c.
　　loss of c.
　　pacemaker c.
　　retrograde arterial c.
　　ventricular c.

Carabelli tube

Carabello sign

CarboMedics
　　C. bileaflet prosthetic heart
　　　　valve
　　C. cardiac valve prosthesis
　　C. top-hat supra-annular
　　　　valve
　　C. valve device

Carbo-Seal
　　C. cardiovascular compos-
　　　　ite graft
　　C. graft material

carboxyhemoglobin (HbCO)

carcinoembryonic antigen
　　(CEA)

carcinogen

carcinogenicity

carcinoid
　　c. heart disease
　　c. murmur
　　c. plaque
　　c. syndrome
　　c. valve disease

carcinomatous pericarditis

Cardak percutaneous catheter
　　introducer

Cardarelli sign

cardiac
　　c. accident

cardiac *(continued)*
　　c. action potential
　　c. adjustment scale
　　c. allograft
　　c. allograft atherosclerosis
　　c. allograft vasculopathy
　　c. alternation
　　c. amyloidosis
　　c. aneurysm
　　c. antrum
　　c. apex
　　c. arrest
　　c. arrhythmia
　　c. asthma
　　c. atrophy
　　c. auscultation
　　c. automatic resuscitative
　　　　device
　　c. ballet
　　c. balloon pump
　　c. baroreceptor
　　c. blood-pool imaging
　　c. border of dullness
　　c. bronchus
　　c. cachexia
　　c. calculus
　　c. catheter
　　c. catheterization
　　c. chamber
　　c. cirrhosis
　　c. cocktail
　　c. compensation
　　c. competence
　　c. compression
　　c. conduction
　　c. conduction system
　　c. contraction
　　c. contusion
　　c. cooling jacket
　　c. cripple
　　c. crisis
　　c. cushion
　　c. cycle
　　c. death
　　c. decompensation
　　c. decompression
　　c. defibrillation
　　c. depressant
　　c. depressor reflex

cardiac *(continued)*
    c. diastole
    c. dilation
    c. diuretic
    c. dropsy
    c. dyspnea
    c. dysrhythmia
    c. edema
    c. efficiency
    c. enlargement
    c. enzymes
    c. event
    c. examination
    c. failure
    c. fibrillation
    c. fossa
    c. function
    c. functional capacity
    c. gap junction protein
    c. gating
    c. glycogenosis
    c. glycoside
    c. hemoptysis
    c. herniation
    c. heterotaxia
    c. hypertrophy
    c. impulse
    c. incisura
    c. index
    c. infarction
    c. insufficiency
    c. insult
    c. interstitium
    c. ichemia
    c. jelly
    c. leads
    c. liver
    c. lung
    c. mapping
    c. mass
    c. massage
    c. memory
    c. metastasis
    c. monitor
    c. murmur
    c. muscle
    c. muscle wrap
    c. myosin
    c. myxoma

cardiac *(continued)*
    c. neural crest
    c. neurosis
    c. notch
    c. orifice
    c. output
    c. output index
    c. output measurement
    c. pacemaker
    c. patch
    c. perforation
    c. performance
    c. perfusion
    c. polyp
    c. probe
    c. rehabilitation
    c. reserve
    c. resuscitation
    c. retraction clip
    c. rhythm
    c. rhythm disturbance
    c. risk factor
    c. risk index
    c. rupture
    c. sarcoidosis myocarditis
    c. sarcoma
    c. sensory nerve
    c. shadow
    c. shock
    c. shunt
    c. silhouette
    c. sling
    c. souffle
    c. sound
    c. source
    c. standstill
    c. status
    c. stump
    c. surgery
    c. symphysis
    c. syncope
    c. systole
    c. tamponade
    c. telemetry
    c. thrombosis
    c. thrust
    c. transplant
    c. troponin
    c. troponin I assay

cardiac *(continued)*
  c. tumor
  c. tumor plop
  c. ultrasound
  c. valve
  c. valve prosthesis
  c. valvular incompetence
  c. variability
  c. vein
  c. volume
  c. waist
  c. wall hypokinesis
  c. wall thickening
  c. work index

cardiaca
  adiposis c.
  steatosis c.

cardiac-apnea

Cardiac Pacemakers, Inc. (CPI)

Cardiac T
  C. T assay for troponin T
  C. T rapid assay

cardiacwise

cardialgia

cardianastrophe

cardiasthenia

cardiataxia

cardiatelia

CardiData Prodigy system

cardiectasia, cardiectasis

cardiectopia

cardinal vein

cardioacceleration

cardioaccelerator center

cardioactive

cardioangiography

cardioangiology

cardioangioscope
  Sumida c.

cardioarterial

cardioauditory syndrome

cardioballistic

cardiocairograph

Cardio-Care

cardiocele

cardiocentesis

cardiochalasia

cardiocirrhosis

cardioclasis

CardioCoil coronary stent

Cardio-Cool myocardial protection pouch

Cardio-Cuff
  Childs C.

cardiocyte

CardioData
  C. Mark IV computer
  C. MK-3 Holter scanner

cardiodiaphragmatic angle

CardioDiary
  C. heart monitor

cardiodilatin

cardiodilator

cardiodynamics

cardiodynia

cardioembolic
  c. stroke

cardioesophageal
  c. junction
  c. reflux
  c. sphincter

cardiofacial syndrome

Cardioflon suture

Cardiofreezer cryosurgical system

cardiogenesis

cardiogenic
    c. pulmonary edema
    c. shock
    c. syncope

Cardiografin

cardiogram
    apex c.
    esophageal c.
    precordial c.
    ultrasonic c.
    vector c.

cardiograph

cardiographic

cardiography
    Doppler c.
    echo-Doppler c.
    ultrasonic c.
    ultrasound c.
    vector c.

Cardio-Green dye

Cardio-Grip
    C. anastomosis clamp
    C. aortic clamp
    C. ligature carrier
    C. renal artery clamp
    C. tangential occlusion
      clamp
    C. vascular clamp

Cardioguard 4000 electrocardiographic monitor

cardiohemothrombus

cardiohepatic

cardiohepatomegaly

cardioinhibitory
    c. center
    c. syncope
    c. type

cardiokinetic

cardiokymogram

cardiokymograph

cardiokymography

Cardiolite
    C. cardiac perfusion study
    C. stress test

cardiolith

cardiologist

cardiology
    invasive c.

cardiolysis
    Brauer c.

cardiomalacia

Cardiomarker catheter

cardiomediastinal silhouette

cardiomegalia

cardiomegaly
    borderline c.
    false c.
    glycogen c.
    idiopathic c.

cardiomelanosis

Cardiomemo device

Cardiometrics cardiotomy reservoir

cardiometer

cardiometry

cardiomotility

cardiomuscular bradycardia

cardiomyocyte

cardiomyoliposis

cardiomyopathic lentiginosis

cardiomyopathy
    African c.
    alcoholic c.
    anthracycline-induced c.

cardiomyopathy *(continued)*
  apical hypertrophic c.
  atrophic c.
  beer-drinkers' c.
  cobalt c.
  concentric hypertrophic c.
  congestive c.
  constrictive c.
  diabetic c.
  dilated c.
  doxorubicin c.
  drug-induced c.
  end-stage c.
  false c.
  familial hypertrophic ob-
    structive c.
  fibroplastic c.
  genetic hypertrophic c.
  HIV c.
  hypertensive hypertro-
    phic c.
  hypertrophic c. (HCM)
  hypertrophic obstructive c.
    (HOCM)
  idiopathic dilated c.
  idiopathic restrictive c.
  infectious c.
  infiltrative c.
  ischemic c.
  metoprolol dilated c.
  mitochondrial c.
  nephropathic c.
  nonischemic dilated c.
  nonobstructive c.
  obliterative c.
  obstructive hypertrophic c.
  parasitic c.
  pediatric c.
  peripartum c.
  postpartum c.
  primary c.
  rejection c.
  restrictive c.
  right ventricular c.
  secondary c.
  tachycardia-induced c.
  toxic c.
  viral c.
  X-linked dilated c.

cardiomyopexy

cardiomyoplasty
  dynamic c.

cardiomyostimulator

Cardio-Myostimulator SP1005

cardiomyotomy

cardionatrin

cardionecrosis

cardionephric

cardioneural

cardioneuropathy

cardioneurosis

cardio-omentopexy

Cardio-Pace Medical Durapulse
  pacemaker

cardiopalmus

cardiopaludism

cardiopath

cardiopathia nigra

cardiopathic

cardiopathy
  endocrine c.
  infarctoid c.

cardiopericardiopexy
  Beck c.

cardiopericarditis

cardiopexy
  ligamentum teres c.

cardiophobia

cardiophone

cardiophony

cardiophrenia

cardiophrenic angle

cardioplegia
  blood c.

cardioplegia *(continued)*
    cold blood c.
    cold crystalloid c.
    cold potassium c.
    cold sanguineous c.
    c. cooling
    crystalloid potassium c.
    hyperkalemic c.
    normothermic c.
    nutrient c.
    potassium chloride c.
    St. Thomas Hospital c.
    whole blood c.

cardioplegic
    c. arrest
    c. needle
    c. solution

cardiopneumatic

cardiopneumonopexy

Cardiopoint cardiac surgery
   needle

cardiopressor

cardioprotective

cardioptosia

cardioptosis

CardioPulmonary
    C. eXercise

cardiopulmonary
    c. arrest
    c. bypass
    c. exercise text
    c. murmur
    c. reserve
    c. resuscitation
    c. support

CardioPump
    Ambu C.

cardiorespiratory
    c. arrest
    c. murmur

cardiorrhaphy

cardiorrhexis

cardioschisis

cardiosclerosis

cardioscope
    Carlens c.
    Siemens BICOR c.
    Siemens HICOR c.
    c. U system

cardioselective
    c. agent
    c. beta blocker

cardiosis

cardiospasm

Cardioserv defibrillator

cardiosphygmogram

cardiosphygmograph

cardiosplenopexy

cardiosymphysis

CardioSync cardiac synchronizer

cardiotachometer

cardiotachometry

Cardio Tactilaze peripheral angioplasty laser catheter

CardioTec
    C. scan

Cardio-Tel

Cardiotest portable electrograph

Cardiothane 51

cardiotherapy

cardiothoracic
    c. ratio
    c. surgery

cardiothrombus

cardiothymic

cardiothyrotoxicosis

cardiotocography

cardiotomy
  c. reservoir

cardiotonic
  c. drug

cardiotopometry

cardiotoxic
  c. myolysis

cardiotoxicity
  Adriamycin c.
  doxorubicin c.

cardiotoxin

Cardiotrast

cardiovalvotomy

cardiovalvular

cardiovalvulitis

cardiovalvulotome

cardiovalvulotomy

cardiovascular
  c. accident
  c. cannula
  c. clamp
  c. collapse
  c. complication
  c. disability
  c. disease (CVD)
  c. excitatory centers
  c. fitness
  c. function
  c. function assessment
  c. hemodynamics
  c. inhibitory centers
  c. pressure
  c. silk suture
  c. steady state
  c. stylet
  c. syphilis
  c. system
  c. tone

cardioversion
  chemical c.
  direct-current c.
  elective c.

cardioversion (continued)
  electrical c.
  endocavitary c.
  low-energy synchronized c.
  c. paddles
  pharmacological c.
  synchronized DC c.

cardiovert

cardioverted

cardioverter
  automatic implantable c.-
    defibrillator
  implantable c.-defibrillator

cardiovirus

Cardiovit
  C. AT-10 ECG/spirometry
    combination system
  C. AT-10 monitor

CardioWest TAH

carditis
  Coxsackie c.
  Lyme c.
  rheumatic c.
  Sterges c.
  streptococcal c.
  verrucous c.

Carey Coombs short mid-diastolic murmur

carina pl. carinae
  c. not splayed
  c. sharp and mobile
  c. of trachea

carinatum
  pectus c.

Carlens
  C. cardioscope
  C. double-lumen endotra-
    cheal tube

Carmalt forceps

Carmeda BioActive Surface

C-arm fluoroscopy

Carmody valvulotome

carmustine

carneae
trabeculae c.

carnitine

Carolina color spectrum CW
Doppler

caroticovertebral
c. stenosis

carotid
c. angiography
c. arch
c. arteriography
c. artery
c. artery disease
c. artery murmur
c. artery shunt
c.-axillary bypass
c. baroreceptor
c. bifurcation
c. body
c. bruit
c. bulb
c. canal
c.-c. bypass
c. cavernous fistula
c. Doppler
c. duplex scan
c. ejection time
c. endarterectomy
c. massage
c. occlusive disease
c. phonoangiography
c. plaque
c. pulse
c. pulse tracing
c. sheath
c. shudder
c. sinus
c. sinus hypersensitivity
c. sinus massage
c. sinus nerve
c. sinus reflex
c. sinus syncope
c. sinus syndrome
c. sinus test
c. siphon

carotid *(continued)*
c. steal syndrome
c. stenosis
c. stent
c.-subclavian bypass
c. triangle
c. upstroke

carotidynia, carotodynia

Carpenter syndrome

Carpentier
C. annuloplasty
C. annuloplasty ring pros-
thesis
C. pericardial valve
C. ring
C. stent
C. tricuspid valvuloplasty
C.-Edwards aortic valve
prosthesis
C.-Edwards bioprosthesis
C.-Edwards glutaraldehyde-
preserved porcine xeno-
graft prosthesis
C.-Edwards mitral annulo-
plasty valve
C.-Edwards pericardial
valve
C.-Edwards Perimount RSR
pericardial bioprosthesis
C.-Edwards porcine pros-
thetic valve
C.-Edwards porcine supra-
annular valve
C.-Rhone-Poulenc mitral
ring prosthesis

carpopedal spasm

Carrel patch

carrier

Carten mitral valve retractor

Carter
C. equation
C. retractor

cartilage
xiphoid c.

Cartwright
C. heart prosthesis
C. implant
C. valve prosthesis
C. vascular prosthesis

carumonam

Carvallo sign

CAS-8000V general angiography
positioner

Casale-Devereux criteria

cascade
c. phenomenon
renin-angiotensin-aldoster-
one c.

caseated tissue

caseating

caseation
tuberculosis c.

CASE computerized exercise
EKG system

case-control study

Casoni's test

Castaneda
C. anastomosis clamp
C. bottle
C. cannula
C. IMM vascular clamp
C. partial occlusion clamp
C. principle
C. vascular clamp

Castellani
C. bronchitis
C. disease
C. point

Castellino sign

Castillo catheter

Castleman disease

castor bean

Castroviejo needle holder

catabolism
c. of rt-PA

catacrotic
c. pulse
c. wave

catacrotism

catacrotus
pulsus c.

catadicrotic
c. pulse
c. wave

catadicrotism

Cat-a-Kit analyzer

cataire
frémissement c.

catalase

catamenial hemothorax

cataplectic

cataplexy

catatricrotic
c. pulse

catatricrotism

CATCH 22 syndrome

catecholamine
c. action
plasma c.

catenoid

CathTrack catheter locator system

catheter
c. ablation
ACE fixed-wire balloon c.
Achiever balloon dilata-
tion c.
ACS angioplasty c.
ACS balloon c.
ACS Concorde coronary
diltation c.
ACS Endura coronary dila-
tion c.

catheter *(continued)*
>ACS Enhanced Torque 8/
>7.5 F Taper Tip c.
>ACS JL4 French c.
>ACS Mini c.
>ACS Monorel c.
>ACS OTW Lifestream coronary dilatation c.
>ACS OTW Photon coronary dilatation c.
>ACS OTW Solaris coronary dilatation c.
>ACS RX Lifestream coronary diltation c.
>c. adapter
>AL-1 c.
>AL II guiding c.
>Alvarez-Rodriguez cardiac c.
>Alzate c.
>Amcath c.
>Amplatz coronary c.
>Amplatz Hi-Flo torque-control c.
>Amplatz left I, II c.
>Amplatz right coronary c.
>Amplatz right I, II c.
>A2 multipurpose c.
>Angiocath PRN c.
>Angioflow high-flow c.
>angiographic c.
>Angio-Kit c.
>Angiomedics c.
>angiopigtail c.
>angioplasty balloon c.
>angioplasty guiding c.
>angled balloon c.
>angled pigtail c.
>angulated multipurpose c.
>Anthron II c.
>Anthron heparinized antithrombogenic c.
>AR-1 c.
>Arani double-loop guiding c.
>Argyle c.
>Arrow balloon wedge c.
>Arrow-Berman balloon c.

catheter *(continued)*
>Arrow Flex intra-aortic balloon c.
>ArrowGard Blue antiseptic-coated c.
>ArrowGard Blue Line c.
>ArrowGard central venous c.
>Arrow-Howes multilumen c.
>Arrow QuadPolar electrode c.
>Arrow TwinCath multilumen peripheral c.
>arterial embolectomy c.
>c. arteriography
>Asuka PTA over-the-wire c.
>atherectomy c.
>AtheroCath spinning blade c.
>Atlas DG balloon angioplasty c.
>Atlas LP PTCA balloon dilatation c.
>Atlas ULP balloon dilatation c.
>ATRAC-II double-balloon c.
>ATRAC multipurpose balloon c.
>Atri-pace I bipolar flared pacing c.
>Auth atherectomy c.
>autoperfusion balloon c.
>AV Paceport thermodilution c.
>Axiom DG balloon angioplasty c.
>Bailey c.
>bailout autoperfusion balloon c.
>Baim pacing c.
>Baim-Turi monitoring/pacing c.
>Balectrode pacing c.
>balloon c.
>balloon angioplasty c.
>balloon dilatation c.
>balloon embolectomy c.
>balloon-flotation pacing c.
>balloon-imaging c.

catheter *(continued)*
- balloon septostomy c.
- balloon-tipped angiographic c.
- balloon-tipped flow-directed c.
- balloon-tipped thermodilution c.
- balloon valvuloplasty c.
- ball-wedge c.
- Baltherm c.
- Bandit PTCA c.
- Bard balloon-directed pacing c.
- Bardco c.
- Bard electrophysiology c.
- Bard guiding c.
- Bardic cutdown c.
- Baxter angioplasty c.
- Bentson-Hanafee-Wilson c.
- Berenstein occlusion balloon c.
- Berman angiographic c.
- Berman balloon flotation c.
- Bicor c.
- bifoil balloon c.
- Bio-Medicus arterial c.
- bipolar pacing electrode c.
- bird's eye c.
- blade septostomy c.
- Block right coronary guiding c.
- Blue FlexTip c.
- Blue Max triple-lumen c.
- Bonzel Monotrail balloon c.
- Bourassa c.
- brachial c.
- BriteTip c.
- Brockenbrough mapping c.
- Brockenbrough modified bipolar c.
- Brockenbrough transseptal c.
- Bronchitrac L flexible suction c.
- Broviac atrial c.
- Buchbinder Omniflex c.
- Buchbinder Thruflex over-the-wire c.

catheter *(continued)*
- Buerhenne steerable c.
- bullet-tip c.
- bur-bearing c.
- bypass graft c.
- Camino intracranial c.
- Camino microventricular bolt c.
- cardiac c.
- cardiac c.-microphone
- Cardima Pathfinder c.
- Cardiomarker c.
- Cardio Tactilaze peripheral angioplasty laser c.
- Castillo c.
- Cath-Finder c.
- Cathlon IV c.
- Cathmark suction c.
- central venous c.
- central venous pressure (CVP) c.
- Cereblate c.
- Chemo-Port c.
- Clark expanding mesh c.
- Clark helix c.
- Clark rotating cutter c.
- closed end-hole c.
- Cloverleaf c.
- coaxial c.
- Cobra over-the-wire balloon c.
- cobra-shaped c.
- coil-tipped c.
- conductance c.
- Cook arterial c.
- Cook TPN c.
- Cook yellow pigtail c.
- Cordis BriteTip guiding c.
- Cordis Ducor I, II, III c.
- Cordis Ducor pigtail c.
- Cordis guiding c.
- Cordis high-flow pigtail c.
- Cordis Lumelec c.
- Cordis Predator balloon c.
- Cordis Son-II c.
- Cordis Titan balloon dilation c.
- Cordis Trakstar PTCA balloon c.

catheter *(continued)*
    Cordis TransTaper tip c.
    coronary angiographic c.
    coronary sinus thermodilution c.
    coronary seeking c.
    corset balloon c.
    Cournand quadripolar c.
    C. R. Bard c.
    Cribier-Letac c.
    CritiCath thermodilution c.
    Critikon balloon temporary pacing c.
    Critikon balloon thermodilution c.
    Critikon balloon-tipped end-hole c.
    Critikon balloon wedge pressure c.
    cryoablation c.
    cutdown c.
    Cynosar c.
    Dacron c.
    c. damping
    Datascope CL-II percutaneous translucent balloon c.
    decapolar electrode c.
    decapolar pacing c.
    deflectable quadripolar c.
    Deseret flow-directed thermodilution c.
    diagnostic ultrasound imaging c.
    Diasonics c.
    Digiflex high flow c.
    c. dilation
    directional atherectomy c.
    Dispatch over-the-wire c.
    DLP cardioplegic c.
    dog-leg c.
    Doppler c.
    Dorros brachial internal mammary guiding c.
    Dorros infusion/probing c.
    Dotter caged-balloon c.
    double-balloon c.
    double-chip micromanometer c.
    double-J c.

catheter *(continued)*
    double-lumen c.
    double-thermistor coronary sinus c.
    drill-tip c.
    dual balloon perfusion c.
    dual-sensor micromanometric high-fidelity c.
    Dualtherm dual thermistor thermodilution c.
    Ducor balloon c.
    Ducor-Cordis pigtail c.
    Ducor HF c.
    EAC c.
    echo c.
    EchoMark angiographic c.
    EDM infusion c.
    Edwards c.
    EID c.
    eight-lumen manometry c.
    Elecath thermodilution c.
    electrode c.
    El Gamal coronary bypass c.
    El Gamal guiding c.
    Elite guide c.
    embolectomy c.
    c. embolectomy
    c. embolism
    c. embolus
    Encapsulon epidural c.
    end-hole c.
    end-hole balloon-tipped c.
    end-hole #7 French c.
    EndoSonics IVUS/balloon dilatation c.
    Endosound endoscopic ultrasound c.
    Endotak lead transvenous c.
    Enhanced Torque 8F guiding c.
    Eppendorf c.
    Erythroflex hydromer-coated central venous c.
    c. exchange
    expandable access c.
    Explorer 360-degree rotational diagnostic EP c.

catheter *(continued)*

Explorer pre-curved diagnostic EP c.

Express over-the-wire balloon c.

extrusion balloon c.

Falcon single-operator exchange balloon c.

FAST (flow-assisted, short-term) balloon c.

FAST coronary balloon angioplasty c.

FAST right heart cardiovascular c.

fiberoptic c. delivery system

fiberoptic oximeter c.

fiberoptic pressure c.

Finesse guiding c.

Flexguard Tip c.

flotation c.

flow-directed balloon cardiovascular c.

fluid-filled c.

fluid-filled balloon cardiovascular c.

fluid-filled balloon-tipped flow-directed c.

fluid-filled pigtail c.

Fogarty c.

Fogarty adherent clot c.

Fogarty arterial embolectomy c.

Fogarty-Chin extrusion balloon c.

Fogarty graft thrombectomy c.

Fogarty venous thrombectomy c.

Foltz-Overton cardiac c.

Force balloon dilatation c.

Forerunner coronary sinus guiding c.

c. fragment

Franz monophasic action potential c.

French double-lumen c.

French JR4 Schneider c.

French SAL c.

catheter *(continued)*

French shaft c.

Ganz-Edwards coronary infusion c.

Gensini coronary c.

Gensini Teflon c.

Gentle-Flo suction c.

Glidecath hydrophilic-coated c.

Goeltec c.

Goodale-Lubin c.

Gorlin c.

Gould PentaCath 5-lumen thermodilution c.

graft-seeking c.

Grollman pulmonary artery-seeking c.

Groshong double-lumen c.

Grüntzig balloon c.

Grüntzig-Dilaca c.

GTO DVI AtheroCath c.

c.-guided biopsy

c.-guided endoscopic intubation (CAGEIN)

c. guide holder

c. guide wire

guiding c.

Hakko Dwellcath c.

Halo c.

Hancock embolectomy c.

Hancock fiberoptic c.

Hancock hydrogen detection c.

Hancock luminal electrophysiologic recording c.

Hancock wedge-pressure c.

Hartzler ACX II c.

Hartzler balloon c.

Hartzler dilatation c.

Hartzler Excel c.

Hartzler LPS dilatation c.

Hartzler Micro-600 c.

Hartzler Micro II c.

Hartzler Micro XT c.

Hartzler RX-014 balloon c.

headhunter angiography c.

helical-tip Halo c.

helium-filled balloon c.

Helix PTCA dilatation c.

catheter *(continued)*

- hexapolar c.
- Hickman indwelling right atrial c.
- high-flow c.
- high-speed rotation dynamic angioplasty c.
- Hilal modified headhunter c.
- His c.
- hockey-stick c.
- hot-tipped c.
- c. hub
- HydroCath c.
- Hydrogel-coated PTCA balloon c.
- IAB c.
- Illumen-8 guiding c.
- ILUS c.
- Imager Torque selective c.
- imaging-angioplasty balloon c.
- c. impact artifact
- impedance c.
- c.-induced thrombosis
- Infiniti c.
- Inoue balloon c.
- c. instability
- Integra c.
- IntelliCat pulmonary artery c.
- internal mammary artery c.
- Interpret ultrasound c.
- Intimax vascular c.
- intra-aortic balloon c.
- intracardiac c.
- intravascular ultrasound c.
- intravenous pacing c.
- Intrepid balloon c.
- c. introducer
- c.-introducing forceps
- ITC balloon c.
- Jackman coronary sinus electrode c.
- Jackman orthogonal c.
- Josephson quadripolar c.
- Jostra c.
- JL-4, JL-5 c.
- JR-4, JR-5 c.

catheter *(continued)*

- Judkins coronary c.
- Judkins curve LAD c.
- Judkins curve LCX c.
- Judkins curve STD c.
- Judkins guiding c.
- Judkins pigtail left ventriculography c.
- Judkins torque control c.
- Katzen long balloon dilatation c.
- Kensey atherectomy c.
- King guiding c.
- King multipurpose c.
- Konigsberg c.
- Kontron balloon c.
- large-bore c.
- large-lumen c.
- laser c.
- Laserprobe c.
- left coronary c.
- left heart c.
- left Judkins c.
- left ventricular sump c.
- Lehman ventriculography c.
- lensed fiber-tip laser delivery c.
- Levin c.
- Leycom volume conductance c.
- Lifestream coronary dilation c.
- long ACE fixed-wire balloon c.
- Longdwel Teflon c.
- Long Skinny over-the-wire balloon c.
- Lo-Profile II c.
- low-speed rotation angioplasty c.
- Lumaguide c.
- Lumelec pacing c.
- Mallinckrodt angiographic c.
- c. manipulation
- manometer-tipped c.
- Mansfield Atri-Pace 1 c.

catheter *(continued)*

Mansfield orthogonal electrode c.
Mansfield Scientific dilatation balloon c.
Mansfield-Webster c.
c. mapping
mapping/ablation c.
Marathon guiding c.
marker c.
McGoon coronary perfusion c.
McIntosh double-lumen c.
Medi-Tech balloon c.
Medi-Tech steerable c.
Medtronic balloon c.
memory c.
Metras c.
Mewissen infusion c.
Micor c.
Micro-Guide c.
micromanometer c.
Microsoftrac c.
Micross dilatation c.
midstream aortogram c.
Mikro-Tip micromanometer-tipped c.
Millar Doppler c.
Millar MPC-500 c.
Millar pigtail angiographic c.
Millennia PTCA c.
Miller septostomy c.
Mini-Profile c.
Mitrage over-the-wire balloon c.
Molina needle c.
monofoil c.
monometer-tipped c.
Monorail imaging c.
MS Classique balloon dilatation c.
MTC c.
Mullins transseptal c.
multiaccess c. (MAC)
multielectrode impedance c.
multilumen c.
multiflanged Portnoy c.

catheter *(continued)*

Multiflex c.
multilayer design c.
multiplex c.
multipolar c.
multipurpose c.
Multipurpose-SM c.
multisensory c.
MVP c.
Mylar c.
Namic c.
NC Bandit c.
Nestor guiding c.
NIH cardiomarker c.
NIH left ventriculography c.
NIH marking c.
nonflotation c.
nontraumatizing c.
NoProfile balloon c.
Norton flow-directed Swan-Ganz thermodilution c.
Novoste c.
Numed intracoronary Doppler c.
Nycore angiography c.
Nycore pigtail c.
octapolar c.
Olbert balloon c.
Olympiz II PTCA dilatation c.
Omniflex balloon c.
one-hole angiographic c.
Opta 5 c.
optical fiber c.
Opticath oximeter c.
Optiscope c.
Oracle Focus PTCA c.
Oracle Micro intravascular ultrasound c.
Oracle Micro Plus PTCA c.
Oreopoulos-Zellerman c.
OTW perfusion c.
other-the-wire PTCA balloon c.
Owens balloon c.
Owens Lo-Profile dilatation c.
oximetric c.
pacemaker c.

catheter *(continued)*
  Paceport c.
  Pacewedge dual-pressure
    bipolar pacing c.
  pacing c.
  Park blade septostomy c.
  P.A.S. Port c.
  c. patency
  Pathfinder c.
  Pathfinder mini c.
  PA Watch position-monito-
    ring c.
  pediatric pigtail c.
  Peel-Away c.
  PE-MT balloon dilatation c.
  PE-Plus II balloon dilata-
    tion c.
  Percor-Stat-DL c.
  percutaneous intra-aortic
    balloon counterpulsa-
    tion c.
  percutaneous transluminal
    coronary angioplasty c.
  perfusion balloon c.
  Periflow peripheral balloon
    angioplasty-infusion c.
  peripherally-inserted c.
  PermCath c.
  Per-Q-Cath percutaneously
    inserted central venous c.
  pervenous c.
  Phantom V Plus c.
  Picollino Monorail c.
  pigtail c.
  Pilotip c.
  Pinkerton .018 balloon c.
  POC Bandit c.
  Polaris steerable diagnos-
    tic c.
  Positrol II c.
  Predator balloon c.
  preshaped c.
  probe balloon c.
  Probing sheath exchange c.
  Procath electrophysiolo-
    gy c.
  Profile Plus balloon dilata-
    tion c.
  Proflex 5 c.

catheter *(continued)*
  Pro-Flo XT c.
  Pruitt-Inahara balloon-
    tipped perfusion c.
  pulmonary arterial c.
  pulmonary flotation c.
  Q-cath c.
  quadripolar electrode c.
  quadripolar steerable elec-
    trode c.
  Quanticor c.
  Quantum Ranger balloon c.
  QuickFlash arterial c.
  Quinton PermCath c.
  Raaf Cath vascular c.
  radiopaque calibrated c.
  Ranger over-the-wire bal-
    loon c.
  Rashkind septostomy bal-
    loon c.
  recessed balloon septosto-
    my c.
  RediFurl TaperSeal IAB c.
  Rentrop c.
  reperfusion c.
  retroperfusion c.
  Revelation microcatheter
    for EP mapping
  Revelation Tx microcath-
    eter for RF ablation
  RF Ablatr ablation c.
  RF-generated thermal bal-
    loon c.
  right coronary c.
  right heart c.
  right Judkins c.
  Rigiflex TTS balloon c.
  Ritchie c.
  Rodriguez c.
  Rodriguez-Alvarez c.
  Rotablator c.
  Rotacs motorized c.
  rotational dynamic angio-
    plasty c.
  rove magnetic c.
  Royal Flush c.
  Rx perfusion c.
  Rx Streak balloon c.

catheter *(continued)*

Safe-T-Coat heparin-coated thermodilution c.
SafTouch c.
Sarns wire-reinforced c.
SCA-EX ShortCutter c.
Schneider c.
Schoonmaker c.
Schwarten LP balloon c.
SciMed angioplasty c.
Scoop 1, 2 c.
Seldinger cardiac c.
Selecon coronary angiography c.
self-guiding c.
self-positioning balloon c.
Sensation intra-aortic balloon c.
Sentron pigtail angiographic micromanometer c.
Seroma-Cath c.
serrated c.
Shadow over-the-wire balloon c.
shaver c.
Sherpa guiding c.
Shiley c.
SHJR-4 c.
ShortCutter c.
side-hole Judkins right, curve 4 c.
sidewinder percutaneous intra-aortic balloon c.
Silastic c.
Silicore c.
Simmons II, III c.
Simmons-type sidewinder c.
Simplus PE/t dilatation c.
Simpson atherectomy c.
Simpson Coronary AtheroCath c.
Simpson-Robert c.
Simpson Ultra Lo-Profile II c.
Skinny dilatation c.
Skinny over-the-wire balloon c.

catheter *(continued)*

Sleek c.
Slider c.
sliding rail c.
Slinky balloon c.
Slinky PTCA c.
Slow-Trax perfusion balloon c.
Smart position-sensing c.
Smec balloon c.
snare c.
Softip c.
Softouch UHF cardiac pigtail c.
Softrac-PTA c.
Soft-Vu Omni flush c.
Solo c.
Sones Cardio-Marker c.
Sones coronary c.
Sones Hi-Flow c.
Sones Positrol c.
Sones woven Dacron c.
Sonicath imaging c.
Sorenson thermodilution c.
Spectra-Cath STP c.
Spectranetics C rapid-exchange laser c.
Spectranetics VitesseE excimer laser c.
Speedy balloon c.
Spring c.
Sprint c.
Stack perfusion c.
standard Lehman c.
steerable electrode c.
steerable guide wire c.
Steerocath c.
Steri-Cath c.
Stertzer brachial c.
Stertzer guiding c.
straight flush percutaneous c.
Sub-4 small vessel balloon dilatation c.
SULP II balloon c.
Superflow guiding c.
Super-9 guiding c.
Swan-Ganz balloon flotation c.

catheter *(continued)*
    Swan-Ganz bipolar pacing c.
    Swan-Ganz flow-directed c.
    Swan-Ganz Pacing TD c.
    TAC atherectomy c.
    TEC (transluminal endarterectomy) c.
    Teflon c.
    TEGwire balloon dilatation c.
    Tennis Racquet angiographic c.
    Ten system balloon c.
    Terumo SP coaxial c.
    tetrapolar esophageal c.
    thermistor thermodilution c.
    thermodilution balloon c.
    thin-walled c.
    c. tip occluder
    Titan balloon c.
    Torcon NB selective angiographic c.
    Torktherm torque control c.
    Total Cross balloon c.
    Tourguide guiding c.
    TrachCare multi-access c.
    Tracker-18 Soft Stream side-hole microinfusion c.
    Trac Plus c.
    Trakstart balloon c.
    transcutaneous extraction c.
    transluminal angioplasty c.
    transluminal endarterectomy c.
    transluminal extraction c.
    Transport drug delivery c.
    Transport dilatation balloon c.
    transseptal c.
    trefoil balloon c.
    Triguide c.
    triple-lumen balloon flotation thermistor c.
    tripolar w/Damato curve c.
    TTS c.

catheter *(continued)*
    Tyshak c.
    Uldall subclavian hemodialysis c.
    ULP c.
    UltraCross profile imaging c.
    ultra-low profile fixed-wire balloon dilatation c.
    Ultra-Thin balloon c.
    UMI c.
    Uniweave c.
    Uresil embolectomy thrombectomy c.
    USCI c.
    Van Andel c.
    Van Tassel angled pigtail c.
    Variflex c.
    Vas-Cath c.
    vascular access c.
    ventriculography c.
    Ventureyra ventricular c.
    Verbatin balloon c.
    Viggo-Spectramed c.
    Viper PTA c.
    V. Mueller c.
    Voda c.
    waist of c.
    Webster decapolar c.
    Webster halo c.
    Webster orthogonal electrode c.
    wedge pressure balloon c.
    Wexler c.
    c. whip
    c. whip artifact
    Wilton-Webster coronary sinus thermodilution c.
    X-Trode electrode c.
    Z-Med c.
    Zucker multipurpose bipolar c.

catheterization
    antegrade transseptal left heart c.
    bypass graft c.
    cardiac c.
    combined heart c.
    coronary sinus c.

catheterization *(continued)*
    hepatic vein c.
    interventional cardiac c.
    left heart c.
    Mullins modification of transseptal c.
    percutaneous transhepatic cardiac c.
    pulmonary artery c.
    retrograde c.
    right heart c.
    selective cardiac c.
    c. technique
    transseptal left heart c.

catheter-related peripheral vessel spasm

catheter-tip
    c.-t. micromanometer system
    c.-t. spasm

Cath-Finder
    C. catheter
    C. catheter tracking system

Cath-Lok catheter locking device

Cathlon IV catheter

Cathmark suction catheter

Cath-Secure

cat-scratch disease

cauda equina syndrome

caudal

caudally angled balloon occlusion aortography

caudocephalad

caudocranial hemiaxial view

cava
    superior vena c.

caval
    c. cannula
    c. catheter

caval *(continued)*
    c. occlusion clamp
    c. snare
    c. valve

caveola

Caverject injection

cavernoma

cavernous
    c. sinus thrombosis
    c. voice

Caves bioptome

Caves-Schultz bioptome

cave sickness

cavitas
    c. pericardiaca
    c. pericardialis

cavitis

cavity
    pericardial c.

Cavitron ultrasonic surgical aspirator

cavocaval shunt

cavopulmonary
    c. anastomosis
    c. connection

C-bar web-spacer

C-C (convexo-concave) heart valve

cDNA
    human closed DNA

CEA
    carcinoembryonic antigen

cedar
    Western red c.

Cedars-Sinai classification

Ceelen disease

Cegka sign

celer
    pulsus c.

Celemajer method

celerrimus
    pulsus c.

Celestin
    C. bougie
    C. esophageal tube

celiac
    c. artery
    c. disease

cell
    adventitial c.
    ameboid c.
    Anichkov (Anitschkow) c.
    Aschoff c.
    automatic c.
    B c.
    B1 c.
    Beale ganglion c's
    blast c.
    brood c.
    c. button
    Caspersson type B c's
    caterpillar c.
    CD4+ c.
    CD4 c.
    CD5 c.
    CD8 c.
    CD8+ T c.
    chicken-wire myocardial c.
    ciliated c.
    Clara c's
    clear c.
    cribrate c.
    daughter c.
    effector c's
    eukaryotic c.
    flagellate c.
    foam c.
    foamy myocardial c.
    giant c.
    glomerular c.
    glomus c.
    goblet c.
    heart-disease c's
    heart-failure c's
    heart-lesion c's

cell *(continued)*
    HeLa c's
    human aortic endothelial
      c's
    hyperplastic mucus-secret-
      ing goblet c.
    IgE-sensitized c.
    Kulchitsky c.
    Langerhans giant c's
    Langhans c's
    littoral c's
    Marchand c.
    mast c.
    c. membrane
    c. membrane-bound aden-
      ylate cyclase
    mesangial c.
    mesenchymal intimal c.
    metaplastic mucus-secret-
      ing c.
    migratory c.
    mononuclear c.
    mother c.
    multinucleated giant c's
    myointimal c.
    N c.
    nodal c's
    nucleated c.
    oat c.
    P c's
    pacemaker c.
    parent c.
    Pelger-Huët c's
    pericapillary c.
    perithelial c.
    perivascular c.
    pi c.
    polyplastic c.
    progenitor c.
    prokaryotic c.
    pup c.
    Purkinje c's
    RA c.
    resting c.
    rod c's
    Rouget c.
    Sala c's
    sensitized c.
    smooth muscle c.

cell *(continued)*
    c. sorter
    stave c's
    squamous c.
    T c's
    transitional c's
    c. type
    typical small c.
    vacuolated c.
    vasofactive c.
    vasoformative c.
    vascular smooth muscle c's
    wandering c.

cellifugal

cellipetal

cell-mediated immunity

Cellolite material

Cell Saver
    C. S. autologous blood recovery system
    C. S. Haemolite
    C. S. Haemonetics Autotransfusion system

celltrifuge

cellular embolism

cellulicidal

cellulifugal

cellulipetal

cellulitis

cellulose
    oxidized c.

celophlebitis

Cel-U-Jec

Cenflex central monitoring system

center
    cardioaccelerator c.
    cardioinhibitory c.
    cardiovascular excitatory c's
    cardiovascular inhibitory c's

center *(continued)*
    cell c.
    Chemetron HR-1 Humidity C.
    Kronecker c.
    pneumotaxic c.
    vasoconstrictor c.
    vasodilator c.

centerline method of wall motion analysis

central
    c. approach
    c. bradycardia
    c. core wire
    c. cyanosis
    c. fibrous body
    c. splanchnic venous thrombosis
    c. terminal electrode
    c. venous catheter
    c. venous line
    c. venous pressure (CVP)

centriacinar emphysema

centriole

centripetal venous pulse

centronuclear myopathy

centroplasm

centrosome

centrosphere

cephalic
    c. artery
    c. vein

cephalocaudad

cerebral
    c. aneurysm
    c. angiography
    c. apoplexy
    c. arteriosclerosis
    c. beriberi
    c. blood flow
    c. embolus
    c. event
    c. infarction

cerebral *(continued)*
   c. ischemia
   c. perfusion
   c. perfusion pressure
   c. protective therapy
   c. thrombosis
   c. vasculopathy

cerebritis

cerebrocardiac

cerebrovascular
   c. accident (CVA)
   c. disease
   c. event
   c. insufficiency
   c. resistance
   c. syncope
   c. thrombosis

cervical
   c. aortic arch
   c. aortic knuckle
   c. heart
   c. rib syndrome
   c. venous hum

cervicalis
   ansa c.

cervicothoracic
   c. sympathectomy

cGMP
   cyclic guanosine mono-
     phosphate

Chagas heart disease

chagasic myocardiopathy

chagoma

chain
   imaging c.
   light c.
   myosin heavy c.
   myosin light c.
   paratracheal c.
   2-c. urokinase plasminogen
     activator (tcu-PA)

chamber
   anterior c.

chamber *(continued)*
   atrialized c.
   cardiac c.
   c. compression
   false aneurysmal c.
   Fisher-Paykel MR290 water
     feed c.
   c's of the heart
   c. rupture
   c. stiffness

Chamberlain mediastinoscopy

Champ cardiac device

Chandler V-pacing probe

change
   arteriovenous crossing c's
   diagnostic ST segment c.
   E to A c's
   E to I c's
   fibrinoid c's
   Gerhardt c.
   hyaline fatty c.
   hydropic c.
   ischemic ECG c's
   malignancy-associated c's
   myxomatous c.
   nonspecific ST-T wave c's
   QRS c's
   QRS–T c's
   rheologic c.
   serial c's
   ST segment c's
   ST–T wave c's
   trophic c's
   T wave c's

channel
   acetylcholine c.
   blood c's
   calcium c.
   calcium-sodium c.
   central c.
   fast c.
   fast sodium c.
   gated c.
   ion c.
   ligand-gated c.
   lymphatic c.
   marker c.

channel *(continued)*
    membrane c.
    potassium c.
    protein c.
    receptor-operated cal-
        cium c.
    c. retractor
    sarcolemmal calcium c.
    slow c.
    sodium c.
    thoroughfare c.
    transnexus c.
    voltage-dependent cal-
        cium c.
    voltage-gated c.
    water c.

Charcot
    C. sign
    C. syndrome
    C.-Bouchard aneurysm
    C.-Bouchard microaneu-
        rysm
    C.-Leyden crystals
    C.-Marie-Tooth disease
    C.-Weiss-Baker syndrome

Chardack
    C. Medtronic pacemaker
    C.-Greatbatch implantable
        cardiac pulse generator
    C.-Greatbatch pacemaker

charge-coupled device trans-
    ducer

Charles procedure

Charlson comorbidity index

Charnley
    C. drain tube
    C. suction drain

chasmatoplasson

Chassaignac axillary muscle

Chaussier tube

CHD
    coronary heart disease

check-valve sheath

chelation therapy

chelator
    iron c.

chemical
    c. cardioversion
    c. exposure
    c. stimulus

chemiluminescence

chemiotaxis

chemoattractant

chemodectoma

Chemo-Port
    C. catheter
    C. perivena catheter sys-
        tem device

chemoprophylaxis
    secondary c.

chemoceptor

chemokinesis

chemokinetic

chemoreception

chemoreceptor

chemotactic

chemotaxin

chemotaxis
    eosinophilic c.

chemotherapy
    antimycobacterial c.

chemotoxin

cherry angioma

cherry-picking procedure

chest
    alar c.
    barrel-shaped c.
    c. bellows
    blast c.
    c. cage
    cobbler's c.
    c. compression

chest *(continued)*
   c. cuirass
   dirty c.
   dropsy c.
   emphysematous c.
   empyema of c.
   flail c.
   foveated c.
   funnel c.
   keeled c.
   c. leads
   c. and left arm
   noisy c.
   c. pain
   paralytic c.
   c. percussion
   c. percussion and vibration
   phthinoid c.
   pigeon c.
   c. port
   c. PT
   pterygoid c.
   quiet c.
   c. and right arm
   c. roentgenogram
   c. shield
   tetrahedron c.
   c. thump
   c. tightness
   c. tube
   c. wall
   c. x-ray

Cheyne
   C.-Stokes breathing
   C.-Stokes respiration
   C.-Stokes sign

CHF
   congestive heart failure

Chiari syndrome

Chiari-Budd syndrome

Chiba needle

chicken fat clot

chicken-wire myocardial cell

Childs Cardio-Cuff

Chinese restaurant syndrome

chloride ion

choanocyte

choc
   bruit de c.
   c. en dome

cholangitis
   sclerosing c.

Cholestech LDX system with TC
   and Glucose Panel

cholesterol
   c. cleft
   c. embolism
   c. embolization
   c. ester
   c. ester storage disease
   c. pericarditis
   serum c.
   c. thorax
   total plasma c.

Cholesterol-Saturated Fat Index

cholesteryl ester storage disease

cholinergic
   c. agent
   c. receptor
   c. response

cholinesterase inhibitor

chondral

chondralgia

chondriome

chondriosome

chondrocostal

chondroma

chondromitome

chondrosarcoma

chondrosternal

chondrosternoplasty

chondroxiphoid

chorda *pl.* chordae
    elongation of chordae
    flail c.
    ruptured chordae tendi-
      neae
    shortening of chordae
    chordae tendineae cordis
    chordae tendineae

chordal
    c. buckling
    c. length
    c. rupture
    c. transfer

chordalis
    endocarditis c.

chordoplasty

chorea
    amyotrophic c.
    c. cordis
    Huntington c.
    Sydenham c.

chorionic villus sampling

Chorus
    C. DDD pacemaker
    C. RM rate-responsive dual-
      chamber pacemaker

Christmas
    C. blood coagulation factor
    C. disease
    C. factor

chromaffin cell tumor

chromate

chromatin

chromatocinesis

chromatography
    affinity c.
    gas c.

chromatokinesis

chromatophorotropic

chromatoplasm

chromatotaxis

chromic catgut suture

chromium
    c. method

chromoplast

chromoplastid

chronic
    c. aortic stenosis
    c. atrial fibrillation
    c. constrictive pericarditis
    c. endocarditis
    c. hemolytic anemia
    c. hypertensive disease
    c. idiopathic orthostatic
      hypotension
    c. myocarditis
    c. passive congestion
    c. renal failure
    c. respiratory failure
    c. shock
    c. stable angina
    c. tamponade
    c. thromboembolic pulmo-
      nary hypertension
    c. valvulitis

chronicity

Chronocor IV external pacemaker

Chronos 04 pacemaker

chronotropic
    c. effect
    c. incompetence
    c. response
    c. therapy

chronotropism
    negative c.
    positive c.

Church cardiovascular scissors

Churchill
    C. cardiac suction cannula
    C. sucker
    C.-Cope reflex

Churg
- C.-Strauss angiitis
- C.-Strauss syndrome

chylomicron
- c. remnant
- c. remnant receptor

chylomicronemia

chylopericarditis

chylopericardium

chylothorax

chylous
- c. hydrothorax
- c. pericardial effusion

CI
- cardiac index
- coronary insufficiency

cicatricial stenosis

cidal effect

cilia (*plural of* cilium)

ciliary
- c. beat frequency
- c. movement

ciliated epithelial cell

ciliocytophthoria

ciliogenesis

cilium *pl.* cilia

Cimino
- C. arteriovenous shunt
- C.-Brescia arteriovenous fistula

Cimochowski cardiac cannula

cinchonism

cineangiocardiography
- biplane c.
- coronary c.
- left ventricular c.
- radionuclide c.
- selective coronary c.

cineangiocardiography (continued)
- Sones technique for c.

cineangiogram

cineangiograph

cineangiography
- conventional c.

cinearteriography

cinecamera

cinefilm

cinefluorography

cinefluoroscopy

cineloop recording

cine-pulse system

cineradiography

cineventriculogram
- biplane c.

cineventriculography

CineView Plus Freeland system

cinoplasm

Circadia dual-chamber rate-adaptive pacemaker

circadian
- c. event recorder
- c. pattern
- c. rhythm
- c. variation

circannual cycle

circaseptan cycle

circle
- arterial c.
- DataVue calibrated reference c.
- Robinson's c.
- vascular c.
- c. of Vieussens
- c. of Willis

Circon videohydrothorascope

circuit
- aortoiliofemoral c.

circuit *(continued)*
  arrhythmia c.
  bypass c.
  Intertech anesthesia
    breathing c.
  Intertech Mapleson D non-
    rebreathing c.
  Intertech nonrebreathing
    modified Jackson-Rees c.
  macroreentrant c.
  microreentrant c.
  reentrant c.
  shunting c.

circular plane

circulation
  allantoic c.
  assisted c.
  balanced coronary c.
  codominant coronary c.
  collateral c.
  compensatory c.
  coronary c.
  coronary collateral c.
  derivative c.
  extracorporeal c.
  fetal c.
  greater c.
  intervillous c.
  left circumflex-dominant c.
  left-dominant coronary c.
  lesser c.
  peripheral c.
  persistent fetal c.
  placental c.
  portal c.
  pulmonary c.
  right-dominant coronary c.
  sinusoidal c.
  systemic c.
  thebesian c.
  c. time
  c. volume

circulatory
  c. arrest
  c. collapse
  c. compromise
  c. congestion
  c. embarrassment

circulatory *(continued)*
  c. failure
  c. hypoxemia
  c. hypoxia
  c. impairment
  c. overload
  c. support
  c. support system

circulus
  c. arteriosus
  c. arteriosus cerebri
  c. articularis vasculosus
  c. articuli vasculosus
  c. umbilicalis
  c. venosus halleri

circumferential
  c. fiber shortening
  c. wall stress

circumflex (circ, CF, CX)
  c. aortic arch
  c. artery
  c. coronary artery

circumnuclear

circumoral cyanosis

circumvascular

circus
  c.-movement tachycardia
  c. senilis

CirKuit-Gard
  C. device
  C. pressure relief valve

cirrhosis
  biliary c.
  cardiac c.
  congestive c.
  Laënnec c.
  c. of liver
  stasis c.

cirrhotic

cirsenchysis

cirsodesis

cirsoid
  c. aneurysm
  c. varix

cisterna *pl.* cisternae
  cylindrical confronting cisternae
  perinuclear c.
  subsarcolemmal cisternae
  terminal c.

citrovorum rescue

CK
  creatine kinase

CK-MB
  myocardial muscle creatine kinase isoenzyme

CKG
  cardiokymographic
    CKG test

CL
  chest and left arm
    CL lead

Clagett closure

clamp (see also *clip*)
  Acland microvascular c.
  Ahlquist-Durham embolism c.
  Alfred M. Large vena cava c.
  Allis c.
  anastomosis c.
  angled peripheral vascular c.
  aortic aneurysm c.
  aortic occlusion c.
  appendage c.
  Atlee c.
  Atra-grip c.
  Bahnson aortic c.
  Bailey aortic c.
  Beck aortic c.
  Beck miniature aortic c.
  Beck vascular c.
  Beck-Potts c.
  Beck-Potts aortic c.

clamp *(continued)*
  Beck-Potts pulmonic c.
  Berman aortic c.
  Blalock pulmonary c.
  Blalock-Niedner c.
  Blalock-Niedner pulmonic stenosis c.
  Bradshaw-O'Neill aorta c.
  Brock c.
  bulldog c.
  Bunnell-Howard arthrodesis c.
  Calman carotid artery c.
  Calman ring c.
  cardiovascular c.
  Castaneda anastomosis c.
  Castaneda vascular c.
  celiac c.
  coarctation c.
  Cooley anastomosis c.
  Cooley aortic c.
  Cooley coarctation c.
  Cooley iliac c.
  Cooley partial occlusion c.
  Cooley patent ductus c.
  Cooley pediatric c.
  Cooley renal c.
  Cooley vascular c.
  Cooley vena cava catheter c.
  Cooley-Beck c.
  Cooley-Beck vessel c.
  Cooley-Derra anastomosis c.
  Cooley-Satinsky c.
  Crafoord aortic c.
  Crafoord coarctation c.
  Crile c.
  Crutchfield c.
  curved c.
  Davidson vessel c.
  Davis aneurysm c.
  DeBakey aortic aneurysm c.
  DeBakey arterial c.
  DeBakey bulldog c.
  DeBakey coarctation c.
  DeBakey cross-action bulldog c.

clamp *(continued)*

DeBakey patent ductus c.
DeBakey pediatric c.
DeBakey peripheral vascu-
lar c.
DeBakey ring-handled
bulldog c.
DeBakey tangential occlu-
sion c.
DeBakey vascular c.
DeBakey-Bahnson c.
DeBakey-Bahnson vascu-
lar c.
DeBakey-Bainbridge c.
DeBakey-Beck c.
DeBakey-Derra anastomo-
sis c.
DeBakey-Harken c.
DeBakey-Harken auricle c.
DeBakey-Howard c.
DeBakey-Howard aortic
aneurysmal c.
DeBakey-Kay c.
DeBakey-Kay aortic c.
DeBakey-Reynolds anasto-
mosis c.
DeBakey-Satinsky vena ca-
va c.
DeBakey-Semb c.
DeBakey-Semb ligature-car-
rier c.
DeMartel vascular c.
Demos tibial artery c.
Derra aortic c.
Derra vena caval c.
DeWeese vena cava c.
Diethrich shunt c.
dreamer c.
Edwards c.
exclusion c.
Favaloro proximal anasto-
mosis c.
Fogarty-Chin c.
Fogarty Hydrogrip c.
Garcia aorta c.
Gerbode patent ductus c.
Glassman c.
Glover's c.

clamp *(continued)*

Glover auricular-appenda-
ge c.
Glover coarctation c.
Glover patent ductus c.
Glover vascular c.
Grant abdominal aortic
aneurysmal c.
Grant aneurysm c.
Gregory baby profunda c.
Gregory carotid bulldog c.
Gregory external c.
Gross coarctation occlu-
sion c.
Grover c.
Gutgeman c.
Gutgeman auricular appen-
dage c.
Halsted c.
Harken auricle c.
Hartmann c.
Heifitz c.
hemostatic c.
Hendrin ductus c.
Henley vascular c.
Herbert-Adams c.
Hopkins aortic c.
Hufnagel aortic c.
Hufnagel ascending aor-
tic c.
Hume c.
Humphries aortic c.
Hunter-Satinsky c.
Jacobson microbulldog c.
Jacobson modified ves-
sel c.
Jacobson-Potts c.
Jahnke anastomosis c.
Javid carotid artery c.
Johns Hopkins coarcta-
tion c.
Jones thoracic c.
Juevenelle c.
Kantrowitz thoracic c.
Kapp-Beck c.
Kapp-Beck-Thomson c.
Kartchner carotid artery c.
Kay aorta c.
Kay-Lambert c.

clamp *(continued)*
- Kelly c.
- Kindt carotid artery c.
- Lambert aortic c.
- Lambert-Kay c.
- Lambert-Kay aorta c.
- Lambert-Kay vascular c.
- Lee microvascular c.
- Leland-Jones vascular c.
- Liddle aorta c.
- Mason vascular c.
- Mattox aorta c.
- McDonald c.
- metal c.
- metallic c.
- Michel aortic c.
- microvascular c.
- Mixter right-angle c.
- Morris aorta c.
- mosquito c.
- Muller pediatric c.
- Müller vena caval c.
- mush c.
- myocardial c.
- Nichols c.
- Niedner pediatric c.
- noncrushing vascular c.
- Noon AV fistula c.
- occluding c.
- O'Neill c.
- partial occlusion c.
- partially occluding vascular c.
- patch c.
- patent ductus c.
- Pean c.
- pediatric bulldog c.
- pediatric vascular c.
- Pilling microanastomosis c.
- Poppen c.
- Poppen-Blalock c.
- Poppen-Blalock-Salibi c.
- Potts aortic c.
- Potts coarctation c.
- Potts patent ductus c.
- Potts-Nieder c.
- Potts-Satinsky c.
- Potts-Smith aortic occlusion c.

clamp *(continued)*
- Reich-Nechtow c.
- Reinhoff c.
- Reynolds vascular c.
- right-angle c.
- Rochester-Kocher c.
- Rochester-Péan c.
- Rumel c.
- Rumel myocardial c.
- Rumel thoracic c.
- Salibi carotid artery c.
- Sarnoff aortic c.
- Satinsky c.
- Satinsky aortic c.
- Satinsky vascular c.
- Satinsky vena cava c.
- Schmidt c.
- Schumacher aorta c.
- Schumaker aortic c.
- Schwartz c.
- Sehrt c.
- Selman c.
- Selverstone carotid c.
- Shoemaker c.
- side-biting c.
- sponge c.
- spoon c.
- stainless steel c.
- Stille-Crawford c.
- straight c.
- Subramanian c.
- Swan aortic c.
- Thompson carotid artery c.
- tissue occlusion c.
- Trendelenburg-Crafoord c.
- tubing c.
- VascuClamp minibulldog vessel c.
- VascuClamp vascular c.
- vascular c.
- vessel c.
- voltage c.
- Vorse-Webster c.
- Wangensteen anastomosis c.
- Wangensteen patent ductus c.
- Weber aortic c.
- Wister vascular c.

clamp *(continued)*
    Wylie carotid artery c.
    Yasargil carotid c.

clamshell
    c. device
    c. septal occluder
    c. septal umbrella

clandestine myocardial ischemia

clapotement
    bruit de c.

claquement
    bruit de c.
    c. d'ouverture

Clara cells

Clark
    C. classification of malignant melanoma
    C. expanding mesh catheter
    C. helix catheter
    C. oxygen electrode
    C. rotating cutter catheter

clasmatosis

classic angina

classification
    American Heart Association (AHA) c.
    American Heart Association (AHA) stenosis c.
    antiarrhythmic drug c. (Ia, Ib, Ic, II, III, IV)
    Astler-Coller c.
    Braunwald c. (I–IIIB)
    Canadian Cardiovascular Society c.
    Canadian Heart C. (CHC)
    Cedars-Sinai pump failure c.
    Child c.
    Clark c. of malignant melanoma
    Cohen-Rentrop c.
    congestive heart failure c. (I–IV)

classification *(continued)*
    Croften c.
    DeBakey c.
    de Grott c.
    Dexter-Grossman mitral regurgitation c.
    Diamond c.
    Dukes c.
    Efron jackknife c.
    Fontaine c. system (Roman numerals)
    Forrester Therapeutic C. (grades I–IV)
    Fredrickson c.
    Fredrickson hyperlipoproteinemia c.
    Fredrickson, Levy, and Lees c.
    Hannover c.
    Keith-Wagener-Barker c.
    Killip heart disease c.
    Killip pump failure c.
    Killip-Kimball heart failure c.
    KWB c.
    Lev c.
    Lev complete AV block c.
    Levine-Harvey heart murmur c.
    Loesche c.
    Lown c.
    Lown ventricular arrhythmia c.
    Lown ventricular premature beat c.
    Minnesota EKG c.
    New York Heart Association (NYHA) c.
        NYHA angina classification
        NYHA congestive heart failure classification
    Rentrop c.
    round-robin c.
    Shaher-Puddu c.
    Singh-Vaughan Williams antiarrhythmic drug c.
    TIMI (thrombolysis in myocardial infarction) c.

classification *(continued)*
    TNM c.
    Vaughn Williams antiar-
       rhythmic drugs c.
    Yocoub and Radley-
       Smith c.

Classix pacemaker

claudicant

claudication
    buttock c.
    calf c.
    hip c.
    intermittent c.
    jaw c.
    leg c.
    lifestyle-limiting c.
    lower extremity c.
    non–lifestyle-limiting c.
    one-block c.
    thigh c.
    three-block c.
    two-block c.
    two-flights-of-stairs c.
    venous c.

claudicatory

Clauss assay

clavipectoral triangle

clear
    c. cell
    c. cell carcinoma
    c. cell tumor

clearance
    creatinine c.
    drug c.
    gas c.
    c. technique

Clear Tussin 30

cleavage
    abnormal c. of cardiac
       valve

cleft
    c. anterior leaflet
    cholesterol c.
    c. mitral valve

cleft *(continued)*
    Schmidt-Lanterman c's
    Sondergaard c.

clenched fist sign

click
    aortic c.
    aortic ejection c.
    ejection c's
    Hamman c.
    loud c.
    metallic c's
    midsystolic c.
    mitral c.
    c. murmur
    c.-murmur syndrome
    nonejection systolic c.
    pulmonary ejection c.
    c. syndrome
    systolic c's
    systolic ejection c.
    systolic nonejection c.
    valvular c.

clinometry

clinostatic bradycardia

clip (see also *clamp*)
    Adams-DeWeese vena caval
       serrated c.
    Astro-Trace Universal
       adapter c.
    Atrauclip hemostatic c.
    Autostat ligating and he-
       mostatic c.
    Benjamin-Havas fiberoptic
       light c.
    cardiac retraction c.
    crankshaft c.
    Elgiloy-Heifitz aneurysm c.
    Horizon surgical ligating
       and marking c.
    ligation c.
    microbulldog c.
    Miles vena cava c.
    Moretz c.
    microbulldog c.
    Miles vena cava c.
    Moretz c.

clip *(continued)*
    partial occlusion inferior
        vena cava c.
    Scoville-Lewis c.
    Smith's c.
    Sugar's c.
    vascular c.
    vena cava c.

Clip On torquer

ClipTip reusable sensor

clockwise
    c. rotation
    c. rotation of electrical axis
    c. rotation of electrical axis
        on EKG
    c. torque

closed
    c. chest cardiac massage
    c. chest commissurotomy
    c. chest pneumothorax
    c. chest water-seal drain-
        age
    c.-loop delivery
    c.-loop device
    c. transventricular mitral
        commissurotomy

closing snap

clostridial myocarditis

closure
    Clagett c.
    clamshell c.
    double umbrella c.
    King ASD umbrella c.
    nonoperative c.
    patch c.
    percutaneous patent duc-
        tus arteriosus c.
    primary c.
    secondary c.
    transcatheter c.
    umbrella c.
    valve c.

clot
    agonal c.
    agony c.

clot *(continued)*
    antemortem c.
    autologous c.
    blood c.
    c. of blood
    c.-bound thrombin
    chicken fat c.
    currant jelly c.
    fibrin c.
    c. formation
    laminated c.
    c. lysis
    passive c.
    postmortem c.
    c. retraction time

cloth
    Dacron c.

clots and debris

Clot Stop drain

clotting
    c. abnormality
    c. disorder

clouded sensorium

clouding
    hilar c.
    mental c.

Cloverleaf catheter

Clr deficiency

clubbing
    c. cyanosis
    digital c.
    c. edema
    c. of fingernails
    c. of fingers and toes
    c. of fingertips

cluster-of-grapes appearance

CM3 cocktail

CM_5 lead

CMS AccuProbe 450 system

CO
    carbon monoxide
        CO-oximeter

CO *(continued)*
>CO-oximetry
>CO Sleuth
>cardiac output

CO_2
>carbon dioxide
>CO_2 laser

Co-A reductase

Coag-A-mate coagulometer

coagulation
>disseminated intravascular c. (DIC)
>c. factor
>c. forceps
>c. necrosis
>c. protein
>c. thrombosis
>c. time

coagulative myocytolysis

coagulator
>argon beam c.
>Biceps bipolar c.
>Concept bipolar c.

coagulopathy
>consumption c.
>disseminated intravascular c.

coagulum
>c. formation

coalescence

Coanda effect

coapt

coaptation
>c. of valve leaflets

coarctate

coarctation
>c. of aorta
>c. of aorta, adult type
>c. of aorta, infantile type
>c. of aorta, postductal
>c. of aorta, preductal
>c. of aorta, reversed

coarctation *(continued)*
>aortic c.
>juxtaductal c.
>native c.
>c. of pulmonary artery
>reversed c.

coarctectomy

coarse
>c. murmur
>c. thrill

CoA-set fibrin monomer assay

coat
>external c. of vessels
>extraneous c.
>inner c. of vessels
>middle c. of vessels
>outer c. of vessels

coating
>Pro/Pel c.
>Teflon c.

coaxial pressure

cobalt
>c. cardiomyopathy
>c. in tungsten carbide

cobbler's chest

cobblestoning

Cobe
>C. cardiotomy reservoir
>C. 2991 cell processor
>C. double blood pump
>C. gun
>C. Optima hollow-fiber membrane oxygenator
>C. small vessel cannula
>C. Spectra apheresis system
>C. Stockert heart-lung machine

Cobra
>C. catheter
>C. over-the-wire balloon catheter

cobra-head anastomosis

Cochran test

Cockayne syndrome

Cockett procedure

cocktail
  Brompton c.
  cardiac c.
  CM3 c.
  scintillation c.

code
  C. Blue
  ICHD pacemaker c.
  Minnesota c.
  pacing c.

codominant
  c. coronary circulation
  c. system
  c. vessel

coefficient
  capillary filtration c.
  damping c.
  c. of diffusion
  Pearson correlation c.

coenzyme
  c. A
  c. Q
  c. Q10

COER-24 delivery system

coeur en sabot (on x-ray)

Coe virus

coexistent pathology

Cogan syndrome

Cohen-Rentrop classification

cohort
  c. study

coil
  Cook retrievable emboliza-
    tion c.
  c. electrode
  c. embolization

coil (continued)
  Gianturco wool-tufted
    wire c.
  c. stent
  tantalum balloon-expanda-
    ble stent with helical c.
  c.-tipped catheter

coin
  c. artifact
  c. lesion
  c. percussion
  c. sound
  c. test

coincidence detection

cold
  c. agglutinins
  c. blood cardioplegia
  c. crystalloid cardioplegia
  c. exposure
  c. gangrene
  c. ischemic arrest
  c. nodule
  c. potassium cardioplegia
  c. pressor stimulation
  c. pressor test
  c. pressor test (Hines and
    Brown test)
  c. pressor testing maneu-
    ver

cold-induced angina

coldness of extremity

Cole
  C. polyethylene vein strip-
    per
  C.-Cecil murmur

Colin ambulatory BP monitor

collagen
  bovine biodegradable c.
  c. deposition
  endomysial c.
  c.-impregnated knitted Da-
    cron velour graft
  c. plug
  c. vascular screen (test)

collagenolysis

collapse
    cardiovascular c.
    circulatory c.
    hemodynamic c.
    massive c.
    right ventricular diastolic c.
    c. therapy

collapsed lung

collapsing pulse

collar
    circumaortic venous c.
    c. incision
    c. of Stokes
    c. prosthesis

collateral
    antegrade c.
    aortopulmonary c.
    arcade of c.
    bridging c.
    c. circulation
    filled by c.
    c. filling
    filling via c.
    c. flow
    gives c.
    c. hyperemia
    jump c.'s
    left to left c.
    persistent congenital steno-
      sed c.
    rain of c.'s
    receives c.
    c. respiration
    retrograde c.
    right to left c.
    septal c.
    systemic c.
    venous c.
    c. vessel
    c. vessel filling

collateralization
    distal c.
    ventilation c.

collecting duct

collimation

collimator
    Picker Dyna Mo c.
    Sophy high-resolution c.

Collins bicycle ergometer

colloid osmotic pressure

Collostat hemostatic sponge

coloboma, heart anomaly,
    choanal atresia, retardation,
    and genital and ear anoma-
    lies (CHARGE)

Coloplasty wafer

color
    c.-coded flow mapping
    c. Doppler energy
    c. flow Doppler
    c.-flow mapping
    c. power angiography

Colorscan II

color vascular Doppler ultra-
    sound

ColorZone tape

column
    plasma exchange c.

columna *pl.* columnae
    columnae carneae
    columnae carneae cordis

combination beat

combined heart catheterization

comes *pl.* comites

Comfeel Ulcus dressing

comites (*plural of* comes)

Command PS pacemaker

commissural
    c. bundle
    c. fusion
    c. splitting

commissure
    aortic c.

commissure *(continued)*
    fused c.
    scalloped c.
    valve c.

commissurorrhaphy

commissurotomy
    balloon mitral c.
    Brockenbrough transseptal c.
    closed c.
    closed mitral c.
    closed transventricular mitral c.
    mitral balloon c.
    mitral valve c.
    open mitral c.
    percutaneous catheter c.
    percutaneous mitral balloon c.
    percutaneous transatrial mitral c.
    percutaneous transvenous mitral c.
    transventricular mitral valve c.

committed mode pacemaker

commode
    bedside c.

common
    c. atrium
    c. carotid artery
    c. femoral artery
    c. femoral vein
    c. hepatic artery
    c. iliac artery

Commucor A+V Patient Monitor

communication
    arteriovenous c.
    interarterial c.

communicator
    stripping of multiple c's

communis
    atrioventricularis c.

comp
    comparison

compartment
    c. procedure
    c. syndrome
    vascular c.

compartmentalization

compartmentation

compensated
    c. congestive heart failure
    c. edentulism
    c. shock

compensation
    cardiac c.
    depth c.
    electronic distance c.
    time-gain c.

compensatory
    c. circulation
    c. hypertrophy
    c. mechanism
    c. pause
    c. vessel enlargement

competence
    cardiac c.

competent valve

complement system

complementary balloon angioplasty

complete
    c. atrioventricular block
    c. atrioventricular dissociation
    c. AV block
    c. AV dissociation
    c. blood count
    c. heart block
    c. pacemaker patient testing system
    c. transposition of great arteries

completed myocardial infarction

complex
    aberrant QRS c.
    anisoylated plasminogen streptokinase activator c.
    anomalous c.
    anti-inhibitor coagulant c.
    atrial c.
    atrial premature c.
    atrioventricular (AV) junctional escape c.
    atrioventricular (AV) junctional premature c.
    auricular c.
    Battey-avium c.
    capture c.
    biphasic EKG c.
    diphasic EKG c.
    Eisenmenger's c.
    electrocardiographic wave c. (QRS complex)
    equiphasic c.
    frequent spontaneous premature c.
    fusion c.
    fusion QRS c.
    Ghon c.
    Golgi c.
    HLA-DQ gene c.
    HLA-DR gene c.
    interpolated premature c.
    interpolated ventricular premature c.
    isodiphasic c.
    junctional c.
    junctional premature c.
    LIP/PLH c.
    Lutembacher's c.
    MAI c.
    monophasic c.
    monophasic contour of QRS c.
    multiform premature ventricular c.
    normal-voltage QRS c.
    parasystolic ventricular c.

complex *(continued)*
    plasminogen-streptokinase c.
    pleomorphic premature ventricular c.
    polymorphic premature ventricular c.
    preexcited QRS c.
    premature atrial c. (PAC)
    premature AV junctional c.
    premature ventricular c.
    prothrombinase c.
    pore c.
    QRS c.
    QRS–T c.
    QS c.
    Ranke c.
    R-on-T premature ventricular c.
    RS c.
    Shone c.
    sling ring c.
    slurring of QRS c.
    Steidele c.
    streptokinase-plasminogen c.
    supraventricular c.
    synaptonemal c.
    thrombin-antithrombin III c.
    transposition c.
    triphasic contour of QRS c.
    TU c.
    VATER c.
    ventricular c.
    c. ventricular ectopic activity
    ventricular escape c.
    ventricular premature c.
    wide QRS c.
    widening of QRS c.

complexus
    c. stimulans cordis

compliance
    aortic c.
    c. of heart
    left ventricular chamber c.
    left ventricular muscle c.

compliance *(continued)*
  patient c.
  c., rate, oxygenation, and
    pressure index
  ventricular c.

complicated myocardial infarction

complication
  cardiovascular c.
  groin c's
  c. rate

component
  elastic c.
  harmonic c.
  plasma thromboplastin c.

composite valve graft replacement

compound
  antimony c.
  c. cyst
  glycyl c.
  Hurler-Scheie c.
  nitinol polymeric c.

compressed Ivalon patch graft

compressible volume

compression
  c. boot
  cardiac c.
  chest c.
  FemoStop pneumatic c.
  c. gloves
  intermittent pneumatic c.
  c. stockings
  c. Sigvaris stocking
  c. thrombosis

Compression-Decompression
  Active C.-D.

compressor
  Deschamps c.

compromise
  circulatory c.
  side branch c.
  c. systemic circulatory
  vascular c.

Compton
  C. effect
  C. scatter

Compuscan Hittman computerized electrocardioscanner

computed
  c. tomography
  c. tomography angio-
    graphic portography
  c. tomography scanner

computer
  c.-assisted diagnostics
  CardioData Mark IV c.
  digital c.

computerized axial tomography

Comtesse medical support
  stockings

conal septum

Concato disease

concealed
  c. bypass tract
  c. conduction
  c. entrainment
  c. rhythm

concentration
  c.-effect relation
  intracellular calcium c.
  minimum inhibitory c.
  plasma endothelin c.

concentric
  c. hypertrophic cardiomy-
    opathy
  c. left ventricular hypertro-
    phy
  c. remodeling

Concept
  C. bipolar coagulator

concept
  leading circle c.
  solid angle c.

concordance
  atrioventricular situs c.

concordance *(continued)*
  ventriculoarterial c.

concordant
  c. alternans
  c. alternation

Concord line draw syringe

concretio
  c. cordis
  c. pericardii

concussion
  myocardial c.

conductance
  c. catheter
  c. stroke volume
  c. vessel

conduction
  aberrant c.
  aberrant ventricular c.
  accelerated c.
  accelerated AV node c.
  anisotropic c.
  anomalous c.
  antegrade c.
  anterograde c.
  atrioventricular (AV) c.
  AV nodal c.
  c. block
  cardiac c.
  concealed c.
  concealed retrograde c.
  decremental c.
  c. defect
  c. delay
  delayed c.
  c. disturbance
  forward c.
  His-Purkinje c.
  impulse c.
  infranodal c.
  internodal c.
  intra-atrial c.
  intraventricular c.
  intraventricular c. defect
  orthograde c.
  c. pathway
  c. pattern
  preexcitation c.

conduction *(continued)*
  Purkinje c.
  c. ratio (number of P waves
    to number of QRS)
  retrograde c.
  retrograde VA c.
  sinoventricular c.
  supernormal c.
  supranormal c.
  c. system
  c. time
  c. velocity
  ventricular c.
  ventriculoatrial c.

conductive coupling

conduit
  Rastelli c.

cone
  antipodal c.
  arterial c.
  sarcoplasmic c.

coned-down view

configuration
  atrial sensing c.
  dome-and-dart c.
  doughnut c.
  horseshoe c.
  spadelike c.
  spike-and-dome c.
  ventricular sensing c.

congenita
  myotonia c.

congenital
  c. adrenal hyperplasia
  c. anomaly of mitral valve
  c. aortic aneurysm
  c. aortic stenosis
  c. conotruncal anomaly
  c. heart block
  c. heart disease
  c. heart failure
  c. interrupted aortic arch
  c. malformation
  c. mitral regurgitation
  c. mitral stenosis
  c. murmur

congenital *(continued)*
    c. pulmonary arteriovenous
      fistula
    c. single atrium

congenitale
    P c.

congenitally absent pericardium

congestion
    active c.
    chronic passive c.
    circulatory c.
    functional c.
    hypostatic c.
    neurotonic c.
    passive c.
    physiologic c.
    pulmonary venous c.
    venous c.

congestive
    c. cardiomyopathy
    c. cirrhosis
    c. edema
    c. heart failure
    c. heart failure classifica-
      tion (I–IV)
    c. pulmonary disease

conjoined cusp

connection
    accessory arteriovenous c.
    anomalous pulmonary ve-
      nous c.
    cavopulmonary c.
    Damus-Kaye-Stansel c.
    partial anomalous pulmo-
      nary venous c.
    pulmonary venous c.
    systemic to pulmonary c.
    total anomalous pulmonary
      venous c.
    total cavopulmonary c.
    univentricular atrioventri-
      cular c.

connector
    ACS angioplasty Y c.
    Biotronik lead c.

connector *(continued)*
    Cordis c.
    Luer-Lok c.
    Medtronic c.
    unipolar c.
    Y c.

conotruncal
    congenital c. anomaly

conoventricular fold and
   groove

Conradi line

Conradi-Hünermann syndrome

Conray contrast medium

consanguineous

consanguinity

consent
    written informed c.

constant
    c. coupling
    empiric c.
    Gorlin c.
    Hodgkin-Huxley c.

constriction
    occult pericardial c.

constrictive
    c. endocarditis
    c. heart disease
    c. pericarditis
    c. physiology

consumption
    c. coagulopathy
    myocardial oxygen c.
    peak exercise oxygen c.
    ventilatory oxygen c.

continuity equation

continuous
    c. ambulatory peritoneal
      dialysis
    c. arrhythmia
    c. arteriovenous hemofiltra-
      tion
    c. atrial fibrillation

continuous *(continued)*
    c. cyclical peritoneal dialysis
    c.-flow ventilation
    c. heart murmur
    c. loop exercise echocardiogram
    c. pericardial lavage
    c. venovenous hemofiltration
    c.-wave Doppler
    c.-wave Doppler echocardiogram
    c.-wave Doppler imaging
    c.-wave Doppler ultrasound
    c.-wave laser ablation

contour
    c. of heart
    Murgo pressure c's
    ventricular c.

contracta
    vena c.

contracted heart

contractile
    c. amplitude
    c. behavior
    c. element
    c. function
    c. pattern
    c. protein
    c. work index

contractility
    cardiac c.
    c. index
    isovolumetric c.
    left ventricular c.
    myocardial c.
    ventricular c.

contraction
    anodal closure c.
    anodal opening c.
    atrial premature c.
    atrioventricular (AV) junctional premature c.
    automatic ventricular c.
    c. band
    c. band necrosis

contraction *(continued)*
    cardiac c.
    escaped ventricular c.
    Gowers c.
    isometric c.
    isotonic c.
    isovolumic c.
    isovolumetric c.
    isovolumic c.
    junctional premature c.
    nodal premature c.
    c. pattern
    premature c.
    premature atrial c.
    premature junctional c.
    premature nodal c.
    premature ventricular c.
    R-on-T ventricular premature c.
    supraventricular premature c.
    tertiary c's
    ventricular premature c.
    ventricular segmental c.

contractor
    Bailey rib c.
    Bailey-Gibbon rib c.
    Graham rib c.
    rib c.

contracture
    ischemic c. of left ventricle
    Volkmann c.

contralateral vessel

contrast
    c. agent
    angiographic c.
    c.-enhanced echocardiography
    c. echocardiography
    left atrial spontaneous echo c.
    c. material
    c. medium
    c. medium delivery
    negative c.
    c. ratio
    spontaneous echo c.

contrast *(continued)*
  time-to-peak c.
  c. venography
  c. ventriculography

contrast medium
  Amipaque c. m.
  Angio-Conray c. m.
  Angiocontrast c. m.
  Angiovist 282 c. m.
  Angiovist 292 c. m.
  Angiovist 370 c. m.
  carbonated saline solution
    c. m.
  Conray c. m.
  Conray-30 c. m.
  Conray-43 c. m.
  Conray-400 c. m.
  degassed tap water c. m.
  dextrose 5% in water c. m.
  diatrizoate meglumine c. m.
  diatrizoate sodium c. m.
  Diatrizoate-60 c. m.
  hand-agitated c. m.
  Hexabrix c. m.
  hydrogen peroxide c. m.
  Hypaque Meglumine c. m.
  Hypaque Sodium c. m.
  Hypaque-76 c. m.
  Hypaque-M c. m.
  indocyanine green c. m.
  iohexol c. m.
  iopamidol c. m.
  Iopamiron 310 c. m.
  Iopamiron 370 c. m.
  iothalamate meglumine
    c. m.
  iothalamate sodium c. m.
  ioxaglate meglumine c. m.
  Isovue-300 c. m.
  Isovue-370 c. m.
  Isovue-M 300 c. m.
  mannitol and saline 1:1 so-
    lution c. m.
  MD-60 c. m.
  MD-76 c. m.
  Omnipaque c. m.
  Optiray c. m.
  polygelin colloid c. m.
  Renografin-60; -76 c. m.

contrast medium *(continued)*
  Renovist c. m.
  Renovist II c. m.
  SHU-454 c. m.
  sodium bicarbonate solu-
    tion c. m.
  sodium chloride 0.9% c. m.
  sonicated meglumine so-
    dium c. m.
  sonicated Renografin-76
    c. m.
  sorbitol 70% c. m.
  Thorotrast c. m.
  Ultravist c. m.
  Urografin-76 c. m.
  Vascoray c. m.
  ZK44012 c. m.

control
  axial c.
  damping c.
  feedback c.
  gain c.
  time-gain c.
  time-varied gain c.
  torque c.
  c. wire

controlled ventricular response

ControlWire guidewire

contusion
  cardiac c.
  myocardial c.

conus
  c. artery
  c. arteriosus
  c. cordis
  c. ligament

conventional cineangiography

conversion
  pressure c.
  c. spontaneous

convertin

convexoconcave disk pros-
  thetic valve

cooing
  c. murmur

cooing *(continued)*
    c. sign

Cook
    C. arterial catheter
    C. deflector
    C. flexible biopsy forceps
    C. FlexStent
    C. intracoronary stent
    C. pacemaker
    C. retrievable embolization coil
    C. TPN catheter
    C. yellow pigtail catheter

cookie
    Gelfoam c.

Cooley
    C. anastomosis clamp
    C. aortic clamp
    C. atrial retractor
    C. cardiac tucker
    C. coarctation clamp
    C. Dacron prosthesis
    C. dilator
    C. forceps
    C. iliac clamp
    C. intrapericardial anastomosis
    C. modification of Waterston anastomosis
    C. neonatal instruments
    C. partial occlusion clamp
    C. patent ductus clamp
    C. pediatric clamp
    C. prosthesis
    C. renal clamp
    C. retractor
    C. scissors
    C. sump tube
    C. U suture
    C. valve dilator
    C. vascular clamp
    C. vascular forceps
    C. vena cava clamp
    C. vena cava catheter clamp
    C. Vital microvascular needle holder
    C. woven Dacron graft

Cooley *(continued)*
    C.-Baumgarten aortic forceps
    C.-Beck clamp
    C.-Beck vessel clamp
    C.-Bloodwell-Cutter valve
    C.-Bloodwell mitral valve prosthesis
    C.-Cutter disk prosthetic valve
    C.-Derra anastomosis clamp
    C.-Merz sternum retractor
    C.-Pontius sternal blade
    C.-Satinsky clamp

cooling
    c. blanket
    cardioplegia c.
    core c.
    topical c.

cool-tip laser

Coombs
    C. direct test
    C. indirect test
    C. murmur
    C. test

Coons Super Stiff long tip guidewire

Cooper ligament

Cooperman event probability

coordinate system

COPD
    chronic obstructive pulmonary disease

Cope
    C. biopsy needle
    C. needle introducer cannula

Copeland technique

copper
    c. wire arteries
    c. wire effect
    c.-wiring

cor
- c. adiposum
- c. arteriosum
- c. biloculare
- c. bovinum
- c. dextrum
- c. en cuirasse
- c. hirsutum
- c. juvenum
- c. mobile
- c. pendulum
- c. pseudotriloculare bi-atriatum
- c. pulmonale
- c. pulmonale, acute
- c. pulmonale, chronic
- c. sinistrum
- c. taurinum
- c. tomentosum
- c. triatriatum
- c. triatriatum dexter
- c. triloculare
- c. triloculare biatriatum
- c. triloculare biventriculare
- c. venosum
- c. villosum

coral thrombus

Coratomic
- C. implantable pulse gener-ator
- C. pacemaker
- C. prosethetic valve
- C. R wave inhibited pace-maker

Cordis
- C. Ancar pacing leads
- C. Atricor pacemaker
- C. bioptome
- C. Brite Tip guiding cathe-ter
- C. Chronocor IV pacemaker
- C. connector
- C. Ducor I, II, III catheter
- C. Ducor pigtail catheter
- C. -Ducor-Judkins
- C. Ectocor pacemaker
- C. electrode

Cordis *(continued)*
- C. fixed-rate pacemaker
- C. Gemini cardiac pace-maker
- C. guiding catheter
- C. Hakim pump
- C. -Hakim shunt
- C. high flow pigtail catheter
- C. lead conversion kit
- C. Lumelec catheter
- C. Multicor II pacemaker
- C. Omni Stanicor Theta transvenous pacemaker
- C. pacemaker
- C. pacing lead
- C. Predator balloon cathe-ter
- C. radiopaque tantalum stent
- C. Sentron transducer
- C. Sequicor II pacemaker
- C. sheath
- C. Son-II catheter
- C. Stanicor unipolar ven-tricular pacemaker
- C. Synchrocor pacemaker
- C. Theta Sequicor DDD pulse generator
- C. Titan balloon dilatation catheter
- C. Trakstar PTCA balloon catheter
- C. TransTaper tip catheter
- C. Ventricor pacemaker

cordis
- accretio c.
- adipositas c.
- angina c.
- annuli fibrosi c.
- apex c.
- ataxia c.
- atrium c.
- bulbus c.
- chordae tendineae c.
- chorea c.
- concretio c.
- Conus c.
- crena c.
- delirium c.

cordis *(continued)*
 diastasis c.
 ectasia c.
 ectopia c.
 hypodynamia c.
 ictus c.
 incisura apicis c.
 malum c.
 myasthenia c.
 myofibrosis c.
 myopathia c.
 palpitatio c.
 pulsus c.
 steatosis c.
 trepidatio c.
 tumultus c.

cordy pulse

core
 c. of atheroma
 c. cooling
 c. temperature

Core-Vent implant

Cor-Flex
 C.-F. guidewire
 C.-F. wire guide

corkscrew arteries

Corlon angiocatheter

Cormed
 C. ambulatory infusion
  pump
 C. pump

cornea
 arcus corneae
 arcus lipoides corneae

corneal arcus

Cornelia de Lange syndrome

Cornell
 C. exercise protocol
 C. voltage
 C. voltage-duration product
  criteria

Corometrics
 C.-Aloka echocardiograph
  machine

Corometrics *(continued)*
 C. Doppler scanner

coronal
 c. cuts
 c. plane
 c. slice

coronarism

coronaritis

coronary
 c. anatomy
 c. aneurysm
 c. angiographic catheter
 c. angiography
 c. angioplasty
 c. arterial reserve
 c. arteriography
 c. arteriosclerosis
 c. arteritis
 c. artery
 c. artery anomaly
 c. artery atherosclerosis
 c. artery bypass graft
  (CABG)
 c. artery bypass grafting
  surgery
 c. artery disease
 c. artery dissection
 c. artery dominance
 c. artery ectasia
 c. artery lesion
 c. artery malformation
 c. artery obstruction
 c. artery occlusion
 c. artery probe
 c. artery-right ventricular
  fistula
 c. artery spasm
 c. artery stenosis
 c. artery thrombosis
 c. atherectomy
 c. atheroma
 c. atherosclerosis
 c. bifurcation
 c. blood flow
 c. blood flow, regional
 c. blood flow measurement
 c. blood flow velocity

coronary *(continued)*
  c. bypass graft patency
  c. bypass surgery
  café c.
  c. care unit (CCU)
  c. collateral circulation
  c. cushion
  c. cusp
  c. disease, three-vessel
  c. embolism
  c. endarterectomy
  c. event
  c. failure
  c. flow reserve
  c. flow reserve technique
  c. heart disease
  c. insufficiency
  c. macroangiopathy
  c. microangiopathy
  c. microvascular disease
  c. nodal rhythm
  c. occlusive disease
  c. ostial dimple
  c. ostial stenosis
  c. ostium
  c. perfusion pressure
  c. prognostic index
  c. reflex
  c. resistance vessel
  c. revascularization
  c. ring
  c. roadmapping
  c. rotational ablation
  c. rotational atherectomy
  c. seeking catheter
  c. sclerosis
  c. sinus
  c. sinus blood flow
  c. sinus catheterization
  c. electrogram
  c. sinus retroperfusion
  c. sinus rhythm
  c. sinus thermodilution
  c. spastic angina
  c. steal
  c. steal mechanism
  c. steal phenomenon
  c. steal syndrome
  c. stenosis

coronary *(continued)*
  c. stenting
  c. sulcus
  c. thrombolysis
  c. thrombosis
  c. vascular reserve
  c. vascular resistance
  c. vascular turgor
  c. vasodilation
  c. vasodilator reserve
  c. vasomotion
  c. vasospasm
  c. vein
  c. venous pressure

COROSKOP C cardiac imaging system

COROSKOP Plus cardiac imaging system

corpus
  c. coccygeum

corrected
  c. dextrocardia
  c. sinus node recovery time
  c. transposition of great arteries
  c. transposition of the great vessels

correction
  Bonferroni c.
  Yates c.

Correra line

corridor procedure

Corrigan
  C. disease
  C. pulse
  C. sign

corset balloon catheter

Corvisart
  C. disease
  C. facies

Coryllos
  C. raspatory
  C. retractor

Cosgrove
C. mitral valve replacement
C. retractor

Cosmos
C. pulse generator pace-
maker
C. 238 DDD pacemaker
C. II DDD pacemaker
C. II pulse generator

costarum
arcus c.

costochondral
c. junction
c. syndrome

costochondritis

costoclavicular maneuver

costophrenic
c. angle
c. sulci

costosternal

costotome
Tudor-Edwards c.

costovertebral angle

cotransport

cottage loaf appearance (on
x-ray)

cottonoid patty

cough
aneurysmal c.
decubitus c.
c.-thrill
trigeminal c.

Coulter counter for platelet
count

Coumadin

coumadinization

Coumel tachycardia

count
blood c.

count *(continued)*
complete blood cell c.
(CBC)
differential blood c.
end-diastolic c.
end-systolic c.
first shock c.
needle, sponge, and instrument c.
platelet c.
c. rate
red blood cell c. (RBC)
reticulocyte c.
second through fifth
shock c.
shock c.
total patient shock c.
touch shock c.
white blood cell c. (WBC)

counteroccluder

counterpressor
Acland-Buncke c.

counterpulsation
balloon c.
c. balloon
enhanced c.
intra-aortic balloon (IAB) c.
intra-arterial c.
percutaneous intra-aortic
balloon c. (PIBC)

countershock
electrical c.
unsynchronized c.

countertransport

coupled
c. beats
c. pulse
c. rhythm
c. suturing

couplet
ventricular c.

coupling
arterial c.
conductive c.
constant c.

coupling *(continued)*
    electromechanical c.
    excitation-contraction c.
    fixed c.
    intercellular c.
    c. interval
    variable c.
    ventriculoarterial c.

Cournand
    C. cardiac device
    C. catheter
    C. dip
    C. needle
    C. quadripolar catheter
    C.-Grino angiography needle
    C.-Potts needle

course of the vessel

couvercle

coved ST segments

cove plane

Cover-Strip wound closure strips

coving of ST segments

coxsackievirus

CPI
    Cardiac Pacemakers, Inc.
        CPI Astra pacemaker
        CPI automatic implantable defibrillator
        CPI DDD pacemaker
        CPI endocardial defibrillation/rate-sensing/ pacing lead
        CPI Endotak SQ electrode lead
        CPI Endotak transvenous electrode
        CPI L67 electrode
        CPI Maxilith pacemaker
        CPI Microthin DI, DII lithium-powered programmable pacemaker

CPI *(continued)*
        CPI Minilith pacemaker
        CPI pacemaker
        CPI porous tined-tip bipolar pacing lead
        CPI-PRx pulse generator
        CPI RPx implantable cardioverter-defibrillator
        CPI Sentra endocardial lead
        CPI Sweet Tip lead
        CPI tunneler
        CPI Ultra II pacemaker
        CPI 910 ULTRA II pacemaker
        CPI Ventak AICD device
        CPI Ventak Prx cardioverter-defibrillator
        CPI Vista-T pacemaker

CPK
    creatine phosphokinase

cpm
    counts per minute

CPR
    cardiopulmonary resuscitation
        closed chest CPR
        cough CPR
        simultaneous compression-ventilation CPR

C protein

cps
    cycles per second

CR
    chest and right arm
        CR lead

Craoford
    C. aortic clamp
    C. coarctation clamp
    C. forceps
    C. thoracic scissors
    C. tunneler
    C.-Cooley tucker

Crafoord *(continued)*
    C.-Sellor hemostatic for-
      ceps
    C.-Senning heart-lung ma-
      chine

Cragg
    C. Convertible wire
    C. endoluminal graft
    C. Endopro system
    C. FX wire
    C. infusion wire

Craig test

cramp
    calf c's

Crampton test

cranial
    c. arteritis
    c. and caudal angulations
    c. angulation, anteroposte-
      rior x-ray projection with
    c. view

craniocardiac reflex

crankshaft clip

crash
    c. induction of anesthesia
    c. technique

crassamentum

Crawford
    C. aortic retractor
    C. graft inclusion technique
    C. suture ring
    C. technique for thoraco-
      abdominal aneurysm
    C.-Cooley tunneler

C. R. Bard catheter

crease
    ear lobe c.

creatine kinase (CK)
    CK/AST ratio
    CK isoenzymes
      CK-BB fraction (CK_1)
      CK-MB fraction (CK_s)
      CK-MM fraction (CK_3)

creatine phosphokinase (CPK)
    CPK isoenzymes
      CPK-MB
      CPK-MM
    CPK-BB bands
    CPK, MB positive
    MB enzymes of CPK
    myocardial band enzymes
      of CPK (CPK-MB)

creatinine
    c. clearance

Creech
    C. aortoiliac graft
    manner of C.
    C. technique

creeping thrombosis

crena *pl.* crenae
    c. cordis

crenulated tantalum wire

creola bodies

crescendo
    c. angina
    c.-decrescendo murmur
    c. murmur
    c. sleep

crest
    cardiac neural c.
    infundibuloventricular c.
    mitochondrial c's
    supraventricular c.
    terminal c. of right atrium
    vagal neural c.

CREST syndrome

Cribier
    C. method
    C.-Letac aortic valvulo-
      plasty balloon
    C.-Letac catheter

cri-du-chat syndrome

Crile
    C. clamp
    C. forceps

Crile *(continued)*
  C. hemostat
  C. tip occluder

crimp

crimper

crimping

crinophagy

crisis *pl.* crises
  anaphylactic c.
  cardiac c.
  hypertensive, c.
  myasthenic c.
  sickle cell c.
  thoracic c.

Crisp aneurysm

crisscross
  c. atrioventricular valve
  c. fashion
  c. heart
  c. heart malposition

crista
  cristae mitochondriales
  mitochondrial cristae
  c. supraventricularis
  c. terminalis
  c. terminalis atrii dextri

criterion *pl.* criteria
  Airlie House c.
  Akaike information c.
  Allen-Brown c.
  Billingham c.
  Bogalusa c.
  Casale-Devereux c.
  Cornell voltage-duration
    product c.
  Dallas c.
  Eagle c.
  Estes EKG c.
  exclusion c.
  Gubner-Ungerleider volta-
    ge c.
  Heath-Edwards c.
  Jones c.
  12-lead voltage-duration
    product c.

criterion *(continued)*
  Penn Convention c.
  pseudodisappearance c.
  Ratliff c.
  Rautaharju ECG c.
  Romhilt-Estes point sco-
    re c.
  Sokolow-Lyon voltage c.
  voltage c.
  Wilks lambda c.

critical
  c. care unit (CCU)
  C. Care ventilator
  c. coupling interval
  c. flicker frequency
  c. flicker fusion
  c. rate

Critikon
  C. automated blood pres-
    sure cuff
  C. balloon temporary pac-
    ing catheter
  C. balloon thermodilution
    catheter
  C. balloon-tipped end-hole
    catheter
  C. balloon wedge pressure
    catheter
  C. catheter
  C. guidewire
  C. pressure infuser

crochetage pattern

Crocq disease

Croften classification

Cross
  C.-Jones disk prosthetic
    valve
  C.-Jones Disk valve pros-
    thesis
  C.-Jones mitral valve

cross
  c. femoral-femoral bypass
  yellow c.

cross-clamp
  aortic c.-c.
  c.-c. time

cross-clamped

cross-clamping
    c.-c. of aorta

crossed embolism

CrossFlex LC coronary stent

crossover
    c. bypass
    c. femoral-femoral bypass

cross-pelvic collateral vessel

cross-sectional
    c.-s. area (CSA)
    c.-s. echocardiography
    c.-s. two-dimensional echo-
        cardiogram

crosstalk
    c. pacemaker

crouposa
    angina c.

Crown-Crisp index

Crump vessel dilator

crunch
    Hamman c.
    Means-Lernan mediastin-
        al c.
    mediastinal c.

cruor

cruris
    angina c.

crus pl. crura
    c. dextrum fasciculi atrio-
        ventricularis
    c. fasciculi atrioventricula-
        ris dextrum
    c. fasciculi atrioventricula-
        ris sinistrum
    left c. of atrioventricular
        bundle
    right c. of atrioventricular
        bundle
    c. sinistrum fasciculi atrio-
        ventricularis

crushing chest pain

Cruveilhier
    C. nodes
    C. sign
    C.-Baumgarten murmur
    C.-Baumgarten sign

crux pl. cruces
    c. cordis
    c. dextrum fasciculi atrio-
        ventricularis
    c. of heart
    c. sinistrum fasciculi atrio-
        ventricularis

cryoablation
    c. catheter
    encircling c.
    encircling endocardial c.

cryocardioplegia

cryocrit

Cryo/Cuff pressure boot

Cryo-Cut microtome

cryofrigitronics

CryoLife single step dilution
    method

CryoLife valve graft

cryoprecipitate

cryopreserved
    c. allograft
    c. heart valve allograft
    c. homograft tissue
    c. homograft valve
    c. human allograft conduit
    c. human aortic allograft
    c. vein

cryoprobe
    DATE c.
    ERBE c.
    MST c.
    Spembly c.

cryosurgery
    map-guided c.

CryoVein saphenous vein allograft

crystalloid
    c. cardioplegic solution
    c. fluid
    c. potassium cardioplegia
    c. prime
    c. prime for heart-lung machine

CT
    computed tomography
        high-resolution CT
        thin-section CT
        ultrafast CT scan

cuff
    antimicrobial catheter c.
    aortic c.
    Astropulse c.
    atrial c.
    blood pressure c.
    Critikon automated blood pressure c.
    Dinamap blood pressure c.
    Finapres finger c.
    finger c.
    Fome c.
    c. plethysmography
    pneumatic c.
    right atrial c.
    c. sign
    c. test

culprit
    c. lesion
    c. lesion angioplasty

culture-negative endocarditis

cupping artifact

cuprophane membrane

curette

Curracino-Silverman syndrome

currant
    c. jelly clot
    c. jelly thrombus

current
    alternating c. (AC)
    axial c.
    bioelectric c.
    c. of injury
    c. of injury, diastolic
    c. of injury, systolic
    diastolic c.
    direct c. (DC)
    fast sodium c.
    K c.
    low-energy direct c. (LEDC)
    membrane c.
    pacemaker c.
    pseudoalternating c.
    pump c.
    radiofrequency c. (RFC)
    range-alternating c.
    systolic c.
    toxin-insensitive c.
    transient inward c.
    transsarcolemmal calcium c.

Curry needle

Curschmann spirals

curve
    AA c.
    A_1A_2 c.
    AH c.
    A_2H_2 c.
    arterial dilution c.
    ascorbate dilution c.
    cardiac output c.
    central intra-aortic pressure c.
    dissociation c.
    dye c.
    dye dilution c.
    Frank-Starling c.
    function c.
    hemoglobin-oxygen dissociation c.
    indicator dilution c.
    indicator dye-dilution c.
    intracardiac dye-dilution c.
    intracardiac pressure c.
    J c.

curve (continued)

Kaplan-Meier event-free survival c.

left ventricular inflow velocity c.

left ventricular pressure-volume c.

oxygen dissociation c.

oxyhemoglobin dissociation c.

pulse c.

Starling c.

thermal dilution c.

thermodilution c.

time activity c. (for contrast agent)

Traube c.

V_2A_2 c.

V_1V_2 c.

venous dilution c.

venous return c.

ventricular function c.

volume-time c.

curved J-exchange wire

curvilinear aortotomy

CUSA

Cavitron ultrasonic surgical aspirator

CUSALap device

Cushing

C. forceps

C. needle

C. pressure response

C. reflex

C. rongeur

C. syndrome

C. triad

C. vein retractor

cushion

atrioventricular canal c.

cardiac c.

coronary c.

endocardial c.

intimal c's

cusp

accessory c.

cusp (continued)

anterior c. of mitral valve

anterior c. of pulmonary valve

anterior c. of tricuspid valve

aortic c.

c's of aortic valve

asymmetric closure of c.

c. billowing

commissural c's

conjoined c.

coronary c.

cuspid c.

c. degeneration

dysplastic c.

c. eversion

c. fenestration

fish-mouth c.

fusion of c.

infundibular c. of tricuspid valve

left c. of aortic valve

left c. of pulmonary valve

marginal c. of tricuspid valve

medial c. of tricuspid valve

c. motion

noncoronary c.

posterior c. of aortic valve

posterior c. of mitral valve

posterior c. of tricuspid valve

c's of pulmonary valve

right c. of aortic valve

right c. of pulmonary valve

semilunar c.

semilunar c's of aortic valve

semilunar c's of pulmonary valve

septal c. of tricuspid valve

septal perforation of c.

c. shots films

cuspis pl. cuspides

c. anterior valvae atrioventricularis dextrae

c. anterior valvae atrioventricularis sinistrae

cuspis *(continued)*
c. anterior valvulae bicus-
pidalis
c. anterior valvulae tricuspidalis
cuspides commisurales
c. medialis valvulae tricuspidalis
c. posterior valvae atrioventricularis dextrae
c. posterior valvae atrioventricularis sinistrae
c. posterior valvulae bicus-
pidalis
c. posterior valvulae tricuspidalis
c. septalis valvae atrioventricularis dextrae

cut and cine film

cutdown
arterial c.
brachial artery c.
c. catheter
femoral c.
c. technique
venous c.

Cutinova Hydro dressing

cutis
c. laxa
c. laxa syndrome
c. marmorata

Cutler-Ederer method

Cutter
C. aortic valve prosthesis
C.-SCDK prosthesis
C.-Smeloff aortic valve
prosthesis
C.-Smeloff cardiac valve
prosthesis
C.-Smeloff disk valve
C.-Smeloff heart valve
C.-Smeloff mitral valve
C.-Smeloff prosthesis

cutter
atherectomy c.
Leather valve c.

cutter *(continued)*
wire c.

cutting device

Cuvier
canal of C.
duct of C.

CVA
cerebrovascular accident
posterior circulation
CVA

c-v systolic wave

CV wave of jugular venous
pulse

CVP
central venous pressure
CVP catheter
CVP line

cyanosis
autotoxic c.
central c.
circumoral c.
c., clubbing, or edema
false c.
hereditary methemoglobi-
nemic c.
late c.
mucous membrane c.
c. of nail beds
peripheral c.
pulmonary c.
c. retinae
shunt c.
systemic c.
tardive c.
tardive pulmonary c.

cyanotic
c. heart defect

Cyberlith
C. multiprogrammable
pulse generator
C. pacemaker

Cybertach
C. 60 bipolar pacemaker
C. automatic-burst atrial
pacemaker

Cybex isokinetic dynamometer

cycle
- asexual c.
- cardiac c.
- cell c.
- circannual c.
- circaseptan c.
- citrate-pyruvate c.
- c.-ergometer
- forced c.
- isometric period of cardiac c.
- Krebs c.
- c. length
- c. length alternans
- c. length alternation
- length of atrial c.
- length of ventricular c.
- c. length window
- c's per second (cps)
- RR c.
- restored c.
- returning c.
- short-long-short c.
- sinus length c.
- Wenckebach c.

cycloergometer
- Mijnhard electrical c.

cyclosis

cylindroid aneurysm

Cynosar catheter

Cyriax syndrome

cyst
- aneurysmal bone c.
- apoplectic c.
- hemorrhagic c.
- locular c.
- loculated c.
- multilocular c.
- pericardial c.
- springwater c.
- Tornwaldt c.
- true c.
- unilocular c.

cytaster

cytobiology

cytocentrum

cytochalasin
- c. B

cytochemism

cytochemistry

cytochylema

cytocidal

cytocide

cytocinesis

cytoclasis

cytoclastic

cytode

cytodieresis

cytofluorimeter

cytogenesis

cytogenic

cytogenous

cytogeny

cytohistogenesis

cytohormone

cytohyaloplasm

cytokinesis

cytologic

cytologist

cytology

cytolymph

cytolysate

cytolysis

cytolysosome

cytolytic

cytomegalovirus

cytometaplasia

cytomitome

cytomorphology

cytomorphosis

cytopathic

cytopathogenesis

cytopathogenetic

cytopathogenic

cytopathogenicity

cytopathologic, cytopathological

cytopathologist

cytopathology

cytophotometer

cytophotometric

cytophotometry

cytophylactic

cytophylaxis

cytophyletic

cytophysics

cytophysiology

cytopigment

cytopipette

cytoplasm

cytoplasmic

cytoplast

cytoreticulum

cytoscopy

cytosiderin

cytoskeletal

cytoskeleton

cytosol

cytosolic

cytosome

cytospongium

cytost

cytostatic

cytostromatic

cytotactic

cytotaxigen

cytotaxin

cytotaxis

cytothesis

cytotoxic

cytotoxicity

cytotropic

cytotropism

D
  D to E amplitude
  D to E slope
  D gate
  D loop
  D point
  D sleep
  D wave
  D1 (diagonal branch #1)
  D_5W
  D5W
  D-5-W

2-D
  two-dimensional
    2-D echocardiogram
    2-D echocardiography
    2-D TEE system Ultra-
      Neb 99

Daae disease

DaCosta syndrome

Dacron
  D. catheter
  D. cloth
  D. conduit
  D. graft
  D. intracardiac patch
  D. mesh
  D. onlay patch-graft
  D. pledget
  D. preclotted tightly woven
    graft
  D. prosthesis
  D. Sauvage graft
  D. Sauvage patch
  D. stent
  D. suture
  D. tape
  D. tube graft

dagger-shaped aortic envelope

DAH
  disordered action of heart

Daig ESI-II

d'airain
  bruit d.

Dale forceps

Dakin
  D. biograft
  D. solution

Dallas
  D. Classification System
  D. criteria

dalton

dam
  left ventricular d.

D'Amato sign

Damian graft procedure

damped

damping
  Accudynamic adjustable d.
  catheter d.
  d. coefficient
  d. control

Damus
  D.-Kaye-Stansel connection
  D.-Kaye-Stansel operation
  D.-Kaye-Stansel procedure
  D.-Stansel-Kaye procedure

dance
  brachial d.
  hilar d.
  hilus d.
  St. Vitus d.

Dandy arterial forceps

Dane particles

Danielson method

Dardik Biograft

darkfield microscopy

Darling disease

Darox cutaneous thoracic patch
  electrode

Dart pacemaker

DASH diet
    dietary approach to pre-
    vent hypertension diet

Dash single-chamber rate-adap-
    tive pacemaker

DASI
    Duke Activity Status Index

Datascope
    D. balloon
    D. DL-II percutaneous
    translucent balloon cathe-
    ter
    D. intra-aortic balloon
    pump
    D. System 90 intra-aortic
    balloon pump
    D. System 90 balloon pump

DataVue calibrated reference
    circle

DATE cryoprobe

Datex ETCO$_2$ multigas analyzer

daughter

DaunoXome

Davidson
    D. pneumothorax appa-
    ratus
    D. protocol exercise test
    D. retractor
    D. scapular retractor
    D. thoracic trocar
    D. vessel clamp

Davies
    D. disease
    D. endomyocardial fibrosis
    D. myocardial fibrosis

Davis
    D. aneurysm clip
    D. bronchoscope
    D. clamp
    D. forceps
    D. rib spreader
    D. sign

Davol pacemaker introducer

DBP
    diastolic blood pressure

DBPC
    dual balloon perfusion
    catheter

DC
    direct current
        DC cardioversion
        DC defibrillator
        DC electrical shock
    dual-chamber

DCA
    directional coronary ather-
    ectomy

DCFM
    Doppler color flow map-
    ping

DCI-S automated coronary anal-
    ysis system

DCM
    dilated cardiomyopathy

DCS (distal coronary sinus)

DDAVP
    desmopressin acetate
        DDAVP injection
        DDAVP Nasal

ddC
    zalcitabine

dD/dt (derived value on apex
    cardiogram)

DDD
    dual-mode, dual-pacing,
    dual-sensing
        DDD mode
        DDD pacing
        DDD pacemaker

DDDR pacing

DD genotype

ddI
    didanosine

D-dimer

DDI
    DDI mode pacemaker
    DDI pacing

DDIR pacing

DDS
    dapsone

DE
    dobutamine echocardiography

dead
    d. space:tidal volume ratio
    d. time

de-aired
    d. graft

de-airing
    d. maneuver
    d. procedure

D-E amplitude of mitral valve

Deane tube

dearterialization
    hepatic d.

death
    aborted sudden cardiac d.
    activation-induced cell d.
    apoptotic cell d.
    brain d.
    cardiac d.
    cell d.
    ischemic sudden d.
    late d.
    programmed cell d.
    sudden d.
    sudden cardiac d. (SCD)
    voodoo d.

Deaver retractor

DeBakey
    D. aortic aneurysm clamp
    D. arterial clamp
    D. arterial forceps
    D. Autraugrip forceps
    D. ball valve prosthesis
    D. blade

DeBakey *(continued)*
    D. bulldog clamp
    D. chest retractor
    D. classification
    D. clamp
    D. coarctation clamp
    D. cross-action bulldog
        clamp
    D. dissecting forceps
    D. endarterectomy scissors
    D. graft
    D. heart pump oyxgenator
    D. patent ductus clamp
    D. pediatric clamp
    D. peripheral vascular
        clamp
    D. rib spreader
    D. ring-handled bulldog
        clamp
    D. tangential occlusion
        clamp
    D. technique for thoracoabdominal aneurysm
    D. tissue forceps
    D. tunneler
    D.-type aortic dissection
    D. valve scissors
    D. vascular clamp; forceps
    D. Vasculour-II vascular
        prosthesis
    D. Vital needle holder
    D.-Bahnson forceps
    D.-Bahnson vascular clamp
    D.-Bainbridge clamp
    D.-Bainbridge forceps
    D.-Balfour retractor
    D.-Beck clamp
    D.-Colovira-Rumel thoracic
        forceps
    D.-Cooley cardiovascular
        forceps
    D.-Cooley Deaver-type retractor
    D.-Cooley dilator,
    D.-Cooley forceps,
    D.-Cooley retractor
    D.-Cooley valve dilator
    D.-Crafoord vascular clamp
    D.-Creech aneurysm repair

DeBakey *(continued)*
    D.-Creech manner
    D.-Derra anastomosis
      clamp
    D.-Derra anatomosis for-
      ceps
    D.- Diethrich coronary ar-
      tery forceps
    D.- Diethrich vascular for-
      ceps
    D.-Harken auricular clamp
    D.-Howard aortic aneurys-
      mal clamp
    D.-Kay aortic clamp
    D.-Kelly hemostatic forceps
    D.-McQuigg-Mixter bron-
      chial clamp
    D.-Metzenbaum scissors,
    D.-Mixter thoracic forceps
    D.-Péan cardiovascular for-
      ceps
    D.-Potts scissors
    D.-Rankin hemostatic for-
      ceps
    D.-Reynolds anastomosis
      forceps
    D.-Satinsky vena cava
      clamp
    D.-Semb forceps
    D.-Semb ligature-carrier
      clamp
    D.-Surgitool prosthetic
      valve
debilis
    pulsus d.
Debove
    D. membrane
    D. treatment
debris
    atheromatous d.
    calcific d.
    calcium d.
    gelatinous d.
    grumous d.
    pultaceous d.
    valve d.
debt
    oxygen d.

debubbling procedure

debulking
    pre-stent d.
    plaque d.
    d. procedure

decannulated

decannulation

decapolar
    d. electrode catheter
    d. pacing catheter

decay
    pressure d.

deceleration
    early d.
    late d.
    d. time
    variable d.

decerebrate posturing

declamping
    d. shock
    d. shock syndrome

decollement

decompensate

decompensated congestive
    heart failure

decompensated shock

decompensation
    cardiac d.
    hemodynamic d.

decompress

decompression
    cardiac d.
    d. of heart
    d. of pericardium
    d. of ventricle
    d. sickness

deconditioning

decortication
    arterial d.

decortication *(continued)*
    d. of heart

decreased
    d. breath sounds
    d. respiration

decrement

decremental
    d. atrial pacing
    d. conduction
    d. element

decrescendo murmur

decrudescence

decrudescent arteriosclerosis

decubitus
    Andral d.
    d. angina
    angina pectoris d.
    d. cough
    d. ulcer

Dedo
    D.-Jako microlaryngoscope
    D.-Pilling laryngoscope

deductive echocardiography

de-endothelialization

de-energization
    myocyte d.

deep
    d. chest therapy
    d. Doppler velocity interrogation
    d. hypothermia circulatory arrest (DHCA)
    d. sleep
    d. tendon reflex (DTR)
    d. venous insufficiency (DVI)
    d. venous thrombosis (DVT)

de-epicardialization

deer-antler vascular pattern

Defares rebreathing method

defecation syncope

defect
    acquired ventricular septal (AVSD) d.
    aortic septal d.
    aorticopulmonary septal d.
    atrial ostium primum d.
    atrial septal d. (ASD)
    atrioseptal d.
    atrioventricular canal d.
    atrioventricular conduction d.
    atrioventricular septal d.
    A-V conduction d.
    clamshell closure of atrial septal d.
    conduction d.
    contiguous ventricular septal d.
    cyanotic heart d.
    endocardial cushion d. (ECD)
    extrafusion d.
    filling d.
    fixed perfusion d.
    Gerbode d.
    humoral immune d.
    iatrogenic atrial septal d.
    inferoapical d.
    infundibular septal d.
    infundibular ventricular septal d.
    interatrial septum d.
    interventricular conduction d.
    interventricular septal (IVSD) d.
    intra-atrial conduction d.
    intraluminal filling d.
    intraventricular conduction d.
    linear d.
    lucent d.
    luminal d.
    match d.
    membranous ventricular septal d.

defect *(continued)*
> muscular ventricular septal d.
> napkin-ring d.
> nonuniform rotational d.
> obstructive ventilatory d.
> ostium primum d.
> ostium secundum d.
> panconduction d.
> partial AV canal d.
> perfusion d.
> peri-infarction conduction (PICD) d.
> perimembranous ventricular septal d.
> postinfarction ventriculoseptal d.
> primum atrial septal d.
> reversible ischemic d.
> reversible ischemic neurologic d. (RIND)
> reversible perfusion d.
> scintigraphic perfusion d.
> secundum and sinus venosus d.
> secundum atrial septal d.
> secundum-type atrial septal d.
> septal d.
> sinus venosus atrial septal d.
> supracristal ventriculoseptal d.
> Swiss cheese d.
> T cell d.
> transcatheter closure of atrial transient perfusion d.
> transient perfusion d.
> ventilation/perfusion d.
> ventricular septal d. (VSD)
> ventriculoseptal d. (VSD)

defervescence

defibrillate

defibrillated

defibrillation
> Antiarrhythmics versus Implantable Defibrillation

defibrillation *(continued)*
> cardiac d.
> d. paddles
> d. patch
> d. shock
> d. single pulse
> d. threshold

defibrillator
> AICD-B cardioverter-d.
> AICD-BR cardioverter-d.
> AID-B d.
> automatic external d. (AED)
> automatic implantable d. (AID)
> automatic implantable cardioverter-d. (AICD)
> automatic internal d.
> automatic internal cardioverter d. (AICD)
> automatic intracardiac d.
> Birtcher d.
> Cadence implantable cardioverter-d.
> Cadet V-115 implantable cardioverter-d.
> Cambridge d.
> Cardioserv d.
> cardioverter-d.
> CPI automatic implantable d.
> CPI PRX implantable cardioverter-d.
> CPI Ventak PRX cardioverter-d.
> DC (direct current) d.
> Endotak nonthoracotomy implantable cardioverter-d.
> external d.
> external cardioverter-d. (ECD)
> Guardian ATP 4210 implantable cardioverter-d.
> Heart Aid 80 d.
> Hewlett-Packard d.
> d. implant
> implantable cardioverter-d. (ICD)

defibrillator *(continued)*
    Intec implantable d.
    Intermedics RES-Q implantable cardioverter-d.
    IPCO-Partridge d.
    Jewel pacer-cardioverter-d.
    Lifepak d.
    LT V-105 implantable cardioverter-d.
    Marquette Responder 1500 multifunctional d.
    Medtronic external cardioverter-d.
    Medtronic PCD implantable cardioverter-d.
    nonthoracotomy lead implantable cardioverter-d.
    ODAM-d.
    pacer-cardioverter-d.
    d. paddles
    programmable cardioverter-d. (PCD)
    Res-Q ACD implantable cardioverter-d.
    Siemens Siecure implantable cardioverter-d.
    smart d.
    subpectoral implantation of cardioverter-d.
    Telectronics ATP implantable cardioverter-d.
    Transvene nonthoracotomy implantable cardioverter-d.
    d. unit
    Ventak d.
    Ventritex Cadence implantable cardioverter-d.
    Zoll PD1200 external d.

deficiency
    acetylcholinesterase d.
    acid maltase d.
    ADA d.
    adenosine deaminase d.
    alpha-1 antitrypsin d.
    Apo A-1 d.
    Clr d.
    cystathionine synthase d.

deficiency *(continued)*
    dopamine beta-hydroxylase d.
    enzymatic d.
    Factor III d.
    Factor VIII d.
    Factor IX d.
    Factor X d.
    fibrinogen d.
    galactosidase d.
    glucosidase d.
    hexosaminidase d.
    homogentisic acid oxidase d.
    HRF d.
    hydroxylase d.
    17-hydroxylase d.
    17-hydroxylase d. syndrome
    magnesium d.
    maltase d.
    nutritional d.
    Owren factor V d.
    protein-calorie d.
    protein S d.
    selenium d.
    surfactant d.
    thiamin d.
    vasopressor d.
    vitamin B-12 d.

deficit
    oxygen d.
    pulse d.
    peripheral pulse d.
    reversible intermittent or ischemic neurologic d. (RIND)
    transient neurological d.
    visual field d.

definition
    Lagrangian d.

deflated profile

deflectable quadripolar catheter

deflection
    delta d.
    H d.

deflection *(continued)*
   His bundle d.
   intrinsic d.
   intrinsicoid d.
   Q–S d.
   RS d.

deflector
   Cook d.

deformans
   arteritis d.
   endarteritis d.

deformity
   buttonhole d.
   cervical spine d.
   gooseneck d.
   gooseneck outflow tract d.
   hockey-stick d.
   hockey-stick tricuspid
     valve d.
   joint d.
   parachute d. of mitral valve
   parachute-type d.
   pigeon-breast d.
   rolled edge d.
   shepherd's crook d.

degeneration
   atheromatous d.
   ballooning d.
   cardiomyopathic d.
   cusp d.
   fibrinoid d.
   glassy d.
   hydropic d.
   Mönckeberg's d.
   mucoid medial d.
   myocardial cellular d.
   myofibrillar d.
   myxomatous d.
   Quain fatty d.
   spinocerebellar d.

DeGimard syndrome

deglutition
   d. apnea
   d. mechanism
   d. murmur
   d. pneumonia
   d. syncope

Degos disease

degranulation
   goblet d.

degrees of heart block

Dehio test

dehisced

dehiscence
   annular d.
   bronchial d.
   sternal d.

dehydrogenase
   alpha-hydroxybutyrate d.
   branched chain alpha ke-
     toacid d.
   glucose-6-phosphate d.
     (G6PD)
   hydroxybutyrate d.
   lactate d.
   lactic d.
   lactic acid d.
   pyruvate d.

Deklene suture

DeKock two-way bronchial
  catheter

Delaborde tracheal dilator

de Lange syndrome

delay
   conduction d.
   intraventricular conduc-
     tion d.

delayed
   d. afterdepolarization
   d. conduction

Delbet sign

deletion
   22q11 d.

delimitation

delirium
   d. cordis
   postcardiotomy d.

delirium *(continued)*
 toxic d.

delivery
 closed-loop d.
 contrast medium d.
 oxygen d.
 d. wire

Del Mar Avionics
 D. M. A. Scanner
 D. M. A. three-channel re-
  corder

Delmege sign

Delorme thoracoplasty

Delphian node

Delrin
 D. frame of valve prosthe-
  sis
 D. frame of valve prosthe-
  sis, Dacron-covered
 D. heart valve

Delta
 D. pacemaker
 D. TRS pacemaker

delta
 d. deflection
 d. wave

DeltaTrac II metabolic monitor

deltopectoral groove

Deltran disposable transducer

delux
 Ohio d.

demand
 myocardial oxygen d.
 d. mode of pacemaker
 d. pacemaker
 d. pacemaker battery
 d. pulse generator
 d. pulse generator unit

Demarquay sign

DeMartel
 D. scissors

DeMartel *(continued)*
 D. vascular clamp
 D.-Wolfson anastomosis
  clamp

dementia
 multi-infarct d.

Demos tibial artery clamp

de Musset sign

denatured homograft

dendritic lesion

denervated

dengue fever

Denhardt solution

denivelation

dense
 d. hemiplegia
 d. thrill

densitogram
 ear d.

densitometry
 video d.

density
 echo d.
 hydrogen d.
 proton d.
 spin d.

density-exposure relationship
 of film

Denucath

denucleated

denudation
 endothelial d.

denude

denuding

Denver
 D. Pak
 D. pleuroperitoneal shunt

deoxygenated

2-deoxyglucose
F-18 2-d. (FDG)

deoxyribonuclease
human recombinant d.

deoxyribonucleic acid (DNA)

dependence
use d.

dependency
ventilator d.

dependent
d. beat
d. edema
d. rubor

deplasmolysis

deplasmolyze

depletion
glycogen d.
volume d.

deployment
stent d.

depolarization
alternating, failure of response, mechanical, to
electrical d. (AFORMED)
atrial d.
atrial premature d.
cardiac d.
diastolic d.
His bundle d.
His bundle–distal coronary
sinus atrial d. (H-DCSA)
His bundle–middle coro-
nary sinus atrial d. (H-
MCSA)
myocardial d.
rapid d.
transient d.
ventricular d.
ventricular premature d.
(VPD)

depolarize

deposition
calcium oxalate d.
collagen d.
mitochondrial calcium d.

depressant
cardiac d.
myocardial d. factor

depressed
d. blood count
d. chest wall
d. level of consciousness,
d. reflexes
d. sternum
d. systolic pressure

depression
aldosterone d.
downhill ST segment d.
downsloping ST segment d.
horizontal ST segment d.
junctional d.
marked ST segment d.
myocardial d.
postdrive d.
P-Q segment d.
reciprocal d.
reciprocal ST d.
ST segment d.
systolic d.
ventricular d.
x d.

depressor
d. reflex

deprivation
sleep d.

Depthalon

depth compensation

de Quervain thyroiditis

Dermalene suture

Dermalon suture

dermatomyositis

dermatosome

derivative
    d. circulation
    ergotamine d's
    hematoporphyrin d. (HPD)
    purified protein d. (PPD)

dermatitis *p.l* dermatitides
    exfoliative d.
    livedoid d.
    stasis d.
    weeping d.

dermatomyositis

dermonecrotic

Derra
    D. aortic clamp
    D. commissurotomy knife
    D. knife
    D. valve dilator
    D. vena cava clamp

desaturation

Desault ligation

descendens
    aorta d.

descending
    d. aorta
    d. necrotizing mediastinitis
        (DNM)
    d. thoracic aneurysm
    d. thoracic aortofemoral-
        femoral bypass

descent
    rapid y d.
    x d.
    y d.

Deschamps compressor

Deseret
    D. angiocatheter
    D. catheter
    D. flow-directed thermodi-
        lution catheter
    D. sump drain

desert fever

desiccation
    mucous d.

designed after natural anatomy

Desilets
    D. introducer
    D. introducer system
    D.-Hoffman catheter intro-
        ducer
    D.-Hoffman sheath

D to E slope on echocardiogra-
    phy

Desnos
    D. disease
    D. pneumonia

d'Espine sign

desquamation
    peribronchial d.

desquamative
    d. alveolitis
    d. interstitial pneumonia
        (DIP)
    d. interstitial pneumonitis
        (DIP)

destruction
    plasmatic vascular d.

desulfatohirudin
    recombinant d.

desynchronized sleep

detection
    automated border d. (ABD)
    automated edge d.
    automatic boundary d.
        (ABD)
    coincidence d.
    echocardiographic auto-
        mated border d.
    edge d.
    manual edge d.
    shunt d.
    single-photon d.

detective quantum efficiency

detector
    ambulatory nuclear d.
    Doppler blood flow d.
    TubeChek esophageal intu-
        bation d.
    VEST ambulatory nu-
        clear d.
    VEST left ventricular func-
        tion d.

detect time

detergent worker's lung

Determann syndrome

determination
    metabolic parameter d.

Detsky
    D. modified risk index
    D. score

deuterosome

devasation
    senile cortical d.

devascularization

DeVega
    D. prosthesis
    D. tricuspid valve annulo-
        plasty

Devereaux-Reichek method

deviation
    abnormal left axis d.
    abnormal right axis d.
    axis d.
    left axis d. (LAD)
    d. on EKG
    right axis d. (RAD)
    standard d.
    ST–T d.
    tracheal d.

device
    abdominal aortic counter-
        pulsation d.
    abdominal left ventricular
        assist d.
    Abiomed Cardiac d.

device (continued)
    ablative d.
    Ablatr temperature con-
        trol d.
    Accutracker blood pres-
        sure d.
    acute ventricular assist d.
    Adams-DeWeese d.
    Aerochamber spacing d.
    AICD plus Tachylog d.
    A-mode echo-tracking d.
    Ancure system d.
    Ange-Med Sentinel ICD d.
    Angio-Seal hemostatic
        puncture closure d.
    arrhythmia control d.
        (ACD)
    Arrow-Clarke thoracentes-
        is d.
    ATL Ultramark 7 echocardi-
        ographic d.
    atrial septal defect single
        disk closure d.
    Baim-Turi cardiac d.
    battery-assisted heart as-
        sist d.
    bioabsorbable closure d.
    BIVAD centrifugal left and
        right ventricular assist d.
    biventricular assist d.
    Block cardiac d.
    bovine collage plug d.
    Brockenbrough cardiac d.
    buttoned d.
    BVM d.
    cage catheter d.
    CarboMedics valve d.
    cardiac automatic resusci-
        tative d.
    Cardiomemo d.
    Cath-Lok catheter lock-
        ing d.
    Champ cardiac d.
    Chemo-Port perivena cath-
        eter system d.
    CirKuit-Gard d.
    clamshell d.
    closed-loop d.
    Cournand cardiac d.

device *(continued)*
  CPI Ventak AICD d.
  CUSALap d.
  cutting d.
  CVIS imaging d.
  DIASYS Novacor cardiac d.
  Digiflator digital inflation d.
  Dinamap automated blood
    pressure d.
  directional atherectomy d.
  displacement sensing d.
  Doppler d.
  double-umbrella d.
  Durathane cardiac d.
  Elecath circulatory sup-
    port d.
  El Gamal cardiac d.
  Emergency Infusion D.
  Encore inflation d.
  Endo Grasp d.
  esophageal detection d.
  extraction atherectomy d.
  FemoStop inflatable pneu-
    matic compression d.
  fiberoptic delivery d.
  Finesse cardiac d.
  Flutter therapeutic d.
  Gensini cardiac d.
  Goetz cardiac d.
  Goodale-Lubin cardiac d.
  GRIP torque d.
  HeartMate implantable ven-
    tricular assist d.
  hemostatic occlusive lever-
    age d.
  hemostatic puncture clo-
    sure d.
  Hershey left ventricular as-
    sist d.
  Hi-Per cardiac d.
  HSRA d.
  ICD-ATP d.
  Ideal cardiac d.
  IMED infusion d.
  In-Exsufflator respiratory d.
  InspirEase d.
  Insuflon d.
  intra-aortic balloon d.
  intracaval d.

device *(continued)*
  Kendall Sequential Com-
    pression d.
  King cardiac d.
  left ventricular assist d.
    (LVAD)
  Lehman cardiac d.
  Light Talker d.
  Linx-EZ cardiac d.
  Linx guidewire extension
    cardiac d.
  locking d.
  Mediflex-Bookler d.
  MediPort implantable vas-
    cular access d.
  Novacor left ventricular as-
    sist d.
  Perclose d.
  Personal Heart D. (PHD)
  PerDUCER d.
  PET balloon atherecto-
    my d.
  pulsatile assist d.
  right ventricular assist d.
    (RVAD)
  rotational atherectomy d.
  Symbion pneumatic as-
    sist d.
  Thoratec BVAD (biventri-
    cular assist d.) d.
  Thoratec RVAD (right ven-
    tricular assist) d.
  Thoratec ventricular as-
    sist d.
  ventricular assist d. (VAD)
  Williams cardiac d.
  Wizard cardiac d.
  Wizard disposable infla-
    tion d.
  Wolvek fixation d.
  Zucker-Myler cardiac d.
Devices, Ltd. pacemaker
devil's grip
devitalized tissue
DeWeese
  D. caval catheter
  D. vena cava clamp

Dew sign

dexiocardia

Dexon suture

dexter
  bronchus principalis d.

Dexter-Grossman classification
  of mitral regurgitation

dextran
  high molecular weight d.
  low molecular weight d.

Dextran 40:75

dextrocardia
  corrected d.
  false d.
  isolated d.
  mirror-image d.
  secondary d.
  type 1 d.
  type 2 d.
  type 3 d.
  type 4 d.
  d. with situs inversus

dextrocardiogram

dextrogastria

dextrogram

dextroisomer

dextroisomerism

dextroposition
  d. of heart

dextrorotation

dextrorotatory

dextrotransposition (D-transposition)
  d. of great arteries

dextroversion
  d. of heart

dextrum
  atrium d.

dextrum (continued)
  cor d.

DFA
  direct fluorescent antibody

D/Flex
  D. filter

DFP
  diastolic filling pressure

DFT
  defibrillation threshold

2DFT
  two-dimensional Fourier
    transform

3DFT
  three-dimensional Fourier
    transform
    3DFT magnetic reso-
      nance angiograph

DHCA
  deep hypothermia circula-
    tory arrest

Diabetes Mellitus Insulin Glucose Infusion in Acute Myocardial Infarction (DIGAMI)

diabetic
  d. cardiomyopathy
  d. coma
  d. diet
  d. gangrene
  d. nephropathy
  d. neuropathy
  d. phthisis
  d. retinopathy
  d. ulcer

diabeticorum
  necrobiosis lipoidica d.

diable
  bruit de d.

diacylglycerate pathway

diacylglycerol
  d. lipase

diagnostic
  d. ST segment changes

diagnostic *(continued)*
    d. ultrasound imaging catheter

diagnostics
    computer-assisted d.

diagonal
    d. artery
    d. branch

diagram
    Dieuaide d.
    ladder d.
    pressure-volume d.
    vector d.
    Wiggers d.

diakinesis

Dialog pacemaker

dialysis
    continuous ambulatory peritoneal d. (CAPD)
    continuous cyclical peritoneal d. (CCPD)
    peritoneal d.
    renal d.

diameter
    anteroposterior thoracic d.
    aortic d.
    aortic root d.
    artery d.
    internal d.
    left anterior internal d. (LAID)
    left ventricular internal d.
    left ventricular internal diastolic d.
    luminal d.
    minimal luminal d.
    right ventricular internal d. (RVID)
    stenosis d.
    stretched d.
    total end-diastolic d.
    total end-systolic d.
    transverse cardiac valve d.

Diamond
    D. classification

Diamond *(continued)*
    D.-Forrester table
    D.-Lite titanium instruments

diamond
    d.-coated bur
    d. ejection murmur
    d.-shaped murmur
    d.-shaped tracing

diaphoresis

diaphoretic

diaphragm
    dome of d.
    eventration of d.
    d. of stethoscope
    d. pacing system
    d. phenomenon
    d. transducer

diaphragmalgia

diaphragmatic
    d. artery
    d. flutter
    d. hernia
    d. myocardial infarction
    d. pacing
    d. pericardium
    d. phenomenon
    d. pleurisy
    d. respiration

diary
    event d.
    Holter d.

Diasonics
    D. Cardiovue 3400
    D. Cardiovue 6400
    D. Cardiovue SectOR scanner
    D. catheter
    D. transducer

Diasonics/Sonotron Vingmed CFM 800 imaging system

diastasis cordis

diastatic

Diastat vascular access graft

diastem

diastema

diaster

diastole
  atrial d.
  cardiac d.
  early d.
  electrical d.
  late d.
  ventricular d.

diastolic
  d. afterpotential
  d. blood pressure (DBP)
  d. blow
  d. closing velocity
  d. current
  d. current of injury
  d. depolarization
  d. doming
  d. dysfunction
  d. filling
  d. filling period
  d. filling pressure (DFP)
  d. fluttering
  d. fluttering aortic valve
  d. function
  d. gallop
  d. gradient
  d. grunt
  d. heart disease
  d. heart failure
  d. hump
  d. hypertension
  d. motion
  d. murmur
  d. overload
  d. pressure-time index
  d. regurgitant velocity
  d. relaxation
  d. reserve
  d. rumble
  d. shock
  d. stiffness
  d. suction
  d. thrill
  d. upstroke

DIASYS Novacor cardiac device

DiaTAP vascular access button

diathermy

diathesis *pl.* diatheses
  allergic d.
  bleeding d.
  hemorrhagic d.

diatrizoate
  d. meglumine contrast medium
  d. sodium contrast medium
  D.-60 contrast medium

DIC
  disseminated intravascular coagulation
  disseminated intravascular coagulopathy

dichotomization

dichotomy

Dick cardiac valve dilator

dicliditis

diclidostosis

dicrotic
  d. notch
  d. pulse
  d. wave
  d. wave of carotid arterial pulse

dicrotism

dictyokinesis

dictyosome

dideoxynucleoside

dielectrography

diet
  American Heart Association d. (AHA diet)
  anticoronary d.
  balanced d.
  betaine d.

diet *(continued)*
   bland d.
   calorie-restricted d.
   cardiac d.
   crash d.
   DASH d.
   diabetic d.
   fat-free d.
   high-fiber d.
   Karell d.
   Kempner d.
   low cholesterol d.
   low-fat d.
   low in saturated fat d.
   low-methionine d.
   low-salt d.
   low-sodium d.
   no added salt d.
   Ornish d.
   prudent d.
   renal d.
   salt-free d.
   salt-restricted d.
   Sauerbruch-Herrmannsdorfer-Gerson d.

dietary
   d. fat
   d. salt
   d. sodium

Dieterle stain

Diethrich
   D. coronary artery set
   D. coronary artery instruments
   D. shunt clamp

Dieuaide
   D. diagram
   D. sign

difference
   arteriovenous (AV) d.
   arteriovenous oxygen d.
   arteriovenous oxygen content d.
   arteriovenous oxygen d.
   AVD O_2 d.
   pulmonary AV d.
   resting AV d.

difference *(continued)*
   systemic AV d.

differens
   pulsus d.

differential
   d. blood count
   d. blood pressure
   d. bronchospirometry

differentiation
   echocardiographic d.

Diff-Quik stain

diffraction
   x-ray d.

diffuse
   d. alveolar damage
   d. arterial ectasia
   d. bronchopneumonia
   d. emphysema
   d. infiltrative lung disease
   d. interstitial lung disease
   d. interstitial pulmonary fibrosis
   d. intimal thickening
   d. intravascular coagulation
   d. lung injury
   d. paroxysmal slowing
   d. pleurisy
   d. sclerosing alveolitis
   d. ST–T depression

diffusing
   d. capacity
   d. capacity of lung for carbon monoxide

diffusion
   d. capacity
   coefficient of d.
   facilitated d.
   single-breath d.

diffusum
   angiokeratoma corporis d.

dig
   digitalis
      dig effect

dig *(continued)*
   dig level

DIGAMI
   Diabetes Mellitus Insulin
   Glucose Infusion in Acute
   Myocardial Infarction

DiGeorge syndrome

digestion
   lipolytic d.

digestive system vascular disease

Digibind
   D. digoxin immune Fab
   fragments
   D. pneumatonometer

Digidote digoxin immune Fab
fragments

Digiflator digital inflation device

Digiflex high flow catheter

Digipate

digital
   d. averaging
   d. calipers
   d. clubbing
   d. computer
   d. constant-current pacing
   box
   d. endarteropathy
   d. fluoroscopic unit
   d. necrosis
   d. phase mapping
   d. runoff
   d. smoothing
   d. subtraction
   d. subtraction angiography
   (DSA)
   d. subtraction arteriography
   d. subtraction echocardiography
   d. subtraction imaging
   d. subtraction supravalvular aortogram
   d. subtraction supravalvular aortography

digital *(continued)*
   d. subtraction technique
   d. vascular imaging
   d. videoangiography

digitalis
   d. effect
   d. glycoside
   d. intoxication
   d. level
   d. sensitivity
   d.-specific antibody
   d. toxicity

digitalization

digitalize

digitalized

digitalizing dose

digitized subtraction angiography

digitizer
   Bitpad d.

digitoxicity

Digitrapper MKIII sleep monitor

Digitron

digitus
   d. mortuus

digoxigenin-labeled DNA probe

digoxin
   d. effect
   d.-immune Fab
   d. level
   D. RIA Bead
   d.-specific Fab
   d. toxicity

dikaryote

dikaryotic

dilatable lesion

dilatancy

dilatant

dilated cardiomyopathy

dilatation
- aneurysmal d.
- annular d.
- balloon d.
- bootstrap d.
- cardiac d.
- catheter d.
- esophageal d.
- d. of the heart
- idiopathic d.
- idiopathic right atrial d.
- left ventricular d.
- d. of aorta
- d. of aortic root
- d. of pulmonary artery
- d. of ventricular wall
- percutaneous balloon d.
- percutaneous transluminal balloon (PTBD) d.
- poststenotic d.
- poststenotic aortic d.
- reactive d.
- right ventricular d.
- sequential d.
- serial d.
- d. thrombosis
- ventricular d.
- Wirsung d.

dilation (see entries under *dilatation*)

dilator
- Amplatz d.
- aortic d.
- argon vessel d.
- Bakes d.
- Beardsley aortic d.
- Brock cardiac d.
- Brown-McHardy pneumatic d.
- Cooley d.
- Cooley valve d.
- Crump vessel d.
- DeBakey-Cooley d.
- Delaborde tracheal d.
- Derra valve d.
- Dick cardiac valve d.
- Einhorn esophageal d.

dilator *(continued)*
- Encapsulon vessel d.
- Garrett d.
- Garrett valve d.
- Gerbode valve d.
- Gohrbrand cardiac d.
- Hegar d.
- Henley d.
- Hiebert vascular d.
- Hohn vessel d.
- Jackson-Mosher d.
- Jackson-Trousseau d.
- Lucchese mitral valve d.
- Maloney mercury-filled esophageal d.
- mitral d.
- Mullins d.
- myocardial d.
- Plummer water-filled pneumatic esophageal d.
- Savary-Gilliard esophageal d.
- Scanlan vessel d.
- d. and sheath technique
- Sippy esophageal d.
- Steele bronchial d.
- Tubbs mitral valve d.
- Tucker d.
- valve d.
- vein d.
- vessel d.
- wire-guided oval intracostal d.

dilator-sheath

dimension
- aortic root d.
- end-diastolic d.
- left atrial d.
- left ventricular end-diastolic d.
- left ventricular end-systolic d.
- left ventricular internal diastolic d.
- left ventricular internal end-diastole d.
- left ventricular internal end-systole d.

dimension *(continued)*
  left ventricular internal d.
  left ventricular systolic d.
  right ventricular d.

dimer
  excited d's

dimple
  blind coronary d.
  coronary ostial d.

Dinamap
  D. automated blood pressure device
  D. blood pressure cuff
  D. blood pressure monitor
  D. monitor
  D. system
  D. ultrasound blood pressure manometer

diode
  light-emitting d. (LED)
  Zener d.

dip
  "a" d.
  Cournand d.
  midsystolic d.
  d. phenomenon
  septal d.
  type I d.
  type II d.

dip-and-plateau pattern

diphasic
  d. complex
  d. complex on EKG
  d. P wave
  d. T wave

diplasmatic

diplocardia

diplococci

diplodiatoxicosis

Diplos
  D. M pacemaker
  D. M 05 pacemaker

diplosome

diplotene

dipole theory

dipyridamole
  d. echocardiography
  d. echocardiography test
  d. handgrip test
  d. infusion test
  d. thallium-201 cardiac perfusion study
  d. thallium imaging
  d. thallium-201 scintigraphy
  d. thallium scan
  d. thallium scan ventriculography

direct
  d. cardiac massage
  d. cardiac puncture
  d. current (DC)
  d. embolism
  d. excitation
  d. fluorescent antibody (DFA)
  d. Fourier transformation imaging
  d. insertion technique
  d. laryngoscopy
  d. lead
  d. mapping sequence
  d. mechanical ventricular actuation
  d. murmur
  d. respiration

direct-current
  d.-c. cardioversion
  d.-c. shock ablation

directional
  d. atherectomy device
  d. coronary atherectomy

dirty
  d. chest
  d. film
  d. necrosis

dirty-lung appearance

disability
  cardiovascular d.

disarticulation
  Burger technique for sca-
    pulothoracic d.

disc (see entries under *disk*)

discontinuity
  atrial-axis d.

discordance
  atrioventricular d.
  ventriculoarterial d.

discordant
  d. alternans
  d. alternation

discrete
  d. coronary lesion
  d. subvalvular aortic steno-
    sis

disease
  Acosta d.
  acquired heart d.
  acromegalic heart d.
  acyanotic heart d.
  Adams d.
  Adams-Stokes d.
  Addison d.
  airspace d.
  alcoholic heart muscle d.
  amyloid heart d.
  aortic aneurysmal d.
  aortic thromboembolic d.
  aortic valve d.
  aortic valvular d. (AVD)
  aortoiliac obstructive d.
  aortoiliac obstructive val-
    vular d.
  aortoiliac occlusive d.
  aortoiliac vascular d.
  apple picker's d.
  arrhythmogenic right ven-
    tricular d.
  arterial occlusive d.
  arteriosclerotic cardiovas-
    cular d. (ASCVD)

disease *(continued)*
  arteriosclerotic heart d.
    (ASHD)
  arteriosclerotic peripheral
    vascular d.
  arteriosclerotic vascular d.
    (ASVD)
  asymptomatic left main d.
    (ALMD)
  atherosclerotic aortic d.
  atherosclerotic carotid ar-
    tery d.
  atherosclerotic coronary
    artery d. (ASCD)
  atherosclerotic pulmonary
    vascular d.
  aviators' d.
  Ayerza d.
  Bamberger-Marie d.
  Bannister d.
  Banti d.
  barometer-maker's d.
  Bazin d.
  Beau d.
  Becker d.
  Behçet d.
  beryllium d.
  biliary d.
  Binswanger d.
  blue d.
  Boeck d.
  Bornholm d.
  Bostock d.
  Bouillaud d.
  Bouveret d.
  branch d.
  Bright d.
  Brill-Zinsser d.
  Buerger d.
  Bürger-Grütz d.
  Buschke d.
  Busse-Buschke d.
  caisson d.
  California d.
  carcinoid heart d.
  carcinoid valve d.
  cardiovascular d.
  carotid artery d.
  carotid occlusive d.

disease *(continued)*
- carotid vascular d.
- Castellani d.
- Castleman d.
- cat-scratch d.
- Ceelen d.
- celiac d.
- cerebrovascular d.
- Chagas d.
- Chagas heart d.
- Charcot-Marie-Tooth d.
- cholesterol ester storage d.
- Christmas d.
- chronic hypertensive d.
- chronic obstructive pulmonary d. (COPD)
- chronic peripheral arterial d. (CPAD)
- Concato d.
- congenital heart d.
- constrictive heart d.
- Cori d.
- coronary artery d. (CAD)
- coronary heart d. (CHD)
- coronary occlusive d.
- Corrigan d.
- Corvisart d.
- Crocq d.
- cyanotic congenital heart d.
- cytomegalic inclusion d.
- Daae d.
- Darling d.
- Davies d.
- Degos d.
- Desnos d.
- diastolic heart d.
- diffuse d.
- digestive system vascular d.
- Döhle d.
- Duroziez d.
- Ebstein d.
- eccentric plaque d.
- effusive-constrictive d.
- Eisenmenger d.
- electrical d.
- elevator d.
- Emery-Dreifuss d.

disease *(continued)*
- endomyocardial d.
- end-stage cardiopulmonary d.
- end-stage liver d.
- end-stage renal d.
- eosinophilic endomyocardial d.
- Epstein d.
- Erb-Goldflam d.
- Erdheim d.
- extracranial cardiac d.
- extracranial carotid arterial d.
- extracranial vascular d.
- Fabry d.
- Fallot d.
- fibrocalcific rheumatic d.
- flint d.
- Fothergill d.
- Friedländer d.
- Friedreich d.
- functional cardiovascular d.
- functional valve d.
- Gairdner d.
- gannister d.
- gastroesophageal reflux d. (GERD)
- Gaucher d.
- Gerhardt d.
- global cardiac d.
- glycogen storage d.
- Goldflam d.
- Goldflam-Erb d.
- Goldstein d.
- graft occlusive d.
- granulomatous d.
- Graves d.
- Hamman d.
- hand-foot-and-mouth d.
- Hand-Schüller-Christian d.
- hard metal d.
- heart d.
- Heberden's d.
- Heller-Döhle d.
- hematologic d.
- hepatic d.
- Heubner d.

disease *(continued)*
    Hodgkin d.
    Hodgson d.
    Horton d.
    Huchard d.
    Hutinel d.
    hyaline membrane d.
    hypereosinophilic heart d.
    hypertensive arteriosclerotic heart d.
    hypertensive cardiovascular d. (HCVD)
    hypertensive heart d.
    hypertensive pulmonary vascular d.
    iliac atherosclerotic occlusive d.
    immune-mediated d.
    inflammatory aneurysmal d.
    intrastent recurrent d.
    intrinsic d.
    iron storage d.
    Isamberg d.
    ischemic heart d. (ISH)
    ischemic myocardial d.
    Kawasaki d.
    Keshan d.
    Kikuchi d.
    kinky-hair d.
    Krishaber d.
    Kugelberg-Welander d.
    Kussmaul d.
    Kussmaul-Maier d.
    large-vessel d.
    latent coronary artery d.
    latent ischemic heart d.
    left anterior descending coronary artery d.
    left main d.
    left main coronary artery d.
    left main equivalent d.
    Legionnaire d.
    Lemierre d.
    Lenègre d.
    Letterer-Siwe d.
    Lev d.
    Lewis upper limb cardiovascular d.

disease *(continued)*
    Libman-Sacks d.
    Little d.
    Löffler d.
    Lucas-Championnière d.
    luetic d.
    lupus-associated valve d.
    Lutembacher d.
    Lutz-Splendore-Almeida d.
    Lyme d.
    Majocchi d.
    maple bark d.
    McArdle d.
    metastatic d.
    Mikity-Wilson d.
    Milton d.
    Mitchell's d.
    mitral valve d.
    Mondor d.
    Monge d.
    Morgagni d.
    Morquio-Brailsford d.
    Moschcowitz d.
    moyamoya d.
    multivalvular d.
    multivessel d.
    multivessel coronary artery d.
    myocardial d.
    necrotizing arterial d.
    neoplastic d.
    Niemann-Pick d.
    nonatherosclerotic coronary artery d.
    nonoperable d.
    occlusive d.
    occlusive peripheral arterial d.
    one-vessel coronary arterial d.
    Opitz's d.
    organic heart d. (OHD)
    organic valve d.
    Osler d.
    Osler-Weber-Rendu d.
    Owren d.
    Paget d.
    Patella d.
    pericardial d.

disease *(continued)*
    peripartal heart d.
    peripheral arterial d.
    peripheral atherosclero-
      tic d.
    peripheral vascular d.
      (PVD)
    pigeon-breeder's d.
    Pick d.
    Plummer d.
    pneumatic hammer d.
    polysaccharide storage d.
    Pompe d.
    Posadas-Wernicke d.
    primary electrical d.
    primary myocardial d.
    primary collagen vascu-
      lar d. (PCVD)
    primary pulmonary paren-
      chymal d.
    pulmonary heart d.
    pulmonary valve d.
    pulmonary vascular ob-
      structive d.
    pulmonary veno-occlusive
      d. (PVOD)
    pulseless d.
    Quincke d.
    ragpicker's d.
    ragsorter's d.
    Raynaud d.
    Refsum d.
    Reiter d.
    renal artery d.
    renal parenchymal d.
    Rendu-Osler-Weber d.
    restrictive airways d.
    restrictive heart d.
    restrictive lung d.
    rheumatic heart d. (RHD)
    rheumatic mitral valve d.
    rheumatic valvular d.
    right coronary artery d.
    Roger d.
    Rokitansky d.
    Rosai-Dorfman d.
    Rougnon-Heberden d.
    Roussy-Lévy d.
    Rummo d.

disease *(continued)*
    Sandhoff d.
    San Joaquin Valley d.
    Schaumann d.
    Schönlein d.
    scleroderma heart d.
    Shaver d.
    Shoshin d.
    single-vessel heart d.
    sinoatrial d.
    sinus node d.
    slim d.
    Sly d.
    Steinert d.
    Still d.
    Stokes-Adams d.
    Sylvest d.
    symptomatic left main d.
      (SLMD)
    Takayasu d.
    Takayasu-Ohnishi d.
    Tangier d.
    Taussig-Bing d.
    Tay-Sachs d.
    Thomsen d.
    three-vessel coronary ar-
      tery d.
    thromboembolic d.
    thyrocardiac d.
    thyrotoxic heart d.
    transplant coronary ar-
      tery d.
    traumatic heart d.
    tricuspid valve d.
    triple coronary artery d.
    triple-vessel d.
    TWAR d.
    two-vessel coronary ar-
      tery d.
    Uhl d.
    valvular heart d. (VD)
    van den Bergh d.
    Vaquez d.
    vasculo-Behçet d.
    veno-occlusive d.
    vertebrobasilar occlusi-
      ve d.
    vibration d.
    von Recklinghausen d.

disease *(continued)*
    von Willebrand d.
    Weber-Christian d.
    Weil d.
    Weir Mitchell's d.
    Wenckebach d.
    Werlhof d.
    Whipple d.
    Wilkie d.
    Wilson d.
    Wilson-Kimmelstein d.
    Winiwarter-Buerger d.

disintegration rate

disk
    cervical d.
    d.-cage valve
    Eigon d.
    intercalated d.
    intervertebral d.
    Molnar d.
    optic d.
    d. oxygenation
    d. oxygenator
    d. poppet
    d. spring

dismutase
    superoxide d.

disobliteration
    carotid d.

disorder
    acid-base d.
    autoimmune d.
    clotting d.
    endocrine d.
    genetic d.
    glycosphingolipid d.
    iatrogenic d.
    lymphocytic infiltrative d.
    mendelian d.
    movement d.
    neurological d.
    neuromuscular d.
    panic d.
    single-gene d.

disordered action of heart

disorganization
    segmental arterial d.

Dispatch over-the-wire catheter

dispersing electrode

dispersion
    QT d.
    QT/QTc d.
    temporal d.

dispira

dispireme

displacement
    d. sensing device
    late systolic d.

disruption
    plaque d.
    traumatic aortic d.

dissecans
    pneumonia d.

dissected
    d. tissue arm
    d. free

dissecting
    d. abdominal aortic aneu-
      rysm
    d. aneurysm
    d. aorta
    d. aortic aneurysm
    d. hematoma

dissection
    aortic d.
    arterial d.
    blunt d.
    coronary artery d.
    DeBakey-type aortic d.
    epiphenomena of d.
    finger d.
    intimal d.
    sharp d.
    spiral d.
    spontaneous coronary ar-
      tery d.
    Stanford-type aortic d.
    therapeutic d.

dissection *(continued)*
  thoracic aortic d.
  type A aortic d.
  type B aortic d.

dissector
  Holinger d.
  Jannetta d.
  Lemmon intimal d.
  Penfield d.
  Spacemaker balloon d.
  sponge d.

disseminata
  tuberculosis miliaris d.

disseminated
  d. intravascular coagulation
  d. intravascular coagulopathy
  d. lupus erythematosus
  d. polyarteritis
  d. tuberculosis

dissociation
  atrial d.
  atrioventricular d.
  auriculoventricular d.
  AV d.
  complete atrioventricular d.
  d. curve
  electromechanical d.
  electromyocardial d.
  incomplete atrioventricular d.
  interference d.
  interference atrioventricular d.
  d. by interference
  intracavitary pressure-electrogram d.
  isorhythmic d.
  isorhythmic atrioventricular d.
  longitudinal d.

dissolution

Distaflex balloon

distal
  d. anastomosis
  d. circumflex marginal artery
  d. convoluted tubule
  d. coronary sinus
  d. ectasia
  d. runoff
  d. splenorenal shunt
  d. stenosis

distance
  half-power d.
  Mahalanobis d.

distant
  d. breath sounds
  d. heart sounds

distensibility
  ventricular d.

distention
  atrial presystolic d.
  jugular venous d. (JVD)
  d. of neck veins

distortion
  pincushion d.

distress
  respiratory d.

distribution
  blood volume d.
  Boltzmann d.
  stocking-glove d.
  volume of d.

distributive shock

disturbance
  cardiac rhythm d.
  conduction d.
  electrolytic d.
  rhythm d.

Dittrich
  D. plugs
  D. stenosis

diurese

diuresed

diuresis
loop d.

diuretic
d. agent
cardiac d.
high-ceiling d.
indirect d.
loop d.
osmotic d.
potassium-sparing d.
potassium-wasting d.
thiazide d.
d. therapy

diurnal rhythm

divarication

diversity
antigen-binding d.

diver's syncope

diverticulectomy
Harrington esophageal d.

diverticulum *pl.* diverticula
Heister's d.
Zenker d.

divided respiration

diving
d. air embolism
d. goiter
d. reflex

division
cell d.
cell d., direct
cell d., indirect
equational d.
maturation d.
reduction d.
vascular ring d.

divisional heart block

dizziness

DKS
Damus-Kaye-Stansel
Damus-Kaye-Stansel
connection

DKS *(continued)*
Damus-Kaye-Stansel
operation
Damus-Kaye-Stansel
procedure

DL
double lumen
QuickFurl DL

D-looping

D-loop transposition of the
great arteries

DLP
DLP cardioplegic catheter
DLP cardioplegic needle

DMI
Diagnostic Medical Instruments
DMI analyzer
diaphragmatic myocardial
infarction

DMPE (^{99m}Tc-bis-dimethylphos-
phonoethane)

DMVA
direct mechanical ventricular actuation

DNA
deoxyribonucleic acid
DNA cloning
human cloned DNA
DNA probe
DNA sequencing
DNA switch

DNM
descending necrotizing mediastinitis

DNR
do not resuscitate

dobutamine
d.-atropine stress echocardiography
d. echocardiography
d. holiday
d. stress echocardiography
d. stress test

DOC
DOC exchange technique
DOC guidewire extension
DOC-2000 demand oxygen
controller

Docke murmur

docking wire

dock wire

Dodd perforating vein

Dodge
D. area-length method
D. area-length method for
ventricular activity
D. area-length method for
ventricular volume
D. method for ejection fraction
D. method for calculating
left ventricular volume

DOE
dyspnea on exertion

dog-leg catheter

Döhle (Doehle)
D. disease
D. inclusion bodies
D.-Heller aortitis

doigt
d. mort

dolens
phlegmasia alba d.
phlegmasia cerulea d.

dolichoectatic aneurysms

dolichol

dolichostenomelia

dolore
angina pectoris sine d.

domain
time d.

dome
d. of atrium

dome (continued)
d.-and-dart configuration
on cardiac catheterization
d. of diaphragm
d. excursion

dome-shaped

dominance
coronary artery d.
mixed d.
right ventricular d.
shared coronary artery d.

dominant

doming
diastolic d.
d. of leaflets
d. of valve
systolic d.
tricuspid valve d.

domino procedure

Donders pressure

Donne corpuscles

donor
d. organ, appropriately
sized and matched
d. organ ischemic time
d.-specific transfusion

do not resuscitate (DNR)

dopexamine

Doppler
D. auto-correlation technique
D. blood flow detector
D. blood pressure
D. cardiography
Carolina color spectrum
CW D.
carotid D.
D. catheter
color D.
D. color flow imaging,
transesophageal
D. color flow mapping

Doppler *(continued)*
  D. color jet
  D. continuity equation
  continuous-wave D.
  D. coronary catheter
  D. device
  D. echocardiography
  D. effect
  D. fetal heart monitor
  D. fetal stethoscope
  D. FloWire
  D. flow probe
  D. guidewire
  D. imaging
  D. interrogation
  D. IntraDop
  D. measurement
  D. pressure gradient
  pulsed D.
  pulsed D. echocardiography
  quantitative D.
  D. recording
  D. shift
  D. signal
  D. spectral analysis
  D. study
  D. tissue imaging
  D. transducer
  D. transesophageal color flow imaging
  D. ultrasonography
  D. ultrasound
  D. velocimetry
  D. velocity probe
  D. waveform analysis
  D.-Cavin monitor

dopplered

dopplergram

Doppler-tipped angioplasty guidewire

Dopplette monitor

Doptone monitoring

d'orange
  peau d.

Dorendorf sign

Dorian rib stripper

dormescent jerks

Dorros
  D. brachial internal mammary guiding catheter
  D. infusion/probing catheter

dorsalis pedis pulse

dorsi
  latissimus d.

DORV
  double-outlet right ventricle

dosage regimen

dose
  digitalizing d.
  loading d.
  nonpressor d's
  priming d.
  radiation absorbed d. (RAD)
  tracer d.

dosing
  trough d.

Dos Santos needle

Dotter
  D. caged-balloon catheter
  D. coaxial catheter
  D. effect
  D. Intravascular Retrieval Set
  D. technique
  D.-Judkins technique
  D.-Judkins technique in percutaneous transluminal angioplasty

dottering effect

double
  d. aortic arch
  d. aortic stenosis
  d.-balloon
  d.-balloon catheter

double *(continued)*
- d.-balloon valvotomy
- d.-balloon valvuloplasty
- d. bubble flushing reservoir
- d.-barrelled aorta
- d.-chain rt-PA
- d.-chip micromanometer catheter
- d.-disk occluder
- d.-dummy technique
- d. extrastimulus
- d.-flanged valve sewing ring
- d.-inlet ventricle
- d.-J catheter
- d.-J stent
- d. lumen
- d.-lumen catheter
- d.-lumen endobronchial tube
- d. lung transplant
- d.-outlet left ventricle
- d.-outlet left ventricle malposition
- d.-outlet right ventricle
- d.-outlet right ventricle malposition
- d. pleurisy
- d. pneumonia
- d. product
- d.-sandwich IgM ELISA
- d.-shock sound
- d. tachycardia
- d. triangular test
- d. umbrella
- d.-thermistor coronary sinus catheter
- d.-umbrella closure
- d.-umbrella device
- d. ventricular extra stimulus
- d. voice
- d.-wire technique

doubling time

doughnut
- d. configuration
- d. sign

Douglas
- D. bag

Douglas *(continued)*
- D. bag collection method
- D. bag spirometer
- D. bag technique

Dow
- D. Corning tube
- D. method (for cardiac output)

Down
- D. flow generator
- D. syndrome

downgoing Babinski

downhill
- d. esophageal varices
- d. ST segment depression

down-regulation

downsloping ST segment depression

downstream
- d. sampling method
- d. venous pressure

downward sloping

doxorubicin cardiotoxicity

Doyen
- D. elevator
- D. rib hook
- D. rib elevator
- D. rib rasp; raspatory

Doyle vein stripper

dP/dt
- upstroke pattern on apex cardiogram

$dPdt_{MAX}$-end-diastolic volume

DPM
- digital phase mapping

DPTI
- diastolic pressure-time index

DR
- dual-chamber rate-responsive

Drager Volumeter

drag forces

drain
Charnley suction d.
Clot Stop d.
Deseret sump d.
Relia-Vac d.

drainage
anomalous pulmonary venous d.
closed chest water-seal d.
partial anomalous pulmonary venous d.
percussion and postural d.
postural d.
pulmonary venous d.
Snyder Surgivac d.
Thoracoseal d.
Thora-Drain III chest d.
total anomalous pulmonary venous d.
underwater seal d.
water-seal d.

Drapanas mesocaval shunt

drapeau
bruit de d.

dreamer clamp

dressing
Comfeel Ulcus d.
Cutinova Hydro d.
jacket-type chest d.
Kaltostat wound packing d.
stent d.
Veingard d.
Vigilon d.
wet-to-dry d.

Dressler
D. beat
D. syndrome

Dr. Gibaud thermal health support

drift

drill-tip catheter

drip
heparin d.

Dripps–American Surgical Association score

drive
d. cycle length
respiratory d.
d. trains
ventricular d.

dromograph

Dromos pacemaker

dromotropic effect

drop
falling d.
d. heart
Rondec D's

dropout
septal d.

dropped beat

dropsy
cardiac d.
d. chest
d. of pericardium

drug
d. abuse
d.-associated pericarditis
cardiotonic d.
d. clearance
d. delivery reservoir
d.-induced cardiomyopathy
d.-induced lupus erythematosus
d.-induced pericarditis
pressor d.
d.-refractory tachycardia
d.-resistant tachyarrhythmia
sympathomimetic d.
vasoactive d.

Drummond
marginal arteries of D.
D. marginal artery
D. sign

dry pericarditis

Drysdale corpuscles

DSA
   digital subtraction angiography

DSAS
   discrete subvalvular aortic stenosis

DSE
   digital subtraction echocardiography
   dobutamine stress echocardiography

DSI-III screw-in lead pacemaker

DTAF-F
   descending thoracic aorto-femoral-femoral
      DTAF-F bypass

D-TGA
   D-transposition of great arteries

DTPA
   diethylenetriamine pentaacetic acid (pentetic acid)
   technetium bound to DTPA

DTR
   deep tendon reflex

dual
   d. balloon perfusion catheter
   d.-chamber pacemaker
   d.-chamber pacing
   d.-chamber rate-responsive
   d.-demand pacemaker
   d. echophonocardiography
   d.-mode
   d.-pacing
   d.-sensing
   d.-sensor micromanometric high-fidelity catheter

duality

Dualtherm dual thermistor thermodilution catheter

Du Bois-Reymond law

Duchenne sign

Duckworth phenomenon

Ducor
   D. balloon catheter
   D. HF catheter
   D.-Cordis pigtail catheter

duct
   d. of Botallo
   collecting d.
   d. of Cuvier
   medullary collecting d.
   thoracic d.

ductal cell carcinoma

ductulus

ductus
   d. Arantii
   d. arteriosus
   d. bump
   patent d. arteriosus
   d. persistent
   d. reversed
   d. thoracicus
   d. venosus

Duffield cardiovascular scissors

Duguet siphon

Duke
   D. Activity Status Index (DASI)
   D. bleeding time
   D. Carcinoid Database
   D. treadmill prognostic score
   D. University Clinical Cardiology Study

Dukes classification

dullness
   absolute cardiac d.
   area of cardiac d.
   border of cardiac d.
   cardiac border of d.
   Gerhardt d.

dullness *(continued)*
    percussion d.
    tympanitic d.

dumoffii
    Legionella dumoffii

Dumont thoracic scissors

Duncan
    D. multiple range test
    D. syndrome

Dunham fans

Dunlop thrombus stripper

Dunnett test

DuoCet

Duostat rotating hemostatic
    valve

duplex
    d. imaging
    d. pulsed-Doppler ultraso-
        nography
    pulsus d.
    d. scanning
    d. ultrasound

dupp

Duracep biopsy forceps

Duraflow heart valve

Duran annuloplasty ring

Durapulse pacemaker

Durathane cardiac device

duration
    action potential d.
    d. of EKG wave
    d. of exercise
    d. of expiration
    half-amplitude pulse d.
    d. of inspiration
    d. of P wave
    d. of QRS
    monophasic action poten-
        tial d.
    pulse d.

Durham tube

Duromedics
    D. bileaflet mitral valve
    D. valve prosthesis,

Duroziez
    D. disease
    D. murmur
    D. sign
    D. symptom

durus
    pulsus d.

duskiness

dusky

duty factor

Duval-Crile lung forceps

DVI
    deep venous insufficiency
    DVI pacing
    DVI Simpson Atherocath

DVT
    deep venous thrombosis

dwarfism
    aortic d.

dyad

dyaster

dye
    Cardio-Green d.
    d. curve
    d. cuvette
    d. dilution curve
    d. dilution method
    d. dilution technique
    flashlamp excited pulsed d.
    Fox green d.
    indocyanine green d.
    d. injection
    d. laser
    radiocontrast d.
    Unisperse blue d.

Dymer
    D. excimer delivery probe
    D. excimer delivery system

dynamic
    d. aorta
    d. cardiomyoplasty
    d. exercise
    fluid d's
    d. frequency response
    funnel d.
    d. intracavitary obstruction
    left ventricular-left atrial
        crossover d's
    d. murmur
    d. pressure
    d. range
    d. relaxation

Dynamic Y stent

dynamite heart

dynamometer
    bicycle d.
    Cybex isokinetic d.

DynaPulse 5000 A

dyne
    d. seconds

dynein

dysarteriotony

dysarthria

dysautonomia
    familial d.

dysbetalipoproteinemia

dyscontrol

dyscrasia
    blood d.

dysfibrinogenemia

dysfunction
    diastolic d.
    endothelial d.
    focal ventricular d.
    global ventricular d.
    intellectual d.
    left ventricular d. (LVD)
    mitral valve d. (MVD)
    papillary muscle d.

dysfunction *(continued)*
    regional myocardial d.
    sinus node d.
    valvular d.
    ventricular d.

dysfunctional myocardium

dysgenesis
    gonadal d.

dysgeusia

dyskaryosis

dyskaryotic

dyskinesia
    d. intermittens
    d. regional

dyskinesis
    anterior wall d.
    anteroapical d.
    left ventricular d.
    posteroinferior d.

dyskinetic

dyslipidemia
    atherogenic d.
    Fredrickson d.

dyslipoproteinemia

dysmodulation

dysnystaxis

dyspeptica
    angina d.

dysphagia
    arrhythmogenic right ven-
        tricular d.
    contractile ring d.
    d. inflammatoria
    d. lusoria
    d. nervosa
    d. paralytica
    pulmonary valve d.
    sideropenic d.
    d. spastica
    vallecular d.
    d. valsalviana
    ventricular d.

dysphasia

dysphasic

dysplasia
   arrhythmogenic right ven-
      tricular d.
   atriodigital d.
   bronchopulmonary d.
   ectodermal d.
   fibromuscular d.
   fibrous d.
   polyostotic fibrous d.
   right ventricular d.
   ventriculoradial d.

dysplastic

dyspnea
   cardiac d.
   effort d.
   episodic d.
   d. on exertion (DOE)
   exertional d.
   functional d.
   inspiratory d.
   Monday d.
   nocturnal d.
   nonexpansional d.
   one-flight exertional d.
   orthostatic d.
   paroxysmal d.
   paroxysmal nocturnal d.
   psychogenic d.
   renal d.
   rest d.

dyspnea *(continued)*
   d. scale
   sighing d.
   d. target
   Traube d.
   two-flight exertional d.

dyspneic

dyspneoneurosis

dysreflexia
   autonomic d.

dysrhythmia
   cardiac d.

Dysschwannian syndrome

dyssynchronization

dyssynchrony
   thoracoabdominal d.

dyssynergia
   d. regional
   d. segmental

dyssynergic myocardial segment

dyssynergy

dysstole

dystrophic calcification

dystrophin

dystrophinoplaty

dysvascular

E
    E to A changes
    E to F slope
    E greater than A
    E to I changes
    E point
    E point on echocardiogram
    E point to septal separa-
      tion (EPSS)
    E sign
    E wave
    E wave to A wave (E/A)

E/A
    E wave to A wave

EAC
    expandable access catheter

EAD
    early afterdepolarization

EAE
    effective arterial elastance

Eagle
    E. criteria
    E. equation
    E. medium
    E. spirometer

ear
    e. densitogram
    e. oximeter

earlobe crease

early
    e. afterdepolarization
      (EAD)
    e. deceleration
    e. diastolic murmur
    e.-peaking systolic murmur
    e. rapid repolarization

EAT
    ectopic atrial tachycardia

Eaton
    E. agent
    E. agent pneumonia
    E.-Lambert syndrome

E:A wave ratio

EBDA
    effective balloon-dilated
      area

EBL
    estimated blood loss

Ebstein
    E. angle
    E. cardiac anomaly
    E. disease
    E. sign

EBV
    Epstein-Barr virus

ECA
    external carotid artery

E-CABG
    endarterectomy and coro-
      nary artery bypass graft-
      ing

ECAD
    extracranial carotid arterial
      disease

ECC
    edema, clubbing, and cya-
      nosis

eccentric
    e. atrial activation
    e. hypertrophy
    e. ledge
    E. locked rib shears
    e. monocuspid tilting-disk
      prosthetic valve
    e. narrowing
    e. plaque disease
    e. stenosis

eccentricity index

ecchymosis *pl.* ecchymoses

ecchymotic mask

ECD
    endocardial cushion defect

ECD *(continued)*
    external cardioverter-defib-
      rillator
    extracranial cardiac dis-
      ease
ECG
    electrocardiogram
    electrocardiograph
    electrocardiography
      ambulatory ECG
      Micro-Tracer portable
        ECG
      ECG rhythm strip
      ECG signal-averaging
        technique
      ECG-synchronized digi-
        tal subtraction angio-
        gram
      ECG triggering unit
echo
    amphoric e.
    atrial e.
    e. beat
    bright e.
    e. catheter
    e. delay time
    e. density
    e. guidance
    e. intensity
    linear e.
    metallic e.
    motion display e.
    nodus sinuatrialis e.
    NS e.
    pericardial e.
    e. probe
    e. ranging
    e. reverberation
    scattered e.
    e. score
    smokelike e.
    specular e.
    transcutaneous e.
    transesophageal e.
    e. transponder electrode
      catheter
    ventricular e.
    e. zone

echoaortography

echocardiogram
    akinesis on e.
    ambulatory Holter e.
    anterior left ventricular
      wall motion e.
    apical e.
    apical five-chamber view e.
    apical four-chamber view e.
    apical left ventricular wall
      motion on e.
    apical two-chamber view e.
    B bump on anterior mitral
      valve leaflet e.
    cardiac output e.
    continuous loop exercise e.
    continuous wave Dop-
      pler e.
    contrast-enhanced e.
    cross-sectional two-dimen-
      sional e.
    2-D e.
    D to E slope on e.
    E point on e.
    echo-free space on e.
    echo intensity disappear-
      ance rate on e.
    Feigenbaum e.
    four-chamber e.
    15-lead e.
    hypokinesis on e.
    inferior left ventricular wall
      motion on e.
    intracoronary contrast e.
    intraoperative cardioplegic
      contrast e.
    lateral left ventricular wall
      motion on e.
    late systolic posterior dis-
      placement on e.
    left ventricular long-axis e.
    long-axis parasternal
      view e.
    meridian e.
    M-mode e.
    Ochsner-Mahorner e.
    parasternal long-axis
      view e.

echocardiogram *(continued)*
    parasternal short-axis
      view e.
    postcontrast e.
    posterior left ventricular
      wall motion on e.
    postexercise e.
    postinjection e.
    postmyocardial e.
    precontrast e.
    preinjection e.
    premyocardial e.
    right ventricular short-ax-
      is e.
    septal wall motion on e.
    short-axis view e.
    signal-averaged e.
    subcostal short-axis view e.
    subxiphoid view of e.
    two-chamber e.
    ventricular wall motion e.

echocardiograph
    Acuson e.
    Biosound Surgiscan e.

echocardiographic
    e. assessment
    e. automated border detec-
      tion
    e. automated boundary de-
      tection system
    e. differentiation
    e. scoring system
    e. transducer

echocardiography
    adenosine e.
    A-mode e.
    any-plane e.
    baseline e.
    bicycle e.
    B-mode e.
    color flow Doppler e.
    continuous-wave Dop-
      pler e.
    contrast e.
    cross-sectional e.
    2-D e.
    deductive e.

echocardiography *(continued)*
    digital subtraction e. (DSE)
    dipyridamole e.
    dobutamine e. (DE)
    dobutamine-atropine
      stress e.
    dobutamine stress e. (DSE)
    Doppler e.
    Doppler e., color
    dyskinesis on e.
    ergonovine e.
    esophageal e.
    exercise e.
    exercise stress e.
    high-frequency epicardial e.
    interventional e.
    meridian e.
    mitral valve e.
    M-mode e.
    myocardial contrast e.
    myocardial perfusion e.
    paraplane e.
    pharmacologic stress e.
    pulmonary valve e.
    pulsed Doppler e.
    pulsed-wave (PW) Dop-
      pler e.
    quantitative two-dimen-
      sional e.
    real-time three-dimension-
      al e.
    resting e.
    sector scan e.
    signal-averaged e.
    stress e.
    stress-injected sestamibi-
      gated SPECT e.
    supine bicycle stress e.
    three-dimensional e.
    transesophageal e. (TEE)
    transesophageal contrast e.
    transesophageal dobuta-
      mine stress e.
    transthoracic e. (TTE)
    treadmill e.
    two-dimensional e.

echodense
    e. mass

echodense *(continued)*
    e. structure

echodensity
    linear e.
    superimposed e.

echo-Doppler cardiography

echoendoscope
    Olympus GIF-EUM2 e.

echo-free space

EchoGen emulsion

echogenicity

echogenic
    e. plaque
    e. mass

echogram

echography
    A-scan e.

echo-guided ultrasound

echolucent
    e. plaque

EchoMark angiographic catheter

echophonocardiography
    combined M-mode e.
    dual e.

echophony

echo-planar imaging

echoreflective

echoreflectivity

echoscanner

echoscope

echo-signal shape

echo-spared area

Echovar Doppler system

echovirus
    e. myocarditis

Eck fistula

ECLS
    extracorporeal life support

ECMO
    extracorporeal membrane
        oxygenation
    ECMO pump

ECS
    extracellular-like, calcium-
        free solution
    ECS cardioplegic solution

ectasia
    alveolar e.
    annuloaortic e.
    aortoannular e.
    artery e.
     e. cordis
    coronary artery e.
    diffuse arterial e.
    distal e.
    hypostatic e.
    papillary e.
    vascular e.

ectasis

ectatic
    e. aneurysm
    e. emphysema

ectobiology

ectoblast

ectocardia

ectocardiac

ectocardial

Ectocor pacemaker

ectocytic

ectodermal dysplasia

ectolysis

ectonuclear

ectopia
    e. cordis

ectopia *(continued)*
    e. cordis abdominalis
    e. cordis pectoral
    e. lentis

ectopic
    e. atrial tachycardia
    e. beat
    e. impulse
    e. pacemaker
    e. rhythm
    e. ventricular beat

ectoplasm

ectoplasmatic

ectoplast

ectoplastic

ectopy
    asymptomatic complex e.
    atrial e.
    bursts of ventricular e.
    high density ventricular e.
    supraventricular e.
    ventricular e.

ectosphere

ECT pacemaker

ED
    emergency department

EDA
    end-diastolic area

eddy
    e. sounds
    e. sounds of patent ductus
        arteriosus

edema
    acute pulmonary e.
    acute cardiogenic pulmon-
        ary e.
    alveolar e.
    angioneurotic e.
    ankle e.
    bland e.
    boggy e.
    brawny e.
    brown e.

edema *(continued)*
    cardiac e.
    cardiogenic pulmonary e.
    cardiopulmonary e.
    cerebral e.
    chronic pulmonary e.
    circumscribed e.
    clubbing, cyanosis, and e.
        (CCE)
    congestive e.
    dependent e.
    fingerprint e.
    flash pulmonary e.
    florid pulmonary e.
    focal e.
    hereditary angioneurotic e.
    high-altitude pulmonary e.
    idiopathic cyclic e.
    interstitial e.
    e. of lung
    localized e.
    lymphatic e.
    Milton e.
    mucosal e.
    myocardial e.
    neurogenic pulmonary e.
    nonpitting e.
    paroxysmal pulmonary e.
    passive e.
    pedal e.
    periodic e.
    periorbital e.
    peripheral e.
    perivascular e.
    pitting e.
    postanesthesia pulmon-
        ary e.
    postcardioversion pulmon-
        ary e.
    presacral e.
    pretibial e.
    pulmonary e.
    Quincke e.
    sacral e.
    stasis e.
    subpleural e.
    tense e.
    terminal e.
    trace e.

edema *(continued)*
  vasogenic e.
  venous e.
  woody e.

edematous

edentulism
  compensated e. (false teeth)

Eder-Puestow wire

edge
  e. detection
  leading e.
  shelving e.
  trailing e.

edge-detection method

EDHF
  endothelium-derived hyperpolarizing factor

Edmark
  E. mitral valve
  E. monophasic waveform

EDM infusion catheter

EDP
  end-diastolic pressure

EDRF
  endothelium-derived relaxing factor

EDV
  end-diastolic volume

EDVI
  end-diastolic volume index

Edwards
  E. catheter
  E. clamp
  E. heart valve
  E. patch
  E. septectomy
  E. Teflon intracardiac patch prosthesis
  E. woven Teflon aortic bifurcation graft
  E.-Carpentier aortic valve brush

Edwards *(continued)*
  E.-Duromedics bileaflet heart valve
  E.-Tapap arterial graft

EECP
  enhanced external counterpulsation

EEG
  electroencephalogram
  electroencephalograph
  electroencephalography

EF
  ejection fraction
    EF slope,

effect
  Anrep e.
  Bainbridge e.
  band saw e.
  Bayliss e.
  blooming e.
  Bowditch e.
  Brockenbrough e.
  cidal e.
  Coanda e.
  Compton e.
  copper wire e.
  digitalis e.
  digoxin e.
  Doppler e.
  Dotter e.
  dottering e.
  dromotropic e.
  erectile e.
  founder e.
  horse-race e.
  inotropic e.
  jet e.
  late proarrhythmic e.
  mille-feuilles e.
  neurotoxic e.
  nonhemodynamic e.
  potassium sparing e.
  Prinzmetal e.
  proarrhythmic e.
  proto-oncogenic e.
  Rivero-Carvallo e.
  silver wire e.

effect *(continued)*
    snowplow e.
    squeeze e.
    training e.
    Vaughn Williams class e.
    Venturi e.
    Wedensky e.
    Windkessel e.

effective
    e. arterial elastance
    e. balloon-dilated area
    e. circulating blood volume
    e. refractory period
    e. regurgitant orifice
    e. renal blood flow

effector cells

efferent
    e. arteriole
    e. artery

efficacy
    e. of drug therapy
    therapeutic e.
    e. of treatment

efficiency
    detective quantum e.

Effler
    E. double-ended dissector
    E. hiatal hernia repair
    E. ring
    E. tack
    E.- Groves cardiovascular
      forceps
    E.- Groves mode of Allison
      procedure
    E.- Groves operation

effort
    e. angina
    e. dyspnea
    first e.
    e.-induced thrombosis
    e. intolerance
    e. syndrome

effusion
    cholesterol pericardial e.

effusion *(continued)*
    chylous pericardial e.
    hemorrhagic e.
    loculated e.
    malignant e.
    pericardial e.
    pleural e.
    serofibrinous pericardial e.
    silent pericardial e.
    subpleural e.

effusive-constrictive
    e.-c. disease
    e.-c. pericarditis

Efron jackknife classification

eggcrate mattress

Eggleston method

egg-shaped heart

eggshell pattern

egg-yellow reaction

egophony

Ehlers-Danlos syndrome

Ehret phenomenon

ehrlichiosis

Eicken method

EID
    Emergency Infusion Device
      EID catheter

Eidemiller tunneler

eight-lumen manometry catheter

Eigon
    E. CardioLoop recorder
    E. disk

Einhorn esophageal dilator

Einthoven
    E. equation
    E. law
    E. lead
    E. string galvanometer

Einthoven *(continued)*
  E. triangle

E:I ratio

Eisenmenger
  E. complex
  E. disease
  E. reaction
  E. reaction with septal de-
    fects
  E. syndrome
  E. tetralogy
  E. VSD

ejection
  area-length method for e.
    fraction
  basilar half e. fraction
  blunted e. fraction
  BSA (body surface area) e.
    fraction
  digital e. fraction
  Dodge method for e. frac-
    tion
  e. click
  e. fraction (EF)
  e. fraction image
  e. fraction slope
  e. murmur
  e. period
  e. phase
  e. phase indices
  e. rate
  e. shell image
  e. sounds
  e. time
  e. velocity
  global e. fraction
  interval e. fraction
  Kennedy method for calcu-
    lating e. fraction
  left ventricular e. fraction
  one third e. fraction
  regional e. fraction
  resting left ventricular e.
    fraction
  right ventricular e. fraction
    (RVEF)
  systolic e. fraction

ejection *(continued)*
  thermodilution e. fraction

EJK
  external jugular vein

Ejrup maneuver

EKG
  electrocardiogram
  electrocardiograph
  electrocardiography
    baseline EKG
    borderline EKG
    EKG leads I, II, III
    EKG leads V1 through
      V6
    EKG leads aVF, aVL,
      aVR
    Micro-Tracer portable
      EKG
    Minnesota classifica-
      tion of EKG
    EKG monitor strip
    EKG rhythm strip
    EKG silence
    straight-line EKG
    EKG tracing

EKY
  electrokymogram

EI
  EI Gamal cardiac device
  EI Gamal coronary bypass
    catheter
  EI Gamal guiding catheter

Ela
  E. Chorus DDD pacemaker
  E. pacemaker
  E. ventricular pacing lead

elaioplast

E-LAM
  endothelium-leukocyte ad-
    hesion molecule

elastance
  effective arterial e.
  end-systolic e.

elastance *(continued)*
    maximum ventricular e.
        (Emax)

elastase
    leukocyte e.
    neutrophil e.
    Pseudomonas e.

elastic
    e. component
    e. lamina
    e. pulse
    e. recoil
    e. recoil pressure
    e. resistance
    e. stiffness
    e. stockings
    e. tissue hyperplasia

Elastorc catheter guidewire

elbow flexion

ELCA
    excimer laser coronary an-
        gioplasty
        ECLA laser

Elecath
    E. circulatory support de-
        vice
    E. ECMO cannula
    E. pacemaker
    E. switch box
    E. thermodilution catheter

elective cardioversion

electrical
    e. activation abnormality
    e. alternans
    e. alternation of heart
    e. axis
    e. cardioversion
    e. catheter ablation
    e. countershock
    e. diastole
    e. disease
    e. events of the EKG
    e. failure
    e. fulguration
    e. heart position

electrical *(continued)*
    e. injury
    e. potential
    e. systole

electric cardiac pacemaker

electro-acuscope

electrocardiogram (ECG, EKG)
    ambulatory e.
    baseline e.
    Burdick e.
    computerized e.
    Corometrics-Aloka e.
    esophageal e.
    evolutionary changes on e.
    exercise e.
    fetal e.
    flat e.
    flatline e.
    His bundle e.
    intracardiac e.
    intracoronary e.
    3-lead e.
    6-lead e.
    12-lead e.
    16-lead e.
    Micro-Tracer portable e.
    normal resting e.
    orthogonal e.
    postconversion e.
    precordial e.
    pre-exercise resting supine
        e.
    resting e.
    scalar e.
    serial changes in e.
    signal-averaged e.
    stress e.
    stress MUGA e.
    surface e.
    telephone transmission of
        e.
    thallium e.
    three-channel e.
    time domain signal-aver-
        aged e.
    treadmill e.
    unipolar e.
    vector e.

electrocardiograph (ECG, EKG)
  bioimpedance e.
  Cambridge e.
  Marquette e.
  Mingograf 62 6-channel e.

electrocardiographic
  e. leads
  e. transtelephonic monitor
  e. wave
  e. wave complex (QRS complex)

electrocardiography (ECG, EKG)
  ambulatory e.
  esophageal e.
  exercise e.
  exercise stress e.
  fetal e.
  intracardiac e.
  intracavitary e.
  12-lead e.
  precordial e.
  signal-averaged e.

electrocardiophonogram

electrocardiophonography

electrocardioscanner
  Compuscan Hittman computerized e.

electrocautery
  Bovie e.
  needlepoint e.

electrochemical polarization

electrode
  Arzco TAPSUL pill e.
  barbed-hook pacemaker e.
  Bard nonsteerable bipolar e.
  Berkovits-Castellanos hexapolar e.
  Bioplus dispersive e.
  Biotronik IE 65-I pacemaker e.
  bipolar myocardial e.

electrode (continued)
  Bisping e.
  button e.
  Cambridge jelly e.
  e. catheter
  central terminal e.
  Clark oxygen e.
  coil e.
  Cordis e.
  corkscrew-tip pacemaker e.
  CPI Endotak transvenous e.
  CPI L67 e.
  CPI porous tine-tipped bipolar pacing e.
  cutaneous thoracic patch e.
  Darox cutaneous thoracic patch e.
  dispersing e.
  endocardial pacemaker e.
  endocardial placement of e.
  EnGuard PFX lead e.
  epicardial e.
  epicardial patch e.
  esophageal e.
  esophageal pill e.
  exploring e.
  Fast-Patch disposable defibrillation/electrocardiographic e.
  flanged e.
  flanged Silastic tip pacemaker e.
  floating e.
  free end of e.
  e. gel
  Goetz bipolar e.
  hand-held e.
  His bundle e.
  hydrogen e's
  implantable cardioverter e's
  indifferent e.
  intravascular catheter e.
  ion-selective e.
  e. jelly
  J orthogonal e.
  Josephson quadripolar mapping e.

electrode *(continued)*
    J-shaped pacemaker e.
    Laserdish e.
    Lifeline e.
    Mansfield Polaris e.
    Medtronic Transvene e.
    monopolar temporary e.
    multiple point e.
    multipolar catheter e.
    MVE-50 implantable
      myocardial e.
    myocardial e.
    Myowire II cardiac e.
    negative pacemaker e.
    Nyboer esophageal e.
    orthogonal e.
    Osypka Cereblate e.
    pacemaker e's
    pacing e.
    e. pad
    e. paddles
    e. paste
    patch e.
    PE-60-I-2 implantable
      pronged unipolar e.
    PE-85-I-2 implantable
      pronged unipolar e.
    PE-60-KB implantable uni-
      polar endocardial e.
    PE-85-KB implantable uni-
      polar endocardial e.
    PE-60-K-10 implantable uni-
      polar endocardial e.
    PE-85-K-10 implantable uni-
      polar endocardial e.
    PE-85-KS-10 implantable
      unipolar endocardial e.
    permanent pacing e.
    pill e.
    platinum e.
    point e.
    Polaris e.
    positive e.
    precordial e.
    QuadPolar e.
    quadripolar Quad e.
    Quinton e.
    reference e.
    ring e.

electrode *(continued)*
    scalp e.
    screw-in epicardial e.
    sensing e.
    Siemens e.
    Silastic e.
    silent e.
    silver bead e.
    silver–silver chloride e.
    skin e.
    e.-skin interface
    Skylark surface e.
    Soft-EZ reusable e.
    stab-in epicardial e.
    stainless steel e.
    stimulating e.
    Stockert cardiac pacing e.
    subxiphoid e.
    Surgicraft pacemaker e.
    e. system
    Tapcath esophageal e.
    Tapsul pill e.
    target tip e.
    Telectronics pacemaker e.
    temporary pacemaker e.
    temporary pacing e.
    temporary transvenous
      catheter e.
    thermistor e.
    thoracic e.
    three-turn e.
    tined e.
    tine tipped pacemaker e.
    transesophageal e. (TEE)
    transthoracic e.
    Transvene tripolar e.
    transvenous e.
    tripolar defibrillation coil e.
    two-turn e.
    unipolar defibrillation co-
      il e.
    unipolar pacemaker e.
    urethane e.
    USCI Goetz bipolar e.
    USCI NBIH bipolar e.
    Vitatron catheter e.
    Waterston pacing e.
    wire e.

electrodesiccation

electrodispersive skin patch

Electrodyne pacemaker

electrodynogram

electrofluoroscopy

electrogenic

electrogram
  atrial e.
  coronary sinus (CS) e.
  Csos (coronary sinus os-
    tium) e.
  esophageal e.
  fractionated ventricular e.
  Furman Type II e.
  high right atrial (HRA) e.
  His bundle e.
  intra-atrial e.
  intracardiac e.
  intracoronary e.
  right atrial e.
  right ventricular e.
  right ventricular apical e.
  sinus node e.

electrograph
  Cardiotest portable e.

electrography

electrohemostasis

electrokymogram

electrokymography

electrolyte
  e. imbalance
  e. disturbance
  serum e.
  e. therapy

electromagnetic
  e. interference (EMI)

electromanometer

electromechanical
  e. artificial heart
  e. coupling
  e. dissociation
  e. interval

electromechanical *(continued)*
  e. systole

electromyocardial dissociation

electronic
  e. distance compensation
  e. fetal monitor
  e. pacemaker
  e. pacemaker load
  e. scanning

electron volt

electrophoresis
  agarose gel e.
  gradient gel e.
  polyacrylamide gel e.
  protein e.
  sodium dodecylsulfate
    polyacrylamide gel e.

electrophysiologic
  e. mapping
  e. study (EPS)
  e. test

electrophysiological

electrophysiology (EP)
  cardiac e.
  clinical cardiac e.
  intracardiac e.

electrostethograph

electrosurgery

electrovectorcardiogram

electroversion

electrovert

Elema
  Siemens E. AG bicycle er-
    gometer
  E. leads
  E. pacemaker

Elema-Schonander pacemaker

eleoplast

elephant-on-the-chest sensation

elev
  elevated

elevated gradient

Elevath pacemaker

elevation
ST segment e.
transient ST segment e.
e. of enzymes
e. pallor of extremity

elevator
Aufricht e.
Cameron-Haight e.
e. disease
Doyen e.
Freer e.
Friedrich rib e.
Hedblom e.
Lemmon sternal e.
Matson rib e.
Matson-Alexander rib e.
Overholt e.
Penfield e.
Phemister e.
rib e.
Sedillot e.

elfin
e. facies
e. facies syndrome

El Gamal coronary bypass catheter

Elgiloy
E. frame
E.-Heifitz aneurysm clip

elimination half-life

ELISA
enzyme-linked immunosorbent assay
double-sandwich IgM ELISA

ELISPOT test

Elite
E. guide catheter
E. pacemaker

Ellestad
E. exercise stress test

Ellestad (continued)
E. protocol

ellipse
prolate e.

Ellipse compact spacer

ellipsin

ellipsoid

elliptical loop

Ellis sign

Ellis-van Creveld syndrome

Eloesser flap

Elscint tomography system

eluting stent

elution

embarrassment
circulatory e.
respiratory e.

Emax
maximum ventricular elastance

embolectomy
arterial e.
catheter e.
e. catheter
femoral e.
pulmonary e.

emboli (plural of embolus)

embolic
e. abscess
e. aneurysm
e. event
e. gangrene
e. infarct
e. phenomenon
e. pneumonia
e. shower
e. stroke
e. thrombosis

emboliform

embolism
acute pulmonary e.

embolism *(continued)*
  air e.
  amniotic fluid e.
  aortic e.
  arterial e.
  atheromatous e.
  bacillary e.
  bland e.
  bone marrow e.
  capillary e.
  catheter e.
  cellular e.
  cholesterol e.
  coronary e.
  crossed e.
  direct e.
  diving air e.
  fat e.
  gas e.
  hematogenous e.
  infective e.
  miliary e.
  multiple e.
  myxomatous pulmonary e.
  obturating e.
  oil e.
  pantaloon e.
  paradoxical e.
  pulmonary e.
  pyemic e.
  retrograde e.
  riding e.
  saddle e.
  straddling e.
  spinal e.
  submassive pulmonary e.
  trichinous e.
  tumor e.
  venous e.

embolization
  air e.
  bronchial artery e.
  cholesterol e.
  coil e.
  paradoxic e.
  pulmonary e.
  septic e.
  Silastic bead e.
  e. therapy

embolization *(continued)*
  transcatheter e.

embolized foreign material

embolomycotic aneurysm

embolotherapy

embolus *pl.* emboli
  air e.
  bullet e.
  calcific e.
  cancer e.
  catheter e.
  catheter induced e.
  cerebral e.
  coronary artery e.
  fat e.
  femoral e.
  foam e.
  intraluminal e.
  mesenteric e.
  obturating e.
  paradoxic e.
  polyurethane foam e.
  prosthetic valve e.
  pulmonary e.
  retinal e.,
  riding e.
  saddle e.
  straddling e.
  threw an e.
  tumor e.

embouchement

embryocardia
  jugular e.
  e. rhythm

embryologic

embryology

embryoma

EMC virus

emeiocytosis

EMD
    electromechanical dissocia-
    tion

emergency
    e. bailout stent
    hypertensive e.
    E. Infusion Device (EID)
    e. reperfusion

Emerson
    E. pump,
    E. vein stripper

emetine toxicity

EMF
    endomyocardial fibrosis

EMI
    electromagnetic interfer-
    ence
        EMI induced pace-
        maker failure

emiocytosis

emissarium
    e. condyloideum
    e. mastoideum
    e. occipitale
    e. parietale

emissary

empiric
    e. constant
    e. therapy

empyema
    anaerobic e.
    e. benignum
    e. of chest
    interlobar e.
    latent e.
    loculated e.
    e. necessitatis
     e. of pericardium
    pneumococcal e.
    pulsating e.
    putrid e.
    sacculated e.
    streptococcal e.
    thoracic e.

en bloc
    e. b., no-touch technique

en face

encarditis

encased heart

encephalopathy
    hypertensive e.
    metabolic e.

enchylema

encircling
    e. cryoablation
    e. endocardial ventriculot-
    omy

Encor
    E. lead
    E. pacemaker

Encore inflation device

encroachment
    luminal e.

encrustation theory of athero-
    sclerosis

endangiitis

endaortic

endaortitis
    bacterial e.

endarterectomize

endarterectomy
    aortoiliac e.
    aortoiliofemoral e.
    blunt eversion carotid e.
    carotid bifurcation e.
    carotid e.
    carotid eversion e.
    coronary e.
    e. and coronary artery by-
    pass grafting (E-CABG)
    femoral e.
    gas e.
    innominate e.
    laser e.
    manual core e.
    profunda e.
    subclavian e.

endarterectomy *(continued)*
  transluminal e.
  vertebral e.

endarterial

endarteritis
  cerebrospinal e.
  e. deformans
  Heubner specific e.
  infective e.
  e. obliterans
  e. proliferans
  syphilitic e.

endarterium

endarteropathy
  digital e.

endartery

end-diastole

end-diastolic
  e.-d. area
  e.-d. count
  e.-d. dimension
  e.-d. left ventricular pressure
  e.-d. murmur
  e.-d. pressure
  e.-d. velocity
  e.-d. volume
  e.-d. volume index

end-hole
  e.-h. balloon-tipped catheter
  e.-h. #7 French catheter

end-inspiratory crackles

endless-loop tachycardiac

endoaneurysmorrhaphy
  ventricular e.

endoangiitis

endoaortitis

endoarteritis

endoauscultation

endocardiac

endocardial
  e. balloon lead
  e. catheter ablation
  e. cushion
  e. cushion defect
  e. fibroelastosis
  e. fibrosis
  e. flow
  e. mapping
  e. mapping of ventricular
    tachycardia
  e. murmur
  e. resection
  e. to epicardial resection
  e. sclerosis
  e. stain
  e. thickening
  e. tube
  e. vegetation

endocardiopathy

endocarditic

endocarditis
  abacterial thrombotic e.
  acute bacterial e. (ABE)
  acute infective e.
  aortic valve e.
  atypical verrucous e.
  bacteria-free stage of bacterial e.
  bacterial e. (BE)
  e. benigna
  cachectic e.
  e. chordalis
  chronic e.
  constrictive e.
  culture-negative e.
  enterococcal e.
  fungal e.
  gonococcal e.
  gram-negative e.
  green strep e.
  Haemophilus e.
  infectious e.
  infective e.
  isolated parietal e.
  e. lenta
  Libman-Sacks e.

endocarditis *(continued)*
  Löffler e.
  Löffler parietal fibroplas-
    tic e.
  malignant e.
  marantic e.
  methicillin-sensitive right-
    sided e.
  mitral valve e.
  mural e.
  mycotic e.
  native valve e.
  nonbacterial thrombotic e.
  nonbacterial verrucous e.
  noninfective e.
  nosocomial e.
  parietal e.
  e. parietalis fibroplastica
  plastic e.
  polypous e.
  postoperative e.
  prosthetic valve e.
  pulmonic e.
  pustulous e.
  rheumatic e.
  rickettsial e.
  right-side e.
  septic e.
  staphylococcal e.
  streptococcal e.
  subacute bacterial e. (SBE)
  subacute infective e.
  syphilitic e.
  terminal e.
  thrombotic e.
  tricuspid valve e.
  tuberculous e.
  ulcerative e.
  valvular e.
  vegetative e.
  verrucous e.
  viridans e.
endocardium
endocellular
endochrome
Endocoil stent
endocyte

endocytosis

end-of-life pacemaker

endogenous lipid

Endo Grasp device

Endoknot suture

endolumen enlargement

EndoLumina illuminated bougie

endoluminal
  e. delivery
  e. stenting

endolysis

endomitosis

endomitotic

endomyocardial
  e. biopsy
  e. disease
  e. fibroelastosis
  e. fibrosis (EMF)

endomyocarditis

endomysial collagen

endomysium

endonuclear

endonuclease
  restriction e.

endonucleolus

EndoOctopus

endopericardial

endopericarditis

endoperimyocarditis

endoperoxide steal

endophthalmitis

endophlebitis
  e. hepatica obliterans
  proliferative e.

endoplasm

endoplasmic

endopolyploid

endopolyploidy

endoreduplication

endosarc

endosome

endostethoscope

EndoSonics IVUS/balloon dilatation catheter

Endotak
  E. C lead
  E. C lead transvenous catheter
  E. C tripolar pacing/sensing/defibrillation lead
  E. C tripolar transvenous lead
  E. lead system
  E. nonthoracotomy implantable cardioverter-defibrillator

endothelin

endothelial
  e. denudation
  e. dysfunction

endothelialization

endothelin
  e.-1
  e.-2
  e.-3
  e. A, B receptors
  plasma e.

endothelioma

endothelium
  e.-dependent dilator response to substance P
  e.-derived hyperpolarizing factor
  e.-derived nitric oxide
  e.-derived relaxing factor
  e.-leukocyte adhesion molecule

endothelium (continued)
  e.-mediated relaxation

endotoxemia

endotracheal
  e. aspirate
  e. intubation
  e. tube

Endotrol
  E. endotracheal tube
  E. tracheal tube

endovascular

endovasculitis

endovenitis

endovenous

endoventricular circular patch plasty

endpoint
  therapeutic e.

end-pressure artifact

end-stage
  e.-s. cardiomyopathy
  e.-s. cardiopulmonary disease
  e.-s. heart failure
  e.-s. liver disease
  e.-s. renal disease

end-systole

end-systolic
  e.-s. counts
  e.-s. dimension
  e.-s. elastance
  e.-s. force-velocity indices
  e.-s. left ventricular pressure
  e.-s. murmur
  e.-s. pressure-volume relation
  e.-s. stress-dimension relation
  e.-s. volume (ESV)
  e.-s. volume index

end-tidal carbon dioxide

end-to-end

end-to-side suture

energometer

energy
color Doppler e.
e. production
e. resolution
e. supply

Enertrax 7100 pacemaker

Englert forceps

engorgement
venous e.

EnGuard
E. double-lead ICD system
E. pacing and defibrillation
lead system
E. PFX lead electrode

enhanced
e. automaticity
e. external counterpulsa-
tion
e. external counterpulsa-
tion unit
E. Torque 8F guiding catheter

enhancement
leading edge e.
mean contrast e.

Enhancer
Ace Cloud E.
Aerosol Could E.

enhancing lesion

enlargement
atrial e.
biatrial e.
cardiac e.
compensatory vessel e.
endolumen e.
e. of heart
left atrial e. (LAE)
panchamber e.
right atrial e. (RAE)

entangling technique

enterococcal endocarditis

entocyte

entoplasm

entoptic pulse

entosarc

entrain

entrained beat

entrainment
concealed e.
epicardial e.
e. of tachycardia
e. with concealed fusion

entrance
e. block
e. wound

entrapment
popliteal artery e.

EnTre guidewire

entry
air e.
e. site

enucleated

enucleation of subaortic stenosis

envelope
aortic e.
dagger-shaped aortic e.
flow e.
nuclear e.
spectral e.

env gene

enzyme
allosteric modification of e.
angiotensin-converting e.
(ACE)
angiotensin-I converting e.
cardiac e.
glycolytic e's

enzyme *(continued)*
  e. immunoassay (EIA)
  lysosomal e.
  mitochondrial e.'s
  myocardial e.
  phosphodiesterase e.
  proteolytic e.
  sarcoplasmic reticulum-associated glycolytic e's

enzyme-linked immunosorbent assay (ELISA)

eosin
  hematoxylin and e. (H&E)

eosinophil
  e. by-products
  e. cationic protein
  e. chemotactic factors of anaphylaxis (ECF-A)

eosinophilia
  peripheral blood e.
  pulmonary infiltration with e.
  tropical pulmonary e.

eosinophilia-myalgia syndrome

eparterial

EP
  electrophysiology
  EP mapping
  EP study

EPBF
  effective pulmonary blood flow

epicardia

epicardial
  e. attachment
  e. biopsy
  e. defibrillator patch
  e. Doppler flow transducer
  e. electrode
  e. entrainment
  e. fat
  e. fat tag
  e. flow
  e. lead

epicardial *(continued)*
  e. pacemaker electrode
  e. patch cathode
  e. reflection
  e. space
  e. surface
  e. vessel patency

epicardiectomy

epicardium

epimyocarditis

epimysium

epinephrine
  racemic e.

epiphenomena of dissection

episode
  presyncopal e.

episodic dyspnea

Epistat double balloon

epistaxis

epistenocardiaca
  pericarditis e.

Eppendorf
  E. angiocatheter
  E. catheter

EPS
  electrophysiologic study

EPSS
  E point to septal separation

Epstein
  E. disease
  E.-Barr nuclear antigen
  E.-Barr virus

EPT-1000 cardiac ablation system

EPTFE
  expanded polytetrafluoroethylene
    EPTFE graft
    EPTFE vascular sutures

equation
    Bernoulli e.
    Bloch e.
    Brunelli e.
    Carter e.
    continuity e.
    Doppler continuity e.
    Eagle e.
    Einthoven e.
    Fick e.
    Ford e.
    Friedewald e.
    Gorlin e.
    Hagenbauch extension of
       Poiseuille e.
    Holen-Hatle e.
    Krovetz-Gessner e.
    Navier-Stokes e.
    Nernst e.
    regression e.
    Riley-Cournand e.
    Rodrigo e.
    Starling e.
    Teicholz e.
    Torricelli orifice e.

equator
    e. of cell

Equen magnet

equilibration

equilibrium
    e. image
    e. multigated radionuclide
       ventriculography
    e. radionuclide angiogra-
       phy
    voltage e.

equilibrium-gated blood pool
    study

equiphasic complex

equivalency
    left main e.

equivalent
    Abell-Kendall e.
    anginal e.

equivalent *(continued)*
    metabolic e. of task (MET)
       (METs)
    right anterior oblique e.
    ventilation e.
    ventilatory e.

Erb
    E. area
    E. atrophy
    E. point

ERBE cryoprobe

Erben reflex

ERBF
    effective renal blood flow

Erb-Goldflam disease

erbium:YAG laser

Erdheim
    E. cystic medial necrosis
    E. disease

ergastoplasm

ergocardiogram

ergocardiography

ergometer
    arm e.
    Bosch ERG 500 e.
    bicycle e.
    Collins bicycle e.
    Ergoline bicycle e.
    Gauthier bicycle e.
    Monark bicycle e.
    pedal-mode e.
    Siemens-Albis bicycle e.
    Siemens-Elema AG bicy-
       cle e.
    Tunturi EL400 bicycle e.

ergometric studies

ergometry
    bicycle e.

ergonomic vascular access nee-
    dle

ergonovine
    e. challenge

ergonovine *(continued)*
    e. echocardiography
    e.-induced spasm
    e.-induced vasospasm
    e. infusion
    e. maleate provocation angina
    e. provocation test

ergoplasm

ergot alkaloid

ergotamine
    e. derivatives
    Medihaler E.

Erie System

Erlanger sphygmomanometer

ERNA
    equilibrium radionuclide angiography

Erni sign

erosion
    spark e.

ERP
    effective refractory period
    ERP atrial
    ERP ventricular

erythema
    e. marginatum
    e. migrans
    e. multiforme
    e. nodosum
    palmar e.

erythematosus
    disseminated lupus e.
    drug-induced lupus e.
    lupus e.
    systemic lupus e. (SLE)

erythematous maculopapular rash

erythralgia

erythremomelalgia

erythrocyte sedimentation rate (ESR)

erythrocytosis

erythroderma

Erythroflex hydromer-coated central venous catheter

erythrogenin

erythromelalgia

erythropheresis

erythropoietin
    plasma e.

erythroprosopalgia

erythropyknosis

ES
    ejection sounds

ESAT-6 protein

escape
    atrioventricular junctional e.
    e. beat
    e.-capture bigeminy
    e. impulse
    e. interval
    junctional e.
    nodal e.
    e. pacemaker
    e. rhythm
    vagal e.
    ventricular e.
    e. ventricular contraction

Escherich test

ESLD
    end-stage liver disease

Esmarch tourniquet

esophageal
    e. achalasia
    e. adventitia
    e. angina
    e. A-ring
    e. artery
    e. atresia
    e. bougienage

esophageal *(continued)*
  e. B-ring
  e. cardiogram
  e. contraction ring
  e. detection device
  e. dilation
  e. dysmotility
  e. echocardiography
  e. electrocardiography
  e. hiatus
  e. lead
  e. lumen
  e. manometry
  e. motility
  e. obturator airway
  e. pill electrode
  e. reflux
  e. rupture
  e. sling procedure
  e. sound
  e. spasm
  e. speech
  e. sphincter
  e. stricture
  e. tamponade
  e. temperature
  e. temperature probe
  e. transit time
  e. varices
  e. web

ESP
  radiation reduction examination gloves
  end-systolic pressure

ESR
  erythrocyte sedimentation rate

essential
  e. bradycardia
  e. hypertension
  e. tachycardia

EST
  exercise stress test
  extrastimulus testing

ester
  cholesterol e.

Estes
  E. EKG criterion
  E. point system
  E. score
  E.-Romhilt EKG point-score system

estimated blood loss (EBL)

estimated Fick method

Estlander operation

ESV
  end-systolic volume

ESVI
  end-systolic volume index

ESWI/ESVI
  end-systolic wall stress index/end-systolic volume index

ET
  ejection time

E-test

Ethalloy needle

Ethibond suture

Ethicon suture

Ethiflex suture

Ethilon suture

ethmocarditis

etiology

E to F slope on echocardiogram

ETT
  exercise tolerance test
  exercise treadmill test

eucaryon

eucaryosis

eucaryote

eucaryotic

euglobulin clot lysis time

eukaryon

eukaryosis

eukaryote

eukaryotic

eukinesis

eumorphism

eunuchoid voice

Euro-Collins multiorgan perfusion kit

Eustace Smith murmur

eustachian valve

eusystole

eusystolic

euthyroid
    e. sick syndrome

euvolemic

eV
    electron volt

evagination

evaluation
    noninvasive e.

EVAN
    ergonomic vascular access
        needle

Evans
    E. blue dye
    E. forceps
    E. Vital tissue forceps,

Eve method

event
    cardiac e.
    coronary e.
    e. diary
    embolic e.
    intracardiac e.

event *(continued)*
    e. monitor
    e. recorder
    soft e.

eventration

eventration of diaphragm

eversion
    blunt e.
    cusp e.

everting mattress suture

evolutus
    Peptostreptococcus evolutus

evolving myocardial infarction

Ewald tube

Ewart sign

Ewing sign

ex vivo
    e. v. gene transfer

exacerbation of chronic congestive heart failure

excavatum
    pectus e.

exchange
    e. guidewire
    e. transfusion

excimer
    e. cool laser
    e. gas laser
    e. laser coronary angioplasty
    e. vascular recanalization

excisional
    e. biopsy
    e. cardiac surgery

excitability
    supranormal e.

excitable gap

excitation
    anomalous atrioventricular e.

excitation *(continued)*
    direct e.
    premature e.
    reentrant e.
    supranormal e.
    e. wave

excitation-contraction coupling

excited dimers

excitovascular

exclusion criteria

excrescence
    Lambl e's

excretion
    eicosanoid e.

excursion
    decreased valve e.
    dome e.
    respiratory e.

exercise
    active e.
    active assisted e.
    active resistive e.
    ankle e.
    Buerger-Allen e.
    e. capacity
    dynamic e.
    e. echocardiography
    e. electrocardiography
    e. factor
    e. imaging
    e. index
    e. intolerance
    e.-induced angina
    e.-induced arrhythmia
    e.-induced myocardial is-
      chemia
    e.-induced silent myocar-
      dial ischemia
    e.-induced ventricular
      tachycardia
    isometric e.
    isotonic e.
    e. load
    peak e.
    e. prescription

exercise *(continued)*
    e. regimen
    rehabilitation e.
    strenuous e.
    e. stress echocardiography
    e. stress electrocardiogra-
      phy
    e. stress test
    e. study
    submaximal e.
    supine e.
    symptom limited e.
    e. thallium-201 scintigraphy
    e. tolerance
    e. tolerance test
    e. treadmill
    e. treadmill test
    upright e.

exertion
    dyspnea on e. (DOE)
    pain precipitated by e.
    perceived e.

exertional
    e. angina
    e. dyspnea
    e. syncope

exit
    e. block
    e. block murmur
    e. point
    e. wound

exocardia

exocardial murmur

exocellular

exocytosis

exogenous
    e. lipid
    e. obesity

exon

exophthalmica
    tachycardia traumosa e.

exophytic

exoplasm

Exorcist technique

expandable access catheter

expanded
> e. polytetrafluoroethylene
> e. polytetrafluoroethylene vascular graft

expander
> blood e.
> Hespan plasma volume e.
> hetastarch e.
> plasma volume e.
> PMT AccuSpan tissue e.
> Ruiz-Cohen round e.

expansion
> infarct e.
> stent e.

explanted heart

Explorer
> E. 360-degree rotational diagnostic EP catheter
> E. pre-curved diagnostic EP catheter

exploring electrode

Express
> E. balloon
> E. over-the-wire balloon catheter

exsanguinate

exsanguination protocol

exsanguinotransfusion

EXS femoropopliteal bypass graft

exsorption

extended collection device

extender
> Taq e.

extension
> DOC guidewire e.
> infarct e.
> knee e.

extension *(continued)*
> Linx guidewire e.
> LOC guidewire e.

external
> e. cardiac massage
> e. cardioverter-defibrillator
> e. carotid artery
> e. carotid steal syndrome
> e. defibrillator
> e. grid
> e. jugular vein
> e. mammary artery
> e. pacemaker
> e. respiration
> e. rotation, abduction, stress test

externum
> pericardium e.

extirpation of valve

extra-anatomic

extracardiac
> e. conduit
> e. murmur
> e. shunt

extracardial

extracellular
> e. lipid
> e. matrix

extracellular-like, calcium-free solution

extracoronary

extracorporeal
> e. circulation
> e. exchange hypothermia
> e. heart
> e. life support
> e. membrane oxygenator
> e. membrane oxygenator
> e. pump oxygenator

extracranial
> e. cardiac disease
> e. carotid arterial disease

extract
cell-free e.
thyroid e.

extraction
e. atherectomy device
lactate e.
oxygen e.
e. reserve

Extractor three-lumen retrieval balloon

extranuclear

extrapericardial

extrarenal azotemia

extrastimulation
critically times e.
double e.
paired e.
premature e.
single premature e.
triple e.

extrastimulus
e. technique
e. testing

extra-support guidewire

extrasystole
atrial e.
atrioventricular (AV) e.
AV nodal e.
auricular e.
auriculoventricular e.
AV junctional e.

extrasystole *(continued)*
infranodal e.
interpolated e.
junctional e.
lower nodal e.
midnodal e.
nodal e.
nonpropagated junctional e.
premature ventricular e.
retrograde e.
return e.
supraventricular e.
upper nodal e.
ventricular e.

extrasystolic beat

extrathoracic

extravascular
e. granulomatous features
e. lung water

extraventricular

extremitas

extremity
e. ischemia
mottling of e's

exudate
fibrinous e.
retinal e.

eyeball compression reflex

eyeball-heart reflex

eyeless needle

F

F gate
F point of cardiac apex
pulse

f

f wave
f wave of jugular venous
pulse

Fab fragment
antimyosin F. f.

fabric baffle

Fabry disease

face
en f.
moon f.
f. shield

facies *pl.* facies
f. anterior cordis
aortic f.
Corvisart f.
cushingoid f.
f. diaphragmatica cordis
elfin f.
f. inferior cordis
mitral f.
f. mitralis
mitrotricuspid f.
f. pulmonalis cordis
f. sternocostalis cordis
f. pulmonalis dextra/sinis-
tra cordis

facilitated angioplasty

FACT coronary balloon angioplasty catheter

factor
f. I (fibrinogen)
f. II (prothrombin)
f. III (thromboplastin)
f. IV (calcium ions)
f. V (proaccelerin)
f. VI

factor *(continued)*
f. VII (proconvertin)
f. VII SPCA (serum pro-
thrombin conversion ac-
celerator)
f. VIII (antihemophilic factor)
f. VIII:C (von Willebrand
factor)
F. viii:c (porcine)
f. IX (Christmas factor)
f. IX complex (human)
f. IX plasma thromboplas-
tin component (Christmas
factor)
f. X (Stuart factor)
f. Xa
f. XI (plasma thromboplastin antecedent factor)
f. XII (Hageman factor)
f. XIII (fibrin stabilizing factor)
acidic fibroblast growth f.
active-site inhibited f. VIIa
angiogenesis f.
antihemophilic f.
atrial natriuretic f. (ANF)
f. B
basic fibroblast growth f.
blood coagulation f.
C f.
cardiac risk f.
chemotactic f.
Christmas f.
coagulation f.
f. D
duty f.
endothelium-derived hy-
perpolarizing f.
endothelium-derived relaxing f.
exercise f.
extrinsic f's
fibrin-stabilizing blood coagulation f.
fibroblast growth f.
Fletcher f.

211

factor *(continued)*
    granulocyte/macrophage
        colony-stimulating f.
    gravitation f.
    f. H
    Hageman f.
    myocardial depressant f.
    necrosis f.
    N-terminal proatrial natri-
        uretic f.
    f. P
    platelet f. 4
    platelet activating f.
    platelet-aggregating f.
    platelet-derived growth f.
    proatrial natriuretic f.
    Rh f.
    rheumatoid f.
    risk f.
    Stuart-Prower f.
    tissue f.
    transforming growth f.
    vascular endothelial
        growth f.
    von Willebrand f.

facultative bacteria

Faget sign

FAI
    functional aerobic impair-
        ment

failure
    acute congestive heart f.
    backward heart f.
    biventricular heart f.
    cardiac f.
    chronic renal f.
    circulatory f.
    compensated congested
        heart f.
    congestive heart f.
    coronary f.
    decompensated congestive
        heart f.
    diastolic heart f.
    electrical f.
    end-stage heart f.
    florid congestive heart f.

failure *(continued)*
    forward heart f.
    heart f.
    high-output heart f.
    left-sided heart f.
    left ventricular f.
    low-output heart f.
    multisystem organ f.
    myocardial f.
    pacemaker f.
    primary bioprosthetic val-
        ve f.
    pump f.
    refractory congestive
        heart f.
    respiratory f.
    right heart f.
    right-sided heart f.
    right ventricular f.
    systolic heart f.

Falcon single-operator ex-
    change balloon catheter

falling drop

Fallot
    F. disease
    F. pentalogy
    pentalogy of F.
    pink tetralogy of F.
    F. pink tetralogy
    F. tetrad
    tetralogy of F.
    F. triad
    trilogy of F.
    F. trilogy

false
    f. angina
    f. aortic aneurysm
    f. bruit
    f. cardiomegaly
    f. cardiomyopathy
    f. combined hyperlipidemia
    f. cyanosis
    f. dextrocardia
    f. hypercholesterolemia

false-negative

false-positive

falx
    f. septi

FAMAT
    fluorescent antimembrane antibody

familial
    f. abetalipoproteinemia
    f. amyloidosis
    f. cholestasis syndrome
    f. dysautonomia
    f. dyslipidemic hypertension
    f. hypercholesterolemia
    f. hypertrophic cardiomyopathy (FHC)
    f. hypertrophic obstructive cardiomyopathy

family history of heart disease

family history of myocardial infarction

Family Index of Life Events (FILE)

fan
    Dunhan f's

FAP
    femoral artery pressure

Farr test

FAS
    fetal alcohol syndrome

F and R

fascia *pl.* fasciae
    f. adherens
    pectoralis f.
    prepectoral f.
    Scarpa f.

fascial layer

fascicle
    left anterior f.
    left posterior f.

fascicular
    f. beat

fascicular *(continued)*
    f. heart block

fasciculation

fasciculoventricular
    f. bypass fiber
    f. Mahaim fiber

fasciculus
    f. atrioventricularis

fasciotomy
    anterior compartment f.

fashion
    antegrade f.
    retrograde f.

FAST
    flow-assisted, short-term
    FAST balloon flotation catheter
    FAST right heart cardiovascular catheter

fast
    f. channel
    f. Fourier spectral analysis
    f. Fourier transform
    f. low-angle shot
    f. pathway
    f.-pathway radiofrequency ablation
    f. sodium current

Fast-Fit vascular stockings

Fast-Pass
    F. endocardial lead
    F. lead pacemaker

Fast-Patch disposable defibrillation/electrocardiographic electrode

FasTrac
    F. guidewire
    F. hydrophilic-coated guidewire
    F. introducer

fat
    animal f.
    body f.

fat *(continued)*
    dietary f.
    f. embolism
    f. embolism syndrome
    f. emulsion
    epicardial f.
    monounsaturated f.
    polyunsaturated f.
    preperitoneal f.
    properitoneal f.
    saturated f.
    trans f.
    unsaturated f.

fatigability

fat-laden microphages

fatty
    f. acid
    f. degeneration of heart
    f. heart
    f. streak

Fauvel granules

Favaloro
    F. proximal anastomosis
        clamp
    F. saphenous vein bypass
        graft
    F. sternal retractor
    F.-Morse rib spreader

Fc receptors

F-18 2-deoxyglucose uptake on
    PET scan

FE
    slow FE

fear of impending death feeling
    from angina

feature
    extravascular granuloma-
        tous f's

febrile agglutinins

Federici sign

feeder vessel

feeling of impending doom
    prior to MI

feet
    cold f.

Feigenbaum echocardiogram

fêlé
    bruit de pot f.

Fell-O'Dwyer apparatus

felt
    Teflon f. bolster

fem-fem bypass

femoral
    f. approach
    f. arteriography
    f. artery
    f. artery occlusion
    f. artery thrombosis
    f. canal
    f. embolectomy
    f. embolus
    f. endarterectomy
    f.-f. bypass
    f.-f. crossover
    f. perfusion cannula
    f.-peroneal in situ vein by-
        pass graft
    f.-popliteal bypass
    f.-popliteal Gore-Tex graft
    f. pulse
    f.-tibial bypass
    f.-tibial-peroneal bypass
    f. vascular injury
    f. vein
    f. vein occlusion
    f. venous thrombosis
    f. vessel

femoroaxillary bypass

femorodistal bypass

femorofemoral crossover by-
    pass

femorofemoropopliteal

femoropopliteal bypass

femorotibial
f. bypass

FemoStop
F. femoral artery compres-
sion arch
F. inflatable pneumatic
compression device
F. pneumatic compression

fem-pop bypass

fenestrated
f. Fontan operation

fenestration
aortopulmonary f.
baffle f.
cusp f.

FEP-ringed Gore-Tex vascular
graft

Fergie needle

Ferguson
F. forceps
F. needle

Fergus percutaneous introducer kit

Fernandez reaction

ferruginous bodies

ferrule (on pacemaker wires)

FES
fat embolism syndrome
flame emission spectros-
copy

fetal
f. alcohol syndrome (FAS)
f. bradycardia
f. circulation
f. electrocardiography
f. heart rate
f. souffle
f. tachycardia

FF
fibrillation-flutter

FFA
free fatty acids

FFA-labeled scintigraphy

f-f interval

FFP
fresh frozen plasma

FGF
fibroblast growth factor

FH
family history
familial hypercholesterolemia

FHC
familial hypertrophic cardiomyopathy

fiber
accelerating f.
afferent nerve f's
astral f.
atriohisian f.
blocking vagal afferent f's
blocking vagal efferent f's
Brechenmacher f.
bulbospiral f.
bystander f.
cardiac accelerator f.
cardiac depressor f.
cardiac muscle f.
cardiac pressor f.
chromatic f.
chromosomal f.
continuous f.
depressor f.
dietary f.
fasciculoventricular f.
fasciculoventricular Ma-
haim f.
half-spindle f.
His-Purkinje f's
Henle f's
impulse-conducting f.
interzonal f.
James f.
Kent f.

fiber *(continued)*
    Mahaim f.
    mantle f.
    muscle f.
    nodoventricular f.
    parasympathetic nerve f's
    pseudo-Mahaim f.
    Purkinje f.
    f. shortening
    f. shortening velocity (V_{CF})
    sinospiral f.
    sinuspiral f.
    spindle f.
    terminal conducting f. of
      Purkinje
    terminal Purkinje f's
    traction f.
    wavy f.

Fiberlase system

fiberoptic
    f. catheter delivery system
    f. delivery device
    f. pressure catheter

fibric acid

fibrillar collage network

fibrillary waves

fibrillation
    atrial f.
    auricular f.
    cardiac f.
    chronic atrial f.
    continuous atrial f.
    electric f.
    idiopathic f.
    lone atrial f.
    paroxysmal atrial f.
    f. potential
    f. rhythm
    f. threshold
    ventricular f.
    ventricular tachycardia/
      ventricular f.

fibrillation-flutter (FF)
    atrial f.-f.

fibrillatory wave

fibrilloflutter

fibrin
    f. clot
    f. glue
    f. split product
    f. thrombus

fibrinogen
    f. degradation product
    plasma f.
    radio labeled f.
    technetium 99 f.

fibrinogen-fibrin
    f.-f. conversion syndrome
    f.-f. degradation product

fibrinogenolysis

fibrinohematic material

fibrinoid
    f. arteritis
    f. changes
    f. degeneration
    f. necrosis

fibrinolysis
    low-dose f.
    f. of thrombi

fibrinolytic
    early intravenous f. ther-
      apy
    f. reaction
    f. system
    f. therapy

fibrinopeptide A

fibrinoplatelet

fibrinous
    f. adhesion
    f. exudate
    f. pericarditis

fibrin-specific antigen

fibrin-stabilizing blood coagula-
    tion factor

fibroblast growth factor

fibrobullous

fibrocalcification

fibrocalcific lesion

fibroelastoma
  papillary f.

fibroelastosis
  endocardial f.
  endomyocardial f.
  primary endocardial f.

fibrofatty plaque

fibrogenesis

fibroid
  f. heart
  f. lung
  f. phthisis

fibroma
  f. of heart

fibromuscular dysplasia

fibromusculoelastic lesion

fibronectin

fibroplastic
  f. cardiomyopathy
  f. disease

fibroplastica
  endocarditis parietalis f.

fibroproliferative

fibrosa
  intervalvular f.

fibrosarcoma
  f. of heart

fibrosis
  African endomyocardial f.
  biventricular endomyocardial f.
  bundle branch f.
  Davies endomyocardial f.
  diffuse interstitial pulmonary f. (DIPF)
  endocardial f.
  endomyocardial f.
  idiopathic pulmonary f.

fibrosis (continued)
  myocardial f.
  nodal f.
  partial intermixed f.
  perielectrode f.
  perivascular f.
  pulmonary f.
  rheumatic f.
  tropical endomyocardial f.

fibrosum
  pericardium f.

fibrosus
  annulus f.

fibrothorax

fibrotic
  f. mitral valve

fibrous
  f. body
  f. dysplasia
  f. dysplasia of bone
  f. mediastinitis
  f. pericarditis
  f. pericardium
  f. plaque
  f. skeleton
  f. subaortic stenosis

Fick
  F. cardiac output
  F. equation
  F. principle
  F. technique

Fiedler myocarditis

figure
  f. 8 heart
  mitotic f.

figure-of-8 abnormality

figure-of-eight suture

filament
  axial f.
  intermediate f's
  linin f.

filamin

filariasis

FILE
    Family Index of Life Events

Filcard vena cava filter

filiformis
    pulsus f.

filiform pulse

filled by collaterals

filling
    capillary f.
    collateral f.
    f. defect
    diastolic f.
    f. fraction
    f. gallop
    rapid f.
    retrograde f.
    f. rumble
    ventricular f.

filter
    arterial f.
    bandpass f.
    bidirectional four-pole But-
        terworth f.
    bird's nest vena cava f.
    BTF-37 arterial blood f.
    Butterworth bidirectional f.
    caval f.
    D/Flex f.
    Filcard vena cava f.
    Gianturco-Roehm bird's
        nest vena cava f.
    Greenfield f.
    Greenfield IVC f.
    Greenfield vena cava f.
    Hamming-Hahn f.
    heparin arterial f.
    high-pass digital f.
    inferior vena cava f.
    Interface arterial blood f.
    Jostra arterial blood f.
    Kim-Ray Greenfield f.
    K-37 pediatric arterial
        blood f.
    LeukoNet F.
    mediastinal sump f.
    Millipore f.

filter (continued)
    Mobin-Uddin umbrella f.
    Mobin-Uddin vena cava f.
    Re/Flex f.
    Simon nitinol inferior vena
        cava f.
    Simon-nitinol IVC f.
    Swank high-flow arterial
        blood f.
    triple-bandpass f.
    umbrella f.
    vena cava f.
    Vena Tech LGM f.
    Wiener f.
    William Harvey arterial
        blood f.

filtragometry

filtration
    x-ray beam f.

filum
    f. coronarium

fimbrin

final
    f. common pathway
    f. rapid repolarization

Finapres
    F. blood pressure monitor
    F. finger cuff

Finesse
    F. cardiac device
    F. guiding catheter

finger
    f. cuff
    dead f.
    f. dilation
    f. fracture dissection
    waxy f.
    white f.

fingerbreadth

finger-in-glove appearance

fingernail
    watch-crystal f.

fingerprint edema

finned pacemaker lead

Finney mask

Finochietto
  F. forceps
  F. retractor
  F. rib spreader
  F. thoracic scissors
  F.-Geissendorfer rib retractor

FiO$_2$
  forced inspiratory oxygen

firing
  laser f.

first
  f.-degree AV block
  f.-degree heart block
  f. effort
  f.-effort angina
  f. heart sound (S1)
  f. obtuse marginal artery
  f. pass study
  f. shock count
  f.-third filling fraction

Fischer
  F. pneumothoracic needle
  F. sign
  F. symptom

Fisher
  F. exact test
  F. murmur
  F.-Paykel MR290 water-feed chamber

fishhook lead

fish-mouth
  f.-m. cusp
  f.-m. incision
  f.-m. mitral stenosis

fishnet pattern

fission
  binary f.
  cellular f.
  multiple f.

fissiparous

fissuring
  plaque f.

fist percussion

fistula *pl.* fistulae, fistulas
  aortic sinus f.
  aortocaval f.
  aortoenteric f.
  aorto-left ventricular f.
  aorto-right ventricular f.
  arteriovenous f. (AVF)
  A-V Gore-Tex f.
  brachioaxillary bridge graft f.
  Brescia-Cimino A-V f.
  cameral f.
  carotid-cavernous f.
  Cimino-Brescia arteriovenous f.
  congenital coronary f.
  congenital pulmonary arteriovenous f.
  coronary artery-right ventricular f.
  coronary arteriovenous f.
  coronary artery f.
  coronary-cameral f.
  coronary-pulmonary f.
  Eck f.
  enteric f.
  Gore-Tex AF f.
  Gross tracheoesophageal f.
  intrapulmonary arteriovenous f.
  pulmonary arteriovenous f.
  solitary pulmonary arteriovenous f.
  subclavian arteriovenous f.
  traumatic f.

Fitch obturator

fitness
  cardiovascular f.

Fitzgerald
  F. forceps
  F. aortic aneurysm forceps

five-chamber view

fixed-rate
  f.-r. mode
  f.-r. pacemaker
  f.-r. perfusion defect

fixed-wire balloon dilatation system

FL4 guide

Flack node

flagella

flagellar

flagelliform

flagellum

flail
  f. chest
  f. chordae
  f. leaflet
  f. mitral valve
  f. segments

flair valve

flame emission spectroscopy

flame-shaped hemorrhages

flank incision

flap
  Abbe f.
  Eloesser f.
  intimal f.
  Linton f.
  liver f.
  microvascular free f.
  pericardial f.
  scimitar-shaped f.
  Waldenhausen subclavian f.

flapping
  f. sound
  f. tremor
  f. valve syndrome

flare
  wheal and f.

FLASH (fast low-angle shot) cardiac MRI

flashlamp
  f.-excited pulsed dye
  f.-pulsed Nd:YAG laser

flask-shaped heart

flat
  f.-hand test
  f. lined
  f. neck veins
  f. P wave

flattening
  f. of ST segment
  T wave f.

Fleischner syndrome

Fletcher factor

Flex
  F. stent
  F. Tip guidewire

Flexguide intubation guide

Flexguard Tip catheter

flexible
  f. J guide wire
  f. steerable wire

Flexicath silicone subclavian cannula

Flexon steel suture

FlexStent
  Cook F.

Flex-Stent stent

flicker fusion threshold

Flint
  F. murmur

flint
  f. disease

flip
  f. angle
  f. flop of heart
  LDH f.

flipped T wave

floating wall motion study

FloMap
  F. guidewire
  F. velocimeter

floppy
  f. mitral valve
  f. valve syndrome

floppy-tipped guidewire

Flo-Rester
  F. vascular occluder
  F. vessel occluder

Florex medical compression
  stockings

florid
  f. congestive heart failure
  f. pulmonary edema

flotation catheter

fluorescent
  f. antimembrane antibody
    (FAMA)
  f. in situ hybridization
  f. treponemal antibody ab-
    sorption (FTA-ABS)

flow
  f. across orifice
  antegrade diastolic f.
  anterograde f.
  aortic f.
  arterial blood f.
  f. artifact
  f.-assisted, short term
    (FAST)
  blood f.
  cerebral blood f. (CBF)
  chronic reserve f.
  collateral f.
  f. convergence method
  coronary blood f.
  coronary reserve f. (CRF)
  coronary sinus blood f.
  f.-directed balloon cardio-
    vascular catheter
  effective pulmonary blood
    f. (EPBF)
  effective pulmonic f.

flow *(continued)*
  endocardial f.
  f. envelope
  epicardial f.
  forward f.
  Ganz method for coronary
    sinus f.
  great cardiac vein f.
  hepatofugal f.
  hepatopetal f.
  high f.
  high velocity f.
  f. injector
  laminar blood f.
  left-to-right f.
  f.-limiting stenosis
  f. mapping
  f. mapping technique
  mitral valve f.
  myocardial blood f.
  pansystolic f.
  petal-fugal f.
  pulmonary blood f.
  pulmonic output f.
  pulmonic versus system-
    ic f.
  pulsatile f.
  f. rate
  f. ratio (Qp/Qs)
  redistribution of pulmo-
    nary vascular f.
  regional myocardial
    blood f.
  regurgitant systolic f.
  restoration of f.
  retrograde systolic f.
  reversed vertebral blood f.
    (RVBF)
  sluggish f.
  splanchnic blood f.
  systemic blood f.
  total cerebral blood f.
    (TCBF)
  transmitral f.
  transvascular blood f.
  tricuspid valve f.
  turbulent blood f.
  f. velocity
  f. wire

flow *(continued)*
    Wright peak f.

FloWire
    Doppler F.
    F. guidewire

flowmeter
    blood f.
    Doppler ultrasonic f.
    Gould electromagnetic f.
    laser Doppler f.
    Narcomatic f.
    Parks 800 bidirectional
        Doppler f.
    Statham electromagnetic f.
    Transonic f.
    transit time f.
    transit time ultrasonic f.
    ultrasonic f.

flowmetry
    magnetic resonance f.
    pulsed Doppler f.

Flowtron
    F. DVT pump
    F. DVT pump system

flow-volume loop

Floyd loop cannula

fluens
    pulsus f.

fluffy-cuffed tube

fluid
    f. aspiration
    f. challenge
    crystalloid f.
    f. dynamics
    f.-filled balloon-tipped flow-
        directed catheter
    f.-filled pigtail catheter
    f.-filled Pressure monitoring
        guidewire
    f. mechanics
    pericardial f.
    f. therapy

fluorescein angiography

fluorescence
    f.-guided smart laser
    laser-induced arterial f.
    f. polarization
    f. spectroscopy

fluorine-18 deoxyglucose

fluorography
    spot-film fluorescent f.

fluoroscopic
    advanced under f. control
    f. guidance
    f. visualization

fluoroscopy
    biplane f.
    C-arm f.
    kV f.

Fluoro Tip cannula

Fluosol
    F. artificial blood
    F.-DA 20% (oxygen trans-
        port fluid)

flush
    f. aortogram
    f. aortography
    f. and bathe technique
    heparin f.
    heparinized saline f.
    mahogany f.
    malar f.

flushed
    aspirated and f.

flushing
    f. time
    f. of catheter

flutter
    atrial f.
    auricular f.
    coarse atrial f.
    f. cycle length
    diaphragmatic f.
    impure f.
    mediastinal f.
    pure f.

flutter *(continued)*
    f. R interval
    ventricular f.

flutter-fibrillation
    f.-f. waves

fluttering of valvular leaflet

Flutter therapeutic device

flux
    soldering f.
    transmembrane calcium f.

fluxionary hyperemia

Flynt needle

FMA cardiovascular imaging
  system

FMV
    floppy mitral valve

FNA
    fine-needle aspiration

foam
    f. cell
    polyurethane f.
    f. stability test

foamy
    f. macrophage
    f. myocardial cell

focal
    f. block
    f. eccentric stenosis
    f. edema
    f. wall motion abnormality

focus *pl.* foci
    arrhythmia f.
    Assmann f.
    Ghon f.
    Simon foci

fodrin

Foerger airway

Foerster forceps

Fogarty
    F. adherent clot catheter

Fogarty *(continued)*
    F. arterial embolectomy
      catheter
    F. balloon catheter
    F. calibrator
    F. embolectomy catheter
    F. forceps
    F. graft thrombectomy
      catheter
    F. Hydrogrip clamp
    F. occlusion catheter
    F. venous thrombectomy
      catheter
    F.-Chin clamp
    F.-Chin extrusion balloon
      catheter

fold
    bulboventricular f.
    Marshall f.
    Rindfleisch f.
    vestigial f.

Folex PFS

folic acid

Foltz-Overton cardiac catheter

Fontaine classification system
  for peripheral vascular claudication (Roman numerals)

Fontan
    F. atriopulmonary anasto-
      mosis
    F. modification of Norwood
      procedure
    F. operation
    F. operation for tricuspid
      atresia and pulmonary
      stenosis
    F. repair
    F.-Baudet procedure
    F.-Kreutzer procedure
    F.-Kreutzer repair, modified

food
    f. angina

foot
    f. cradle
    trash f.

foot *(continued)*
    f. ulcer

foramen *pl.* foramina
    bulboventricular f.
    Galen f.
    interventricular f.
    Lannelongue f.
    f. of Moro
    f. of Morgagni
    f. ovale, oval f.
    f. of smallest veins of heart
    thebesian f.
    f. secundum
    f. venarum minimarum
        atrii dextri
    f. venae cavae
    Vieussens f.

Force balloon dilatation catheter

force
    atrial ejection f.
    drag f's
    f.-frequency relation
    lateral anterior f.
    left ventricular f's
    f.-length relation
    peak twitch f.
    P terminal f.
    reserve f.
    rest f.
    shear f.
    Starling f's
    Venturi f's

forced
    f. beat
    f. cycle
    f. ischemia-reperfusion
        transition

forceps
    Adson f.
    alligator f.
    Allis f.
    artery f.
    Babcock thoracic tissue-holding f.

forceps *(continued)*
    Bailey aortic valve cutting f.
    Barraya f.
    Bengolea f.
    biopsy f.
    Bloodwell f.
    Boettcher f.
    bronchus f.
    Brown-Adson f.
    Brunschwig f.
    bulldog f.
    Carmalt f.
    coagulation f.
    Cooley f.
    Cooley-Baumgarten aortic f.
    Crafoord f.
    Crafoord-Sellors hemostatic f.
    Crile f.
    Cushing f.
    Dale f.
    Davis f.
    DeBakey arterial f.
    DeBakey Autraugrip f.
    DeBakey dissecting f.
    DeBakey tissue f.
    DeBakey vascular f.
    DeBakey-Bahnson f.
    DeBakey-Bainbridge f.
    DeBakey-Colovira-Rumel thoracic f.
    DeBakey-Cooley f.
    DeBakey-Diethrich vascular f.
    DeBakey-Mixter thoracic f.
    DeBakey-Péan cardiovascular f.
    DeBakey-Semb f.
    Duval lung f.
    Duval-Crile lung f.
    Effler-Groves f.
    Englert f.
    Evans f.
    Fergeson f.
    Finochietto f.
    Fitzgerald f.
    Fitzgerald aortic aneurysm f.

forceps *(continued)*
- Foerster f.
- Fogarty f.
- Foss cardiovascular f.
- Fraenkel f.
- Gemini thoracic f.
- Gerald f.
- Gerbode f.
- Glover f.
- grasping f.
- Halstead f.
- Harken f.
- Harrington thoracic f.
- Harrington-Mixter f.
- Hayes Martin f.
- Heiss artery f.
- hemoclip-applying f.
- Hendrin f.
- Hopkins f.
- Horsley f.
- Iselin f.
- Jacobson f.
- Johns Hopkins f.
- Johnson f.
- Jones IMA f.
- Julian thoracic f.
- Karp aortic punch f.
- Lahey thoracic f.
- Lebsche f.
- Lees artery f.
- Lejune thoracic f.
- Leland-Jones f.
- Leriche f.
- Lillehei valve f.
- Liston-Stille f.
- Love-Gruenwald f.
- Mayo Pean f.
- McNealy-Glassman-Mixter f.
- Mixter f.
- mosquito f.
- Mount-Mayfield f.
- NIH mitral valve f.
- Ochsner f.
- O'Shaughnessy artery f.
- Overholt thoracic f.
- Phaneuf artery f.
- Potts bronchus f.
- Potts bulldog f.
- Potts thumb f.

forceps *(continued)*
- Potts vascular f.
- Potts-Smith tissue f.
- Price-Thomas bronchial f.
- Randall stone f.
- Rienhoff f.
- Rochester-Mixter artery f.
- Ruel f.
- Rumel thoracic f.
- Ruskin f.
- Russian tissue f.
- Samuels f.
- Sarot artery f.
- Satinsky f.
- Sauerbruch f.
- Scholten endomyocardial bioptome and biopsy f.
- Selman vessel f.
- Semb f.
- Singley f.
- Snowden-Pencer f.
- sponge f.
- Stille-Luer f.
- straight-end cup f.
- Thomas-Allis f.
- thumb f.
- tissue f.
- tonsillar f.
- torsion f.
- Tuttle thoracic f.
- up-biting cup f.
- Vanderbilt f.
- Varco thoracic f.
- Westphal f.
- Yasargil artery f.

Ford equation

Forerunner coronary sinus guiding catheter

Forlanini treatment

form
- myocardial infarction in dumbbell f.

forme fruste

formicans
- pulsus f.

formicant pulse

formula *pl.* formulas, formulae
  Bazett f.
  biplane f.
  Bohr f.
  Brozek f.
  Cannon f.
  Einthoven f.
  Fick f.
  Friedewald f.
  Ganz f.
  geometric cube f.
  Gorland f.
  Gorlin f.
  Hakki f.
  Hamilton-Stewart f.
  Janz f.
  f. of Mirsky
  Poiseuille resistance f.
  Sramek f.
  Teichholz f.
  Yeager f.

Forney syndrome

Forrester
  F. syndrome
  F. Therapeutic Classification grades I through IV

fortis
  pulsus f.

forward
  f. conduction
  f. flow of velocity
  f. heart failure
  f. stroke volume (FSV)
  f. triangle method
  f. triangle technique

fossa *pl.* fossae
  antecubital f.
  cardiac f.
  f. ovalis
  oval f. of heart
  f. ovalis cordis
  supraclavicular f.

Foss cardiovascular forceps

Fothergill disease

founder effect

four-beam laser Doppler probe

four-chamber
  f.-c. view
  f.-c. apical view
  f.-c. plane on echocardiography

four-day syndrome

Fourier
  fast F. transform
  F. series analysis
  F. transform
  F. transform analysis
  F. two-dimensional imaging

four-legged cage valve

Fourmentin thoracic index

fourth heart sound (S4)

foveated chest

Fowler
  F. thoracoplasty
  F. position

Fox green dye

fraction
  beta lipoprotein f.
  CPK-MB f.
  ejection f.
  filling f.
  first-third filling f.
  global left ventricular ejection f.
  growth f.
  left ventricular ejection f. (LVEF)
  light pen-determined ejection f.
  MB f.
  MM f.
  regurgitant f.
  rest ejection f.
  right ventricular ejection f.
  shortening f.
  Teichholz ejection f.

fractional
  f. myocardial shortening

fracture
cough f.
outlet strut f.
pacemaker lead f.
plaque f.

Fraenkel
F. forceps
F. nodes

fragility
capillary f.

fragment
f. antigen-binding
antimyosin monoclonal antibody with FAB f.
catheter f.
Digibind digoxin immune Fab f's
Digidote digoxin immune Fab f's
Fab f.

fragmentation
f. myocarditis
f. of myocardium

Framingham Heart study

frank blood

Frank
F. EKG lead placement system
F. XYZ orthogonal lead
F.-Starling curve
F.-Starling mechanism
F.-Starling reserve
F.-Straub-Wiggers-Starling principle

Frankel treatment

Fräntzel murmur

Franzen needle guide

Franz monophasic action potential catheter

frappage

Frater
F. intracardiac retractor

Frater (continued)
F. suture

Fraunhofer zone

Frazier suction tip; tube

Fredrickson
F. classification
F. dyslipidemia
F. hyperlipoproteinemia classification
F., Levy, and Lees classification

free
f. end of electrode
f. fatty acids
f. thyroxine index

free-beam laser

FreeDop
F. portable Doppler unit

freeing up of adhesion

Freer elevator

Freestyle aortic root bioprosthesis

Freitag stent

frémissement cataire

fremitus
auditory f.
friction f.
hydatid f.
pectoral f.
pericardial f.
tactile f.
vocal f.

French
F. double-lumen catheter
F. 5 angiographic catheter
F. JR4 Schneider catheter
F. MBIH catheter
F. paradox
F. SAL catheter
F. scale
F. shaft catheter
F. sheath
F. size

French *(continued)*
    F. sizing of catheter

frequency
    ciliary beat f.
    critical flicker f.
    f. domain imaging
    dynamic f. response
    fundamental f.
    natural f.
    pulse repetition f.
    resonant f.
    f. response
    f. shifter
    f. tracer

frequency-domain analysis

frequens
    pulsus f.

fresh frozen plasma (FFP)

Fresnel zone

Freund
    F. anomaly
    F. operation

Frey-Sauerbruch rib shears

friable wall

friction
    f. fremitus
    f. murmur
    f. rub
    f. sound

Friedewald
    F. approximation
    F. equation
    F. formula

Friedländer disease

Friedman
    F. Splint brace
    F. test

Friedrich
    Friedrich rib elevator
    Friedrich sign

froissement
    bruit de f.

frolement

front wall needle

frontal plane on EKG

frontotemporal

frosted heart

frosting heart

frottement
    bruit de f.

Frouin
    quadrangulation of F.

frozen thorax

FRP
    functional refractory period
        FRP atrial
        FRP ventricular

fruste
    forme f.

frustrate systole

FSV
    forward stroke volume

FTA-ABS
    fluorescent treponemal antibody absorption

fucosidosis

Fukunaga-Hayes unbiased jackknife classification

fulcrum
    left ventricular f.

fulguration
    f. during electrophysiologic study
    electrical f.
    endocavity f.

fully automatic pacemaker

fulminans
    purpura f.

function
    atrial transport f.

function *(continued)*
- cardiac f.
- cardiovascular f.
- contractile f.
- f. curve
- diastolic f.
- exercise LV f.
- global left ventricular f.
- left ventricular f. (LVF)
- left ventricular systolic/ diastolic f.
- left ventricular systolic pump f.
- mitochondrial f.
- myocardial f.
- neurohormonal f.
- parasympathetic f.
- perturbed autonomic nervous system f.
- phagocytic f.
- probability density f.
- pump f.
- regional left ventricle f.
- right ventricular f.
- right ventricular systolic/ diastolic f.
- sigh f.
- sinus node f.
- systolic f.
- ventricular f.
- ventricular contractility f. (VCF)

functional
- f. aerobic impairment (FAI)
- f. assessment
- f. block
- f. capacity classification
- f. cardiovascular disease
- f. classification of CHF
- f. congestion
- f. dyspnea

functional *(continued)*
- f. image
- f. murmur
- f. pain
- f. refractory period (FRP)

fundamental frequency

fundus *pl.* fundi

funduscopic examination

funduscopy

fungal
- f. endocarditis
- f. infection

fungating mass

funic
- f. pulse
- f. souffle

funnel
- f. chest
- f. dynamics
- mitral f.
- vascular f.

Furman Type II electrogram

furrow
- atrioventricular f.
- Schmorl f.

fusiform
- f. aortic aneurysm

fusion
- f. beat
- commissural f.
- f. complex
- critical flicker f.
- entrainment with concealed f.
- f. QRS complex

G

3G4

G5
    G5 massage and percussion machine
    G5 Neocussor percussor

Ga
    gallium

^{68}Ga
    gallium 68

Gabriel Tucker tube

Gad hypothesis

Gaertner phenomenon

Gaillard syndrome

gain
    g. control
    time compensation g.
    time-varied g.

Gairdner disease

Gaisböck syndrome

gaiter perforators

galactophlebitis

galactose

galactosidase deficiency

Galanti-Giusti colorimetric method

Galaxy pacemaker

Galen foramen

Gallagher bipolar mapping probe

Gallavardin
    G. murmur
    G. phenomenon

gallinatum
    pectus g.

gallium (Ga)
    g. 67
    g. 68

gallium (continued)
    g. imaging
    g. scan
    g. scintigraphy

gallop
    atrial g.
    diastolic g.
    filling g.
    fourth heart sound g.
    low frequency g.
    presystolic g.
    protodiastolic g.
    g. rhythm
    S_3 g.
    S_4 g.
    S_7 g.
    summation g. (S_7)
    third heart sound g.
    ventricular g.
    ventricular diastolic g.

gallop, murmur, or rub (GMR)

galop
    bruit de g.

galvanometer
    Einthoven g.
    string g.
    thread g.

Gambro
    G. Lundia Minor hemodialyzer
    G. oxygenator

Gamna-Gandy bodies

ganglion
    Bezold g.
    Bock g.
    Remak g.
    sinoatrial g.
    sinus g.
    stellate g.
    Wrisberg g.

ganglionectomy
    left stellate g.

ganglionic blocker

gangliosidosis

gangrene
  angiosclerotic g.
  cold g.
  diabetic g.
  dry g.
  embolic g.
  Fournier g.
  gas g.
  hot g.
  Raynaud g.

gangrenosa
  angina g.

gannister disease

Ganz
  G. formula
  G.-Edwards coronary infusion catheter

gap
  anion g.
  auscultatory g.
  chromatid g.
  g. conduction phenomenon
  excitable g.
  isochromatid g.
  g. junction
  silent g.

Garcia aorta clamp

gargoylism

garment
  antishock g.
  Jobst pressure g.
  pneumatic antishock g.

garnet
  yttrium-aluminum-g. (YAG)

Garrett
  G. dilator
  G. retractor
  G. vascular dilator

Gärtner
  G. method
  G. tonometer
  G. vein phenomenon

gas
  arterial blood g. (ABG)
  blood g.
  capillary blood g.
  g. chromatography
  g. clearance
  g. clearance method
  g. constant
  g. embolism
  g. endarterectomy
  g. exchange
  g. gangrene

gaseous pulse

gasp reflex

gastrocardiac syndrome

gastroepiploic artery

gate
  acquisition g.
  D g.
  F g.
  H g.
  M g.

gated
  g. blood-pool angiography
  g. blood-pool cardiac wall motion study
  g. blood-pool imaging
  g. blood-pool scanning
  g. blood-pool scintigraphy
  g. blood-pool study
  g. blood-pool ventriculogram
  g. cardiac scan
  g. cardiac blood pool imaging
  g. computed tomography
  g. equilibrium blood pool scanning
  g. equilibrium ventriculography, frame-mode acquisition
  g. equilibrium ventriculography, list-mode acquisition
  g. list mode
  g. nuclear angiogram

gated (continued)
  g. radionuclide angiography
  g. sweep magnetic resonance imaging
  g. system
  g. technique

GateWay Y-adapter rotating hemostatic valve

gating
  cardiac g.
  in-memory g.
  g. mechanism
  g. of heartbeats
  R wave g.
  g. signal

Gaucher disease

gauge
  mercury-in-Silastic strain g.
  pounds per square inch g.
  Silastic strain g.
  strain g.

gaussian

Gauthier bicycle ergometer

gauze
  Teletrast g.
  Xeroform g.
  Surgicel g.

GBPS
  gated blood-pool study

Gc protein

GCS
  graduated compression stockings

GCVF
  great cardiac vein flow

Gd-DTPA
  gadolinium-diethylenetriamine pentaacetic acid
  Gd-DTPA-enhanced MRI

GDP
  guanosine 5'-diphosphate

GEA
  gastroepiploic artery
  GEA graft

Gehan statistic

gel
  aluminum hydroxide g.
  Cann-Ease moisturizing nasal g.
  Dermaflex G.
  EKG g.
  electrode g.
  Lectron II g.
  H.P. Acthar G.

gelatin
  absorbable g.
  g. compression body
  g. compression boot
  g. sponge slurry
  zinc g.

gelatinous debris

Gelfilm

gelfiltration

Gelfoam
  G. cookie
  thrombin-soaked G.
  G. Topical

Gelpi retractor

gelsolin

Gemini
  G. DDD pacemaker
  G. 415 DDD pacemaker
  G. thoracic forceps

gemma

Gen2 pacemaker

gene
  angiotensinogen g.
  beta-myosin heavy-chain g.
  env g.

gene *(continued)*
   g. expression
   gag g.
   human preproendothelin-1 g.
   g. secretor
   g. transcription
   tuple-1 g.
   zinc finger g.

General Electric
   G. E. Advantx system
   G. E. Pass-C echocardiograph machine
   G. E. pacemaker

generation
   thrombin g.

generator
   asynchronous g.
   asynchronous pulse g.
   atrial synchronous pulse g.
   atrial triggered pulse g.
   Aurora pulse g.
   bipolar g.
   Bird neonatal CPAP g.
   Chardack-Greatbatch implantable cardiac pulse g.
   Coratomic implantable pulse g.
   Cordis Theta Sequicor DDD pulse g.
   Cosmos pulse g.
   Cosmos II pulse g.
   CPI-PRx pulse g.
   Cyberlith multiprogrammable pulse g.
   demand pulse g.
   Down flow g.
   fixed-rate pulse g.
   implantable pulse g.
   Intec AID cardioverter-defibrillator g.
   intrapleural pulse g.
   Itrell I unipolar pulse g.
   lithium powered pulse g.
   Maxilith pacemaker pulse g.
   Medtronic pulse g.

generator *(continued)*
   Microlith pacemaker pulse g.
   Minilith pacemaker pulse g.
   multiprogrammable pulse g.
   physiologic g.
   Programalith III pulse g.
   pulse g.
   quadripolar Itrell 2 pulse g.
   standby pulse g.
   Stilith implantable cardiac pulse g.
   Spectrax SXT pulse g.
   subpectoral pulse g.
   tantalum-178 g g.
   Telectronics PASAR antitachycardia pulse g.
   Trilogy DC, DR, SR pulse g.
   ventricular demand g.
   ventricular inhibited pulse g.
   ventricular synchronous pulse g.
   ventricular triggered pulse g.
   Versatrax pulse g.
   Vivalith II pulse g.
   x-ray g.

GenESA closed-loop delivery system

genetic
   g. disorder
   g. heterogeneity
   g. hypertrophic cardiomyopathy
   g. locus
   g. transmission

Gensini
   G. cardiac device
   G. catheter
   G. coronary arteriography catheter
   G. index
   G. score
   G. scoring of coronary artery disease

Gensini *(continued)*
G. Teflon catheter

Gentle-Flo suction catheter

Gentran 40:75

geometry
normal g.
g. of stenosis
ventricular g.

George Lewis technique

George Washington strut

geotrichosis

Gerald forceps

Gerbode
G. annuloplasty
G. defect
G. dilator
G. forceps
G. mitral valvulotome
G. patent ductus clamp
G. sternal retractor
G. valve dilator

Gerdy intra-auricular loop

Gerhardt
G. change
G. syndrome
G. triangle

gestational hypertension

Gey solution

GHB
gamma hydroxybutyrate

Ghon
G. complex
G. focus
G. primary lesion

ghost vessel

giant
g. cell
g. cell aortitis
g. cell arteritis
g. cell carcinoma

giant *(continued)*
g. cell myocarditis
g. v wave
g. a wave

Gianturco
G. stent
G. wool-tufted wire coil
G. Z stent
G.-Roehm bird's nest vena
cava filter
G.-Roubin stent

Gibbon-Landis test

Gibson
G. circularity index
G. murmur
G. rule

Giertz
G. rib guillotine
G. rongeur
G.-Shoemaker rib shears

Gigli saw

Gill I respirator

Gill-Jonas modification of Norwood procedure

giving-up/given-up response

gland
arteriococcygeal g.
carotid g.
coccygeal g.
glomiform g.
intercarotid g.
Luschka g.
vascular g.

glandula
g. glomiformis

glare
veiling g.

Glasgow
G. Coma Scale
G. sign

Glassman clamp

glassy degeneration

Glattelast compression pantyhose

Glenn
  G. anastomosis
  G. operation
  G. procedure
  G. shunt

Glidecath hydrophilic-coated catheter

Glidewire
  G. Gold surgical guidewire

glissonitis

global
  g. amnesia
  g. aphasia
  g. cardiac disease
  g. ejection fraction
  g. hypokinesis
  g. left ventricular ejection fraction
  g. left ventricular function
  g. ventricular dysfunction

globoid heart

globular
  g. heart
  g. thrombus

globulin
  antithymocyte g.
  gamma g.
  lymphocyte immune g.
  rabbit antithymocyte g.
  Rho(D) immune g.

glomectomy

glomic

glomoid

glomus *pl.* glomera
  glomera aortica
  g. coccygeum
  jugular g.
  g. jugulare

glomus *(continued)*
  g. tympanicum
  g. vagale

glossopharyngeal
  g. breathing
  g. neuralgia

glottic atresia

glove
  compression g's
  ESP radiation reduction examination g's

gloved fist technique

Glover
  G. auricular-appendage clamp
  G. coarctation clamp
  G. patent ductus clamp
  G. vascular clamp

Gluck rib shears

glucocorticoid

glucocorticoid-induced hypertension

glue
  fibrin g.

glu-plasminogen

glutamate

glutamic-oxaloacetic transaminase

glutamic oxalotransaminase

glutaraldehyde
  g.-tanned bovine collagen tube
  g.-tanned bovine heart valve
  g.-tanned porcine heart valve

glutathione

glyceraldehyde 3-phosphate

glycocalicine index

glycocalix, glycocalyx

glycogen
  g. cardiomegaly
  g. depletion
  g. loading
  g. phosphorylase
  g. storage disease
  g. synthase

glycogenosis
  cardiac g.

glycolysis

glycolytic enzymes

glycopeptide teicoplanin

glycoprotein
  g. Iib/IIIa receptor
  platelet receptor g.

glycopyrrolate

glycoside
  cardiac g.
  digitalis g.

glycosis

glycosphingolipid disorder

glycosylated hemoglobin

glycosylation of intracellular
  proteins

GM-CSF
  granulocyte/macrophage
    colony-stimulating factor

GMP
  guanosine monophosphate

GMR
  gallop, murmur or rub

GNB
  gram-negative bacilli

goblet
  g. cell
  g. cell degranulation
  g. cell metaplasia

Goeltec catheter

Goethlin test

Goetz
  G. bipolar electrode
  G. cardiac device

Gohrbrand cardiac dilator

Golaski
  G. knitted Dacron graft
  G.-UMI vascular prosthesis

gold (Au)
  g. marker
  g.-195m radionuclide
  g. salt

Goldberg-MPC mediastinoscope

Goldblatt
  G. hypertension
  G. phenomenon

Golden
  S sign of G.

Goldenhar syndrome

Goldflam
  G. disease
  G.-Erb disease

Goldman
  G. cardiac risk index score
  G. index of risk
  G. risk-factor index

Goldscheider percussion

Goldsmith operation

Goldstein hemoptysis

Golgi tendon organs

golgiosome

Golub EKG lead

Gomco thoracic drainage pump

Gomori methenamine silver
  stain

gonococcal endocarditis

Goodale-Lubin
  G.-L. cardiac device

Goodale-Lubin *(continued)*
  G.-L. catheter

Goodpasture syndrome

goose-honk murmur

gooseneck deformity

Goosen vascular punch

Gordon elementary body

Gore-Tex
  G. AV fistula
  G. baffle
  G. bifurcated vascular graft
  G. cardiovascular patch
  G. catheter
  G. graft
  G. jump graft
  G. limb
  G. shunt
  G. soft tissue patch
  G. surgical membrane
  G. tube
  G. vascular graft
  G. vascular implant
  G. vascular prosthesis

Goris background subtraction
  technique

Gorland formula

Gorlin
  G. catheter
  G. constant
  G. equation
  G. formula for aortic valve
    area
  G. hydraulic formula
  G. hydraulic formula for mi-
    tral valve area
  G. method for cardiac out-
    put
  G. pacing catheter
  G. syndrome

GOT
  glutamic-oxaloacetic trans-
    aminase

Gott
  G. butterfly heart valve
  G. shunt
  G.-Daggett heart valve
    prosthesis
  G.-Daggett shunt

Gould
  G. electromagnetic flowme-
    ter
  G. PentaCath 5-lumen ther-
    modilution catheter
  G. Statham pressure trans-
    ducer

gout

gouty phlebitis

Gowers
  G. contraction
  G. sign
  G. syndrome

G6PD
  glucose-6-phosphate dehy-
    drogenase

G proteins

grabbing technique

gracile habitus

Gradational Step exercise
  stress test

grade
  thrombus g.
  g. 1 through 6 murmur
  g. 1 through 6 holosystolic
    murmur

graded exercise stress test

gradient
  aortic outflow g.
  aortic pressure g.
  aortic valve g.
  aortic valve peak instanta-
    neous g.
  arm-leg g.
  atrioventricular g.
  brain-core g.

gradient *(continued)*
coronary perfusion g.
diastolic g.
Doppler pressure g.
electrochemical g.
elevated g.
end-diastolic aortic-left
ventricular pressure g.
g. gel electrophoresis
hemodynamic g.
holosystolic g.
instantaneous g.
intracavitary pressure g.
left ventricular outflow
pressure g.
maximal estimated g.
mean mitral valve g.
mean systolic g.
mitral valve g.
outflow tract g.
peak diastolic g.
peak instantaneous g.
peak pressure g.
peak right ventricular-right
atrial systolic g.
peak systolic g.
peak to peak pressure g.
peak transaortic valve g.
pressure g.
pulmonary artery diastolic
and wedge pressure
(PADP-PAWP) g.
pulmonary artery to right
ventricle diastolic g.
pulmonary outflow g.
pulmonary valve g.
pulmonic valve g.
g. reduction
residual g.
right ventricular to main
pulmonary artery pres-
sure g.
stenotic g.
subvalvular g.
systolic g.
transaortic valve g.
translesional g.
transmitral diastolic g.
transpulmonic g.

gradient *(continued)*
transstenotic pressure g.
transtricuspid valve diastolic g.
transvalvular pressure g.
tricuspid valve g.
ventricular g.

gradient across valve

gradient-recalled acquisition in
the steady state

graduated compression stockings

graft
albumin-coated vascular g.
albuminized woven Dacron
tube g.
aldehyde-tanned bovine carotid artery g.
aorta to left anterior descending saphenous vein
bypass g.
aortic aneurysm g.
aortic tube g.
aortocoronary bypass g.
aortocoronary snake g.
aortofemoral bypass g.
(AFBG)
aortoiliac bypass g.
aortovein bypass g.
arterial g.
araldehyde-tanned bovine
carotid artery g.
autologous fat g.
autologous vein g.
AV Gore-Tex g.
bifurcated vascular g.
biograft
Bionit vascular g.
BioPolyMeric vascular g.
Björk-Shiley g.
bovine allograft
bovine heterograft
bovine pericardial heart
valve xenograft
bypass g.
Carbo-Seal cardiovascular
composite g.

graft *(continued)*
    collagen-impregnated knitted Dacron velour g.
    composite valve g.
    compressed Ivalon patch g.
    Cooley woven Dacron g.
    coronary artery bypass g. (CABG)
    Cragg endoluminal g.
    Creech aortoiliac g.
    cross-leg bypass g.
    CryoLife valvular g.
    cryopreserved human aortic allograft
    Dacron knitted g.
    Dacron onlay patch g.
    Dacron preclotted g.
    Dacron Sauvage g.
    Dacron tightly woven g.
    Dacron tube g.
    Dacron tubular g.
    Dacron velour knitted g.
    deaired g.
    g. dependent
    double velour knitted g.
    Diastat vascular access g.
    Edwards-Tapp arterial g.
    Edwards woven Teflon aortic bifurcation g.
    endothelialization of vascular g.
    EPTFE g.
    expanded polytetrafluoroethylene vascular g.
    EXS femoropopliteal bypass g.
    extracardiac g.
    extrathoracic carotid subclavian bypass g.
    Favaloro saphenous vein bypass g.
    femoral-peroneal in situ vein bypass g.
    femoro-distal vein g.
    FEP-ringed Gore-Tex vascular g.
    GEA g.
    glutaraldehyde-tanned bovine carotid artery g.

graft *(continued)*
    glutaraldehyde-tanned bovine collagen tubes for vascular g.
    glutaraldehyde-tanned porcine heart valve g.
    Golaski knitted Dacron g.
    Gore-Tex bifurcated vascular g.
    Gore-Tex jump g.
    Gore-Tex vascular g.
    Hancock pericardial valve g.
    Hancock vascular g.
    heterograft
    homograft
    Human umbilical vein bypass g.
    HUV bypass g.
    IEA g.
    IMA g.
    Impra bypass g.
    Impra Flex vascular g.
    Impra-Graft microporous PTFE vascular g.
    g. insertion site
    internal mammary artery g. (IMA)
    Ionescu-Shiley pericardial valve g.
    Ionescu-Shiley pericardial xenograft
    Ionescu-Shiley porcine heterograft heart valve g.
    ITA (internal thoracic artery) g.
    jump g.
    Kimura cartilage g.
    kinking of g.
    knitted g.
    knitted Dacron arterial g.
    LIMA (left internal mammary artery) g.
    Lo-Por vascular g.
    lower extremity bypass g.
    mammary artery g.
    mandrel g.
    Meadox g.
    Meadox Microvel g.

graft *(continued)*
  mesenteric bypass g.
  Microknit patch g.
  Microvel double velour g.
  Milliknit vascular g. prosthesis
  modified human umbilical vein g.
  nonvalved g.
  g. occlusion
  g. occlusive disease
  patch g.
  g. patency
  patent g.
  pedicle g.
  pericardial xenograft
  Perma-Flow coronary g.
  Plasma TFE vascular g.
  Poly-Plus Dacron vascular g.
  porcine g.
  porcine xenograft
  portacaval H g.
  preclotted g.
  prosthetic patch g.
  PTFE (polytetrafluoroethylene) g.
  g. rejection
  renal artery bypass g.
  reversed saphenous vein g.
  revision of g.
  saphenous g.
  saphenous vein bypass g.
  Sauvage g.
  Sauvage arterial g.
  Sauvage Bionit g.
  Sauvage vein g.
  SCA-EX 7F g.
  seamless arterial g.
  sequential g.
  Shiley Tetraflex vascular g.
  skip g.
  snake g.
  St. Jude composite valve g.
  straight g.
  straight tubular g.
  subclavian artery bypass g.
  synthetic g.

graft *(continued)*
  Teflon g.
  g. trimmed on the bias
  tube g.
  umbilical vein g.
  unilateral aortofemoral g.
  valved g.
  g. vasculopathy
  Vascutek gelseal vascular g.
  Vascutek knitted vascular g.
  Vascutek woven vascular g.
  vein g.
  vein patch g.
  Velex woven Dacron vascular g.
  velour collar g.
  ventriculoarterial g.
  vertebral artery bypass g.
  Vitagraft vascular g.
  Weavenit patch g.
  Wesolowski bypass g.
  woven Dacron g.
  woven Dacron tube g.
  Y-shaped g.

GraftAssist vein-graft holder

grafting
  endarterectomy and coronary artery bypass g. (E-CABG)
  port-access coronary artery bypass g.

graft-patch

graft-seeking catheter

graftable

Graham
  G. rib contractor
  G. Steell murmur

gram-negative
  g.-n. bacilli
  g.-n. cocci
  g.-n. endocarditis
  g.-n. organism
  g.-n. pericarditis

gram-positive
    g.-p. bacilli
    g.-p. cocci
    g.-p. organism

Gram stain

Grancher
    G. sign
    G. triad

granoplasm

Grant
    G. abdominal aortic aneu-
       rysmal clamp
    G. aneurysm clamp

granulation
    Bayle g's
    cell g's
    g. stenosis

granule
    albuminous g's
    aleuronoid g's
    atrial g's
    azurophil g.
    Babès-Ernst g.
    cytoplasmic g's
    Fauvel g.
    metachromatic g.
    Much g's
    specific atrial g's
    thread g's
    volutin g's

granulocyte/macrophage col-
    ony-stimulating factor (GM-
    CSF)

granulocytopenia

granuloma
    cocci g.
    eosinophilic g.
    sarcoid g.

granulomatosis
    allergic g.
    lymphomatoid g.
    Wegener g.

granuloplasm

grape
    Carswell g's

GRASS
    gradient-recalled acquisi-
       tion in the steady state

Grass S88 muscle stimulator

Gräupner method

Graves disease

gravidocardiac

gravitation factor

gray-scale ultrasound

great
    g. anterior radicular artery
    g. artery
    g. cardiac vein
    g. cardiac vein flow (GCVF)
    g. saphenous vein
    g. vessel

greater
    g. arterial circle of iris
    g. circulation
    g. palatine artery

green
    g. coffee bean
    g. dye curve
    g. strep endocarditis

Greene sign

Greenfield
    G. filter
    G. IVC filter
    G. inferior vena cava filter

Gregg
    G. cannula
    G. phenomenon

Gregory
    G. baby profunda clamp
    G. carotid bulldog clamp
    G. external clamp
    G. forceps

grelot
    bruit de g.

grayout spell

Gricco sign

grid
    external g.

Griesinger sign

GRIP torque device

groaning murmur

Grocco sign

Grocott methenamine silver

groin area

groin complications

Grollman
    G. catheter
    G. pulmonary artery-seek-
        ing catheter

Grönblad-Strandberg syndrome

Grondahl-Finney operation

groove
    arterial g.
    atrioventricular g.
    auriculoventricular g.
    AV g.
    bulboventricular g.
    conoventricular fold and g.
    deltopectoral g.
    Harrison g.
    interatrial g.
    interventricular g.
    interventricular g., anterior
    interventricular g., inferior
    interventricular g., poste-
        rior
    interventricular g. of heart
    terminal g.
    vascular g.
    venous g's
    Waterston g.

Groshong double-lumen cathe-
    ter

Gross
    G. coarctation occlusion
        clamp
    G.-Pomeranz-Watkins re-
        tractor

Grossman
    G. scale
    G. scale for regurgitation
    G. sign

Grover clamp

growth
    accretionary g.
    balanced g.
    g. factor
    g. hormone
    g. retardation

Gruentzig
    G. balloon catheter angio-
        plasty
    G. catheter
    G. Dilaca catheter
    G. femoral stiffening can-
        nula
    G. technique
    G. technique for PTCA

grumous
    g. debris
    g. material

grunt
    diastolic g.
    expiratory g.

G-suit

GTP
    guanosine triphosphate
    guanosine 5'-triphosphate

Guangzhou
    G. BD-1 prosthetic valve

guanine nucleotide modulatable
    binding

guanosine
    g. monophosphate (GMP)
    g. triphosphate (GTP)

guanosine *(continued)*
    g. 5'-diphosphate (GDP)
    g. 5'-triphosphate (GTP)

guanylate cyclase

Guardian
    G. AICD
    G. ATP 4210 implantable
        cardioverter-defibrillator
    G. ICD
    G. pacemaker

guar gum

Gubner-Ungerleider
    G.-U. voltage
    G.-U. voltage criteria

Guéneau de Mussy point

guidance
    echo g.
    fluoroscopic g.

Guidant TRIAD three-electrode
    energy defibrillation system

guide
    ACS LIMA g.
    Amplatz g.
    Amplatz tube g.
    Arani g.
    Cor-Flex wire g.
    FL4 g.
    Flexguide intubation g.
    Franzen needle g.
    movable core straight
        safety wire g.
    Muller catheter g.
    Pilotip catheter g.
    Slick stylette endotracheal
        tube g.
    Slidewire extension g.
    steerable wire g.
    tapered movable core
        curved wire g.
    Tefcor movable core
        straight wire g.
    TEGwire g.
    TrueTorque wire g.
    wire g.

guidelines
    McGoon g.

guider
    NL3 g.

guidewire, guide wire
    ACS g.
    ACS exchange g.
    ACS extra-support g.
    ACS floppy-tip g.
    ACS LIMA g.
    AES Amplatz g.
    Amplatz Super Stiff g.
    Amplex g.
    angiographic g.
    atherolytic reperfusion g.
    Becton-Dickinson g.
    Bentson exchange
        straight g.
    Bentson floppy-tip g.
    catheter g.
    ControlWire g.
    Coons Super Stiff long tip g.
    Cor-Flex g.
    Critikon g.
    Doppler-tipped angioplas-
        ty g.
    Elastorc catheter g.
    EnTre g.
    exchange g.
    extra-support g.
    FasTrac g.
    FasTrac hydrophilic-coa-
        ted g.
    Flex g.
    flexible g.
    Flex Tip g.
    FloMap g.
    floppy g.
    floppy-tipped g.
    FloWire g.
    fluid-filled pressure monito-
        ring g.
    Glidewire Gold surgical g.
    heparin-coated g.
    high torque g.
    Hi-Per Flex g.

guidewire *(continued)*
  Hi-Torque Flex-T g.
  Hi-Torque Floppy g.
  Hi-Torque Floppy exchan-
    ge g.
  Hi-Torque Floppy II g.
  Hi-Torque Floppy interme-
    diate g.
  Hi-Torque Intermediate g.
  Hi-Torque standard g.
  hydrophilic-coated g.
  J g.
  J Rosen g.
  J-tip g.
  J-tipped exchange g.
  g. loop
  Linx exchange g.
  Magic Torque g.
  Magnum g.
  Medi-Tech g.
  Newton g.
  PDT g.
  g. perforation
  Phantom cardiac g.
  Platinum PLUS g.
  Preceder interventional g.
  Premo g.
  Pressure guide g.
  Redifocus g.
  g. reflection
  Reflex SuperSoft steera-
    ble g.
  Roadrunner PC g.
  Rosen g.
  Rotacs g.
  safety g.
  Schwarten LP g.
  Seeker g.
  silk g.
  SOF-T g.
  soft-tipped g.
  Sones g.
  SOS g.
  stainless steel g.
  steerable g.
  steerable angioplastic g.
  straight g.
  Superselector Y-K g.
  TAD g.

guidewire *(continued)*
  Taper g.
  g. technique
  Teflon-coated g.
  Terumo g.
  transluminal coronary an-
    gioplasty g.
  Ultra-Select nitinol PTCA g.
  USCI g.
  USCI Hyperflex g.
  VeriFlex g.
  Wholey Hi-Torque floppy g.
  Wholey Hi-Torque modified
    J-g.
  Wholey Hi-Torque stan-
    dard g.

guiding catheter

guillotine
  Giertz rib g.
  rib g.
  Sauerbruch rib g.

Guisez tube

gum
  g. acacia
  g. elastic bougie introducer
  guar g.
  polacrilex chewing g.
  Stay Trim Diet g.

Gunn crossing sign

Gurvich biphasic waveform

Gutgeman
  G. clamp
  G. auricular appendage
    clamp

guttural
  g. pulse
  g. rales

gymnocyte

gymnoplast

Gyroscan
  ACS G.
  G. HP Philips 15 S whole-
    body system

H
 H gate
 H space
 H spike
 H wave
 H zone

h
 h peak
 h plateau

H1 receptor

Haake water bath

Haber-Weiss reaction

habit
 endothelioid h.
 leukocytoid h.

habitus
 gracile h.

Hadow balloon

HAEC
 human aortic endothelial
 cells

H–Ae interval

Haemolite
 H. autologous blood recov-
 ery system
 Cell Saver H.

Haemonetics
 H. Cell Saver
 H. Cell Saver System

Haemophilus
 H. b conjugate vaccine
 H. endocarditis

Hagar probe

Hageman factor

Hagenbach extension of Poiseuille equation

Haight-Finochietto rib retractor

Haimovici arteriotomy scissors

hair-matrix carcinoma

hairy heart

Hakim-Cordis pump

Hakki formula

Hakko Dwellcath catheter

Halbrecht syndrome

Haldane-Priestley tube

Haldrone

Hale piesimeter

half-amplitude pulse duration

half-life
 biological h.-l.
 elimination h.-l.

half-power distance

half-time
 h.-t. method
 pressure h.-t.

half-value layer

Hall
 H. prosthetic heart valve
 H. sign
 H. valvulotome
 H.-Kaster prosthetic valve

Hallion test

Halo catheter

halogenated
 h. hydrocarbon
 h. hydrocarbon propellant

halo sheathing

Halsted clamp

hamartoma
 myocardial h.

Hamburger test

Hamilton
 H. ventilator
 H.-Stewart formula

Hamman
 H. click

Hamman *(continued)*
  H. crunch
  H. disease
  H. murmur
  H. sign
  H.-Rich syndrome

Hammersmith mitral prosthesis

Hamming-Hahn filter

hammocking of posterior mitral
  valve leaflet

Hampton hump

Ham test

Hancock
  H. bipolar balloon pace-
    maker
  H. embolectomy catheter
  H. fiberoptic catheter
  H. hydrogen detection
    catheter
  H. luminal electrophysio-
    logic-recording catheter
  H. mitral valve prosthesis
  H. modified orifice valve
  H. M.O. II porcine biopros-
    thesis
  H. pericardial valve graft
  H. porcine heterograft
  H. porcine valve
  H. temporary cardiac pac-
    ing wire
  H. vascular graft
  H. wedge-pressure catheter

Hand-Schüller-Christian disease

Hand-E-Vent

hand-foot-and-mouth disease

handgrip
  isometric h.

HANE
  hereditary angioneurotic
    edema

hanging heart

hangout interval

Hank balanced salt solution

Hanley-McNeil method

Hanning window

Hannover classification

hANP
  human atrial natriuretic
    peptide

Hans
  H. Rudolph nonrebreathing
    valve
  H. Rudolph three-way valve

Hantaan virus

haplophase

haplotype
  HLA-DQA1 gene h.
  HLA-DQB1 gene h.

hard
  h. metal disease
  h. pulse

hardening
  h. of arteries

Hare syndrome

Harken
  H. auricular clamp
  H. ball valve
  H. cardiovascular forceps
  H. clamp
  H. forceps
  H. heart needle
  H. prosthesis
  H. prosthetic valve
  H. retractor
  H. rib spreader
  H.-Cooley forceps

harmonic
  h. component
  h. content

harness
  Heart Hugger sternum sup-
    port h.

Harpoon suture anchor

Harris adapter

Harrison groove

harsh
    h. murmur
    h. respiration

Hartmann
    H. clamp
    H. solution

HARTS
    heat-activated recoverable
        temporary stent

Hartzler
    H. ACX II catheter
    H. angioplasty balloon
    H. balloon catheter
    H. dilatation catheter
    H. Excel catheter
    H. LPS dilatation catheter
    H. Micro-600 catheter
    H. Micro II catheter
    H. Micro XT catheter
    H. rib retractor
    H. RX-014 balloon catheter

Harvard pump

HASHD
    hypertensive arterioscle-
        rotic heart disease

Hashimoto thyroiditis

Hassall corpuscles

HAST
    high-altitude stimulation
        test

hat
    bishop's h.

Hatle method

Hayek oscillator

Hb
    hemoglobin

HBT Sleuth

HCl
    hydrochloride

HCM
    hypertrophic cardiomyopa-
        thy

HCTZ
    hydrochlorothiazide

HDL
    high-density lipoprotein

head-down tilt test

headhunter angiography cathe-
    ter

Head paradoxical reflex

head-tilt method

head-up
    h.-u. tilt table test
    h.-u. tilt test

Heaf test

heart
    abdominal h.
    H. Aid 80 defibrillator
    air-driven artificial h.
    Akutsu III total artificial h.
    ALVAD artificial h.
    armored h.
    h. arrest
    artificial h.
    athletic h.
    atrium of h.
    h. attack
    baggy h.
    balloon-shaped h.
    Baylor total artificial h.
    beer h.
    beriberi h.
    Berlin total artificial h.
    h. block
    3:1 h. block
    3:2 h. block
    boat-shaped h.
    bony h.

heart *(continued)*
>   booster h.
>   bovine h.
>   CardioWest total artificial h.
>   cervical h.
>   chaotic h.
>   contour of h.
>   contracted h.
>   crisscross h.
>   crux of h.
>   decortication of h.
>   dextroposition of h.
>   dextroversion of h.
>   dilation of h.
>   h. disease
>   disordered action of h.
>   donor h.
>   drop h.
>   dynamite h.
>   egg-shaped h.
>   electromechanical artificial h.
>   encased h.
>   explanted h.
>   extracorporeal h.
>   h. failure
>   fatty h.
>   fatty degeneration of h.
>   fibroid h.
>   figure 8 h.
>   flask-shaped h.
>   frosted h.
>   frosting h.
>   globoid h.
>   globular h.
>   hairy h.
>   h. and hand syndrome
>   hanging h.
>   Hershey total artificial h.
>   holiday h.
>   Holmes h.
>   horizontal h.
>   H. Hugger sternum support harness
>   hyperthyroid h.
>   hypoplastic h.
>   icing h.
>   intermediate h.

heart *(continued)*
>   intracorporeal h.
>   irritable h.
>   Jarvik-7 artificial h.
>   Jarvik 7-70 artificial h.
>   Jarvik 2000 artificial h.
>   Kolff-Jarvik artificial h.
>   h. laser revascularization
>   H. Laser for TMR
>   left h.
>   Liotta total artificial h.
>   h. loop
>   luxus h.
>   h. massage
>   mechanical h.
>   movable h.
>   h. murmur
>   myocytolysis of h.
>   myxedema h.
>   one-ventricle h.
>   orthotopic biventricular artificial h.
>   orthotopic univentricular artificial h.
>   ox h.
>   paracorporeal h.
>   parchment h.
>   pear-shaped h.
>   pectoral h.
>   pendulous h.
>   Penn State total artificial h.
>   Phoenix total artificial h.
>   h. position
>   postischemic h.
>   pulmonary h.
>   h. pump
>   Quain fatty h.
>   h. rate (HR)
>   h. rate reserve
>   h. rate variability
>   recipient h.
>   h. reflex
>   rheumatism of h.
>   right h.
>   round h.
>   RTV total artificial h.
>   sabot h.
>   semihorizontal h.
>   semivertical h.

heart *(continued)*
    senescent h.
    septation of h.
    skin h.
    snowman h.
    soldier's h.
    h. sounds S_1, S_2, S_3, S_4
    stiff h.
    stone h.
    h. stroke
    superoinferior h.
    suspended h.
    swinging h.
    Symbion/CardioWest 100
        mL total artificial h.
    Symbion Jarvik-7 artifi-
        cial h.
    systemic h.
    tabby cat h.
    h. tamponade
    Taussig-Bing h.
    teardrop h.
    H. Technology Rotablator
    three-chambered h.
    thrush breast h.
    tiger h.
    tiger lily h.
    tobacco h.
    h. tones
    total artificial h.
    h. transplant
    transverse section of h.
    Traubeheart
    triatrial h.
    trilocular h.
    univentricular h.
    University of Akron artifi-
        cial h.
    upstairs-downstairs h.
    Utah total artificial h.
    h. valve
    h. valve prosthesis
    venous h.
    vertical h.
    Vienna total artificial h.
    waist of h.
    wandering h.
    water-bottle h.
    wooden-shoe h.

heartbeat

HeartCard
    H. monitor

heart-hand syndrome

heart-lung
    h.-l. bloc
    h.-l. bypass
    h.-l. machine
    h.-l. resuscitation
    h.-l. transplant

HeartMate
    H. implantable pneumatic
        left ventricular assist sys-
        tem
    H. implantable ventricular
        assist device
    H. LVAD
    H. pump

HEARTrac I Cardiac Monitoring
    system

Heartwire
    H. lead

heat
    h. load
    h. shock protein
    h. stroke

heat-activated recoverable
    temporary stent (HARTS)

heat-expandable stent

Heath-Edwards criteria

heave
    parasternal h.
    precordial h.
    right ventricular h.

heavy metal

Heberden
    H. angina
    H. asthma
    H. nodes

Hegglin syndrome

Heim-Kreysig sign

Heimlich
    H. chest drainage valve
    H. heart valve
    H. maneuver
    H. sign

Heinecke method

Heiner syndrome

Heinz body

helical coil stent

helical-tip Halo catheter

heliox
    helium-oxygen mixture

helium
    h. dilution method
    h. washout

helium-cadmium diagnostic laser

helix *pl.* helices
    amphipathic h.
    H. balloon
    H. PTCA dilatation catheter

Heller-Belsey operation

Heller-Döhle disease

Heller-Nissen operation

helminth

helminthic
    h. myocarditis

Helsinki Heart Study

hemadostenosis

Hemaflex
    H. PTCA sheath with obturator
    H. sheath

hemagglutinin

hemal

hemangiectasia, hemangiectasis

hemangioendothelioma

hemangioma
    sclerosing h.
    strawberry h.

hemangioma-thrombocytopenia syndrome

hemangiomatosis

hemangiopericyte

hemangiosarcoma

Hemaquet
    H. introducer
    H. PTCA sheath with obturator
    H. sheath

Hemashield

hematocelia, hematocoelia

hematocrit

hematogenous
    h. embolism

hematologic disease

hematology rocker

hematoma
    aneurysmal h.
    aortic intramural h.
    dissecting h.
    pelvic h.
    perianal h.
    pulsating h.
    subungual h.

hematopericardium

hematopoiesis

hematopoietic system

hematoporphyrin derivative

hematoxylin-eosin
    h.-e. stain

hematuria

hemautogram

Hemex prosthetic valve

hemiaxial view

hemiazygos vein

hemiblock
    left anterior h.
    left middle h.
    left posterior h.
    left septal h.

hemic
    h. murmur
    h. systole

hemicardia

hemidiaphragm
    tenting of h.

hemi-Fontan
    h.-F. operation
    h.-F. procedure

hemikaryon

hemin

hemisphygmia

hemisystole

hemithorax

hemitruncus

hemizygosity

hemizygous

hemochromatosis

Hemochron high-dose thrombin
    time assay

hemoclip

hemoconcentrator
    Biofilter cardiovascular h.

HemoCue photometer

hemocyanin
    keyhole-limpet h.

hemocytometer

hemodialysis

hemodialyzer
    Gambro Lundia Minor h.

hemodilution

hemodynamic
    h. abnormality
    h. assessment
    h. collapse
    h. gradient
    intraoperative h's
    h. maneuver
    h. measurement
    h. principle
    systemic h's
    h. tolerance
    h. vise

hemodynamically significant
    stenosis

hemodynamic-angiographic
    study

hemodyscrasia

hemofiltration
    continuous arteriovenous h.
    continuous venovenous h.

hemoglobin (Hb)
    glycosylated h.
    pyridoxilated stroma-
        free h.

hemoglobinemia

hemoglobin-oxygen dissociation curve

hemoglobinuria
    paroxysmal nocturnal h.

hemolysis

hemokinesis

hemokinetic

hemolytic anemia

hemoperfusion

hemopericardium

hemopneumopericardium

hemoptysis
    cardiac h.

hemoptysis *(continued)*
    Goldstein h.
    oriental h.

hemopump
    Johnson & Johnson h.
    Nimbus h.

hemorheology

hemorrhage
    arterial h.
    capillary h.
    concealed h.
    external h.
    flame-shaped h.
    internal h.
    parenchymatous h.
    petechial h.
    punctate h.
    reperfusion-induced h.
    splinter h's
    spontaneous h.
    venous h.

hemorrhagic
    h. bronchitis
    h. bronchopneumonia
    h. cyst
    h. fever
    h. pericarditis
    h. pleurisy
    h. sputum
    h. telangiectasia

hemorrheology

hemosiderin

hemosiderin-laden macrophage

hemosiderosis
    essential pulmonary h.
    idiopathic pulmonary h.
    pulmonary h.
    transfusional h.

hemostasis valve

hemostat
    angulated-vein h.
    Kelly h.
    Mayo h.
    microfibrillar collagen h.

hemostat *(continued)*
    mosquito h.
    straight h.

hemostatic
    h. occlusive leverage device
    h. thoracic clamp
    h. puncture closure device

HemoTec activated clotting time monitor

Hemotene fiber

hemothorax *pl.* hemothoraces
    catamenial h.

Hemovac
    Arbrook H.

hen-cluck stertor

Henle
    ascending loop of H.
    H. elastic membrane
    H. fenestrated membrane
    H. loop
    H.-Coenen test

Henoch-Schönlein
    H.-S. purpura
    H.-S. syndrome
    H.-S. vasculitis

Henry-Gauer response

heparin
    h. arterial filter
    beef-lung h.
    h. block
    h. drip
    h. flush
    h. injection
    h. lock
    low-molecular-weight h.

heparin-coated guidewire

heparin-dihydroergotamine

heparin-induced extracorporeal low-density lipoprotein precipitation

heparinization

heparinized saline

hepatic
  h. artery
  h. dearterialization
  h. disease
  h. failure
  h. function
  h. hydrothorax
  h. lipase
  h. sphincter
  h. vein catheterization

hepatis
  porta h.

hepatitis
  h. A
  h. B
  h. C
  h. D
  h. E
  granulomatous h.
  viral h.

hepatization

hepatofugal flow

hepatojugular
  h. reflex
  h. reflux

hepatomegaly

hepatopetal flow

hepatosplenomegaly

hepatotoxicity

Hep-Lock

heptapeptide

hereditary
  h. angioneurotic edema
  h. ataxia
  h. hemorrhagic telangiecta-
    sia
  h. methemoglobinemic cya-
    nosis

heredopathia atactica polyneu-
  ritiformis

Hering
  nerve of H.
  H. phenomenon
  H.-Breuer reflex

Hermansky-Pudlak syndrome

Herner syndrome

herniation
  cardiac h.

herpangina pharyngitis

Hershey total artificial heart

herzstoss

Hespan
  H. plasma volume ex-
    pander

Hess capillary test

hetastarch plasma expander

heterochronicus
  pulsus h.

heterocladic

heterogeneity
  genetic h.

heterogeneous attenuation

heterograft
  bovine h.
  Hancock porcine h.
  porcine h.

heterokaryon

heterokaryosis

heterologous cardiac transplant

heterolysosome

heterometric autoregulation

heterophagosome

heterophagy

heterophyiasis

heteroscedastic

heterotaxia
  cardiac h.

heterotopic
  h. cardiac transplant
  h. heart transplant
  h. stimulus

heterozygosity

heterozygote

heterozygous familial hypercholesterolemia (hFH)

Hetzel forward triangle method

Heubner specific endarteritis

Hewlett-Packard
  H.-P. 78720 A SDN monitor
  H.-P. defibrillator
  H.-P. 5 MHz phased-array
    TEE system
  H.-P. Sonos 1000, 1500,
    5500 ultrasound system

Hexabrix
  H. contrast material

hexapolar catheter

hexaxial reference system

hexokinase reaction

hexosaminidase deficiency

HFEE
  high-frequency epicardial
    echocardiography

hFH
  heterozygous familial hy-
    percholesterolemia

HFJV
  high-frequency jet ventila-
    tion

HFPPV
  high-frequency positive
    pressure ventilation

HFV
  high-frequency ventilation

Hg
  mercury

H_1–H_2 interval

HHT
  heterotopic heart trans-
    plant

hiatus
  h. aorticus
  h. esophageus
  pleuropericardial h.

hibernating myocardium

hibernation
  myocardial h.

HibTITER

Hib-VAX

high
  h. blood pressure
  h. flow
  h. resolution thin section
    computed tomographic
  h. right atrium

high-ceiling diuretic

high-density lipoprotein (HDL)

high-dose steroid

high-efficiency particulate air
  (HEPA)

high-energy
  h.-e. laser
  h.-e. transthoracic shock

high-fiber diet

high-flow catheter

high-frequency
  h.-f. epicardial echocardi-
    ography
  h.-f. jet ventilation
  h.-f. jet ventilator
  h.-f. murmur

high-grade stenosis

high-output heart failure

high-pitched murmur

high-resolution
  h.-r. B-mode ultrasonogra-
    phy
  h.-r. CT

high-risk
  h.-r. angioplasty
  h.-r. phenotype

high-speed
  h.-s. rotational atherectomy
  h.-s. rotation dynamic an-
    gioplasty catheter
  h.-s. volumetric imaging

high-torque wire

Hilal modified headhunter catheter

hilar
  h. adenopathy
  h. clouding
  h. dance
  h. fullness
  h. haze
  h. lymphadenopathy
  h. mass
  h. prominence

Hill
  H. phenomenon
  H. sign

Hillis-Müller maneuver

Hilton sac

hilum
  h. convergence sign
  h. overlay sign

Hines-Brown test

hinge
  annulocuspid h.

Hi-Per
  H. cardiac device
  H. Flex exchange wire

hippocratic
  h. angina
  h. sound

hippocratic (continued)
  h. succussion

hirsutum
  cor h.

Hirulog

His
  H. bundle
  H. bundle ablation
  H. bundle depolarization
  H. bundle electrocardio-
    gram
  H. bundle heart block
  H. canal
  H. catheter
  H. perivascular space
  H. spindle
  H.-Purkinje cells
  H.-Purkinje conduction
  H.-Purkinje fibers
  H.-Purkinje system
  H.-Purkinje tissue
  H.-Tawara node

histiocyte
  cardiac h.
  palisading h.

histiocytoma

histiocytosis

histocompatibility agent B27

Histocryl Blue tissue adhesive

histogram
  DNA h.
  h. mode

histologic

histoplasmic pericarditis

histoplasmosis
  African h.

history
  pack-year smoking h.
  smoking h.

Hi-Torque
  H. Flex-T guidewire

Hi-Torque *(continued)*
  H. floppy exchange guide-
    wire
  H. floppy II guidewire
  H. floppy intermediate
    guidewire
  H. floppy with Propel
  H. standard guidewire

Hitzenberg test

HIV
  human immunodeficiency
    virus
      HIV cardiomyopathy

HIV-1 riboprobe

HIVAGEN test

Hixson-Vernier protocol

HJR
  hepatojugular reflux

HLA
  human leukocyte antigen
    HLA-129
    HLA-A11
    HLA-DQA1 gene haplo-
      type
    HLA-DQB1 gene haplo-
      type
    HLA-DQ gene complex
    HLA-DR gene complex
  human lymphocyte antigen

HLHA
  hypoplastic left heart syn-
    drome

HLT
  heart-lung transplant

HMG-CoA
  hydroxymethylglutaryl co-
    enzyme A
  3-hydroxy-3-methylglutaryl
    coenzyme A
      HMG-CoA reductase in-
        hibitor

hockey-stick
  h.-s. catheter
  h.-s. deformity

hockey-stick *(continued)*
  h.-s. tricuspid valve

HOCM
  hypertrophic obstructive
    cardiomyopathy

Hodgkin
  H. disease
  H.-Huxley constant
  H.-Huxley model
  H.-Huxley theory
  H.-Key murmur

Hodgson disease

Hoffman reflex

Hohn vessel dilator

hoist
  Temco h.

HOLD
  hemostatic occlusive lever-
    age device

holder
  Ayers cardiovascular need-
    le h.
  Berry sternal needle h.
  Björk-Shiley heart valve h.
  blade control wire h.
  Castroviejo needle h.
  catheter guide h.
  Cooley Vital microvascular
    needle h.
  DeBakey cardiovascular
    needle h.
  DeBakey Vital needle h.
  GraftAssist vein-graft h.
  Lewy chest h.
  Marquette 3-channel las-
    er h.
  needle h.
  Vital Cooley microvascular
    needle h.
  Vital Ryder microvascular
    needle h.
  Watson heart valve h.
  wire needle h.

holiday
  dobutamine h.

holiday *(continued)*
  h. heart
  h. heart syndrome

Hollenberg treadmill score

Hollenhorst plaque

Holmes heart

Holmes-Rahe scale

holmium laser

holmium:yttrium-aluminum-gar-
  net (Ho:YAG) laser

holodiastolic
  h. murmur

holography
  ultrasound h.

holoschisis

holosystolic
  h. murmur

Holt-Oram syndrome

Holter
  H. diary
  Marquette 3-channel
    laser H.
  H. monitor
  H. tube

Holzknecht space

Homans' sign

Hombach
  H. lead placement system
  H. placement of leads

homeometric autoregulation

homeokinesis

homeostasis

Homochron monitor

homocladic

homocollateral reconstitution

homocysteine

homocystinuria syndrome

homodimer
  alpha-alpha h.
  beta-beta h.

homogentisic acid oxidase deficiency

homograft
  aortic h.
  denatured h.
  h. valve

homologous cardiac transplant

homomorphic

homoscedastic

homotropism

homozygosity

homozygote

honk
  precordial h.
  systolic h.

honking murmur

Hood-Westaby T-Y stent

hook
  barbed h.
  Bryant mitral h.
  DeBakey valve h.
  Doyen rib h.
  Krayenbuehl vessel h.
  Linton vein h.
  Moldestad vein h.

Hooke law

Hoover sign

Hope
  H. bag
  H. resuscitator
  H. sign

Hopkins
  H. aortic clamp
  H. aortic forceps
  H. aortic occlusion clamp
  H. symptom checklist

Horder spots

Horizon surgical ligating and
   marking clip

horizontal
   h. heart
   h. long-axis view

hormone
   adrenocorticotropic h.
      (ACTH)
   antidiuretic h. (ADH)
   female h.
   growth h.
   mineralocorticoid h.
   natriuretic h.
   parathyroid h.
   syndrome of inappropriate
      antidiuretic h. (SIADH)
   thyroid-stimulating h.

Horner syndrome

horripilation

horse-race effect

Horton
   H. arteritis
   H. disease

hose
   Juzo h.

hospital-acquired infection

host
   humoral h.
   immunocompetent h.
   nonimmunocompromi-
      sed h.

host-generated neutrophils re-
   cruitment

HOT
   hypertension optimal treat-
      ment

hot
   h. gangrene
   h. potato voice
   h. spot

Hotelling T2 test

hot-tip laser probe

Hounsfield unit

hourglass
   h. murmur
   h. pattern
   h. stenosis

Howard method

Howel-Evans syndrome

Howell test

Ho:YAG
   holmium:yttrium-alumi-
      num-garnet
         Ho:YAG laser
         Ho:YAG laser angio-
            plasty

H–Q interval

H–QRS interval

HR
   heart rate

H–R conduction time

HRR
   heart rate reserve

HRV
   heart rate variability

HSRA
   high-speed rotational ath-
      erectomy

HSS
   hypertrophic subaortic ste-
      nosis

HTLV
   human T-cell leukemia/lym-
      phoma virus
   human T-cell lymphotropic
      virus
         HTLV-I
         HTLV-II

HTN
   hypertension

hub
   catheter h.

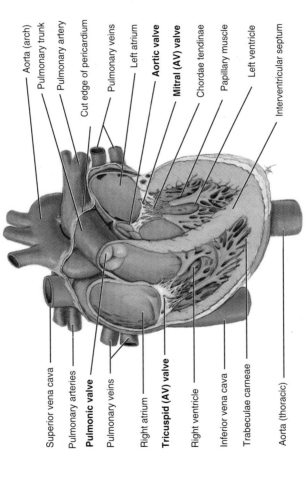

Internal view of the heart showing the chambers. (From Jarvis, C: Physical Examination and Health Assessment. Philadelphia, W. B. Saunders, 1992.)

Aorta (arch)
Pulmonary trunk
Pulmonary artery
Cut edge of pericardium
Pulmonary veins
Left atrium
Aortic valve
Mitral (AV) valve
Chordae tendinae
Papillary muscle
Left ventricle
Interventricular septum

Superior vena cava
Pulmonary arteries
Pulmonic valve
Pulmonary veins
Right atrium
Tricuspid (AV) valve
Right ventricle
Inferior vena cava
Trabeculae carneae
Aorta (thoracic)

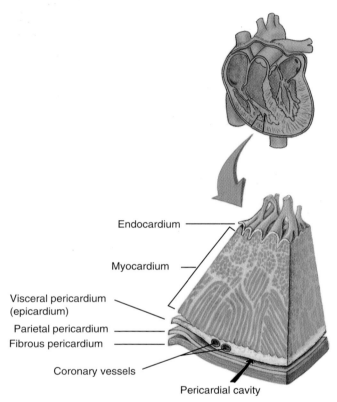

Endocardium

Myocardium

Visceral pericardium
(epicardium)

Parietal pericardium

Fibrous pericardium

Coronary vessels

Pericardial cavity

Layers of the heart wall. (From Applegate, E: The Anatomy and Physiology
Learning System, 2nd ed. Philadelphia, W. B. Saunders Company, 2000.)

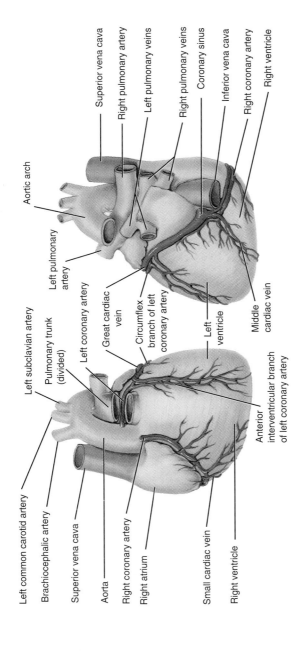

Left common carotid artery

Brachiocephalic artery

Superior vena cava

Aorta

Right coronary artery

Right atrium

Small cardiac vein

Right ventricle

Left subclavian artery

Pulmonary trunk
(divided)

Left coronary artery

Great cardiac
vein

Circumflex
branch of left
coronary artery

Left
ventricle

Anterior
interventricular branch
of left coronary artery

Left pulmonary
artery

Aortic arch

Superior vena cava

Right pulmonary artery

Left pulmonary veins

Right pulmonary veins

Coronary sinus

Inferior vena cava

Right coronary artery

Right ventricle

Middle
cardiac vein

ANTERIOR

POSTERIOR

Blood supply to the myocardium. (From Applegate, E: The Anatomy and Physiology Learning System, 2nd ed. Philadelphia, W. B. Saunders Company, 2000.)

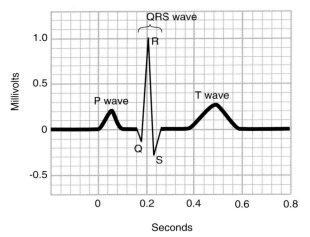

Electrocardiogram. (From Applegate, E: The Anatomy and Physiology Learning System, 2nd ed. Philadelphia, W. B. Saunders Company, 2000.)

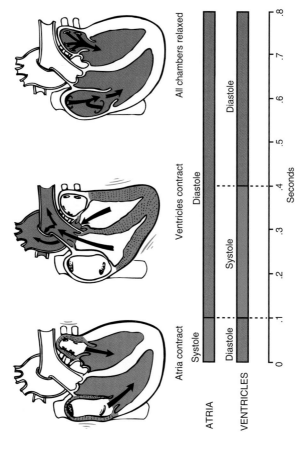

Cardiac cycle. (From Applegate, E: The Anatomy and Physiology Learning System, 2nd ed. Philadelphia, W. B. Saunders Company, 2000.)

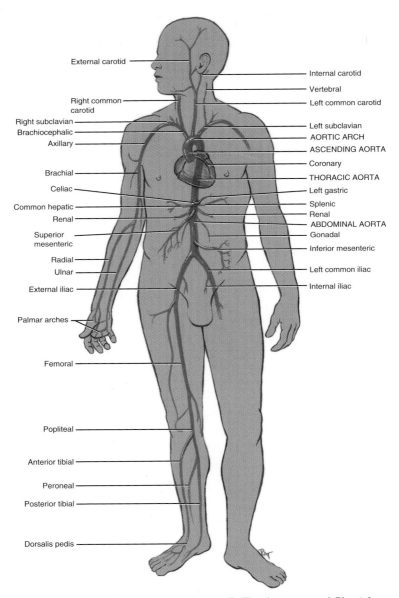

External carotid

Internal carotid

Vertebral

Right common carotid

Left common carotid

Right subclavian

Left subclavian

Brachiocephalic

AORTIC ARCH

Axillary

ASCENDING AORTA

Coronary

Brachial

THORACIC AORTA

Celiac

Left gastric

Common hepatic

Splenic

Renal

Renal

ABDOMINAL AORTA

Superior mesenteric

Gonadal

Inferior mesenteric

Radial

Ulnar

Left common iliac

External iliac

Internal iliac

Palmar arches

Femoral

Popliteal

Anterior tibial

Peroneal

Posterior tibial

Dorsalis pedis

Major systemic arteries. (From Applegate, E: The Anatomy and Physiology Learning System, 2nd ed. Philadelphia, W. B. Saunders Company, 2000.)

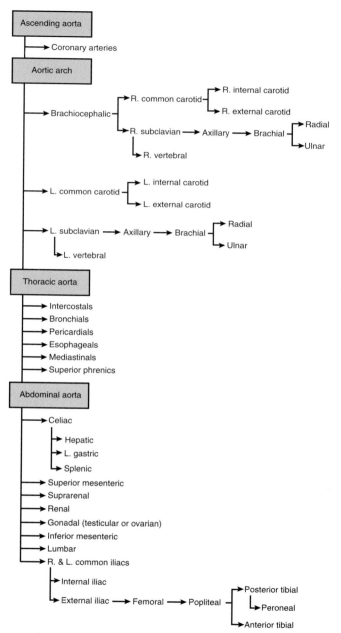

Schematic diagram of the major systemic arteries. (From Applegate, E: The Anatomy and Physiology Learning System, 2nd ed. Philadelphia, W. B. Saunders Company, 2000.)

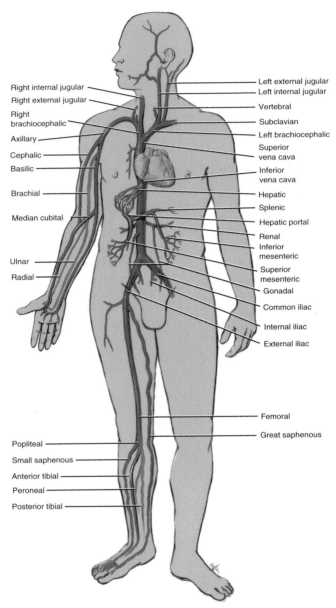

Right internal jugular
Right external jugular
Right brachiocephalic
Axillary
Cephalic
Basilic
Brachial
Median cubital
Ulnar
Radial

Left external jugular
Left internal jugular
Vertebral
Subclavian
Left brachiocephalic
Superior vena cava
Inferior vena cava
Hepatic
Splenic
Hepatic portal
Renal
Inferior mesenteric
Superior mesenteric
Gonadal
Common iliac
Internal iliac
External iliac

Femoral
Great saphenous

Popliteal
Small saphenous
Anterior tibial
Peroneal
Posterior tibial

Major Systemic veins. (From Applegate, E: The Anatomy and Physiology Learning System, 2nd ed. Philadelphia, W. B. Saunders Company, 2000.)

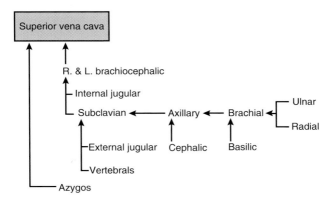

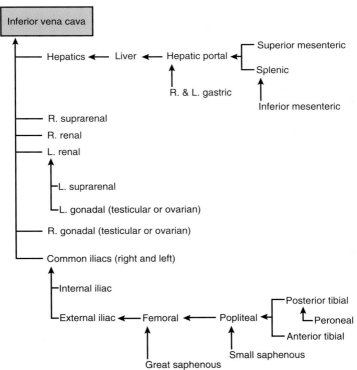

Schematic diagram of the major systemic veins. (From Applegate, E: The Anatomy and Physiology Learning System, 2nd ed. Philadelphia, W. B. Saunders Company, 2000.)

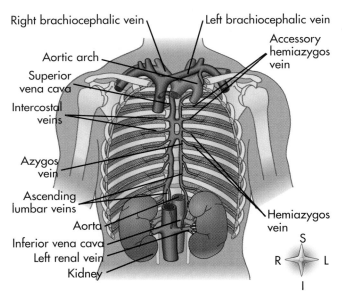

Right brachiocephalic vein

Left brachiocephalic vein

Aortic arch

Accessory hemiazygos vein

Superior vena cava

Intercostal veins

Azygos vein

Ascending lumbar veins

Aorta

Inferior vena cava

Left renal vein

Kidney

Hemiazygos vein

S

R ✦ L

I

Principal veins of the thorax. Smaller veins of the thorax drain blood into the inferior vena cava or into the azygos vein; both are shown here. The hemiazygos vein and accessory hemiazygos vein on the left drain into the azygos vein on the right. (From Thibodeau, GA, Patton KT: Anatomy & Physiology, 4th ed. St. Louis, Mosby, Inc., 1999.)

Huchard
    H. disease
    H. sign

Hufnagel
    H. ascending aortic clamp
    H. caged-ball heart valve
    H. disk heart valve
    H. mitral valve-holding for-
        ceps
    H. prosthetic valve
    H.-Ryder needle holder

Hugenholtz method

Hugger
    Bair H.

Hughes-Stovin syndrome

Hull triad

hum
    cervical venous h.
    venous h.

humming murmur

humming-top murmur

humoral
    h. host
    h. immune defect

hump
    Hampton h.

hunger
    air h.

Hunter
    H. canal
    H. detachable balloon oc-
        cluder
    H. operation
    H. syndrome
    H.-Hurler syndrome
    H.-Satinsky clamp
    H.-Sessions balloon

Hurler syndrome

Hurler-Scheie compound

Hurwitz thoracic trocar

Hustead needle

Hutinel disease

HUTTT
    head-up tilt-table test

HUV
    human umbilical vein
    HUV bypass graft

Huygens principle

H–V
    H. conduction time
    H. interval

hyaline
    h. arterionecrosis
    h. arteriosclerosis
    h. fatty change
    h. membrane disease
    h. thrombus

hyalinosis
    arteriolar h.

hyalomitome

hyaloplasm
    nuclear h.

hyalosome

hyaloserositis
    progressive multiple h.

hyalotome

hybridization
    somatic cell h.

hydraulic
    h. resistance
    h. vein stripper

hydrocarbon
    halogenated h.
    h. toxicity

HydroCath catheter

hydrochloric acid

hydrocyanic acid

Hydrogel-coated PTCA balloon
    catheter

hydrogen
  h. density
  h. electrodes
  h. fluoride
  h. inhalation technique
  h. ion concentration (pH)
  h. peroxide
  h. sulfide

hydrogen-3 mazindol

hydrolase
  lysosomal h's

hydrolysis
  ATP h.
  h. of surfactant

hydropericarditis

hydropericardium

hydroplasma

hydrophilic-coated guidewire

hydropneumopericardium

hydrops pericardii

hydrosphygmograph

Hydro-Splint II

Hydro-T

hydrothorax
  chylous h.
  hepatic h.

hydroxide
  potassium h. (KOH)

hydroxyamphetamine hydro-
  bromide

hydroxybutyrate
  h. dehydrogenase (HBDH)
  gamma h. (GHB)

hydroxylase
  h. deficiency
  17- h. deficiency

hydroxyl radical

hydroxyurea

hyperabduction syndrome

hyperaldosteronism

hyperalimentation

hyperalphalipoproteinemia

hyperammonemia

hyperapobetalipoproteinemia

hyperapolipoprotein B syndrome

hypercalcemia
  familial hypocalciuric h.

hypercalciuria

hypercapnia
  permissive h.

hypercapnic acidosis

hypercarbia

hypercardia

hyperchloremic acidosis

hypercholesterolemia
  false h.
  familial h. (FH)
  heterozygous familial h.
  (hFH)
  polygenic h.
  h. (Types IIa and IIb)

hypercholesterolemic

hyperchromasia

hyperchromatic

hyperchromatin

hyperchromatism

hyperchromatosis

hyperchromia

hyperchylomicronemia

hypercoagulable state

hypercontractile

hypercontractility

hypercyanotic
    h. angina
    h. spell

hyperdiastole

hyperdicrotic

hyperdicrotism

hyperdynamic state

hyperemia
    active h.
    arterial h.
    collateral h.
    exercise h.
    fluxionary h.
    passive h.
    peristatic h.
    reactive h.
    venous h.

hyperemic

hyperemization

hypereosinophilia

hyperesthesia

hyperestrogenemia

hypergammaglobulinemia

hyperglycemia

hyperhomocysteinemia

hyperinflated

hyperinsulinemia

hyperirritability

hyperkalemia

hyperkalemic cardioplegia

hyperkinemia

hyperkinesia

hyperkinesis

hyperkinetic
    h. heart syndrome
    h. pulse
    h. state

hyperlipidemia
    false combined h.
    multiple lipoprotein-type h.
    polygenic h.

hyperlipoproteinemia

hypermagnesemia

hypernatremia

hypernephroma

hyperoxaluria

hyperparathyroidism

hyperphosphatemia

hyperpiesis, hyperpiesia

hyperpietic

hyperplasia
    adrenal h.
    bilateral adrenal h.
    congenital adrenal h.
    elastic tissue h.
    intimal h.
    lymphoid h.

hyperplastica
    arteritis h.

hyperplastic mucus-secreting
  goblet cell

hyperpnea
    isocapnic h.

hyperpolarization

hyperreflexia
    autonomic h.

hyperreninemia

hyperresonance

hyperresonant

hyperresponsiveness

hypersecretion
    mucus h.

hypersensitive carotid sinus
  syndrome

hypersensitivity
  aminosalicylic acid h.
  carotid sinus h.
  h. myocarditis
  h. vasculitis

hyperserotonemia
  vasculocardiac syndrome
    of h.

hypersomnolence

hypersphyxia

hypersystole

hypersystolic

hypertension (HTN)
  accelerated h.
  adrenal h.
  alveolar h.
  arterial h.
  benign intracranial h.
  borderline h.
  chronic thromboembolic
    pulmonary h.
  cuffed h.
  diastolic h.
  essential h.
  familial dyslipidemic h.
  gestational h.
  glucocorticoid-induced h.
  Goldblatt h.
  hypoxic pulmonary h.
  idiopathic h.
  intracranial h.
  kidney Goldblatt h.
  labile h.
  left atrial h.
  malignant h.
  masked h.
  mineralocorticoid-indu-
    ced h.
  neuromuscular h.
  office h.
  h. optimal treatment
  oral contraceptive-indu-
    ced h.
  orthostatic h.
  Page episodic h.
  pale h.

hypertension (continued)
  pediatric h.
  portal h.
  postpartum h.
  pregnancy-induced h.
  pulmonary h.
  recalcitrant h.
  red h.
  renal h.
  renoprival h.
  renovascular h.
  resistant h.
  salt-and-water dependent h.
  secondary h.
  splenoportal h.
  stress-related h.
  systemic vascular h.
  systemic venous h.
  systolic h.
  thromboembolic pulmon-
    ary h.
  venous h.
  white-coat h.

hypertensive
  h. arteriopathy
  h. arteriosclerosis
  h. arteriosclerotic heart
    disease
  h. crisis
  h. emergency
  h. encephalopathy
  h. heart disease
  h. hypertrophic cardiomy-
    opathy
  h. nephropathy
  h. pulmonary vascular dis-
    ease
  h. retinopathy
  h. urgency
  h. vasculopathy

hyperthermia

hyperthyroid heart

hyperthyroidism
  amiodarone-induced h.
  apathetic h.

hypertonica
  polycythemia h.

hypertriglyceridemia

hypertrophic
h. cardiomyopathy
h. obstructive cardiomyopathy (HOCM)
h. subaortic stenosis (HSS)

hypertrophy
asymmetrical septal h.
basal-septal h.
cardiac h.
compensatory h.
concentric left ventricular h.
eccentric h.
isolated septal h.
left ventricular h. (LVH)
lipomatous h.
myocardial h.
myocyte h.
right ventricular h. (RVH)
septal h.
submucosal gland h.
trabecular h.
ventricular h.
volume load h.

hyperuricemia

hyperventilation
alveolar h.
h. maneuver
h. syndrome

hyperviscosity syndrome

hypervitaminosis

hypervolemia

hypervolemic

hypha *pl.* hyphae

hyphemia

hypnagogic hallucinations

hypnalgia

hypnesthesia

hypnic

hypnology

hypnopompic

hypoadrenalism

hypoaldosteronism
hyporeninemic h.

hypoalphalipoproteinemia

hypobaric hypoxia

hypocalcemia

hypocapnia

hypocholesterolemia

hypochondrial reflex

hypodynamia
h. cordis

hypodynamic

hypoechoic

hypofunction

hypoglossal nerve

hypoglycemia

hypoglycemic
h. agent
h. syncope

hypokalemia

hypokalemia-induced arrhythmia

hypokinemia

hypokinesis
anteromesial h.
cardiac wall h.
global h.

hypokinetic pulse

hypomagnesemia

hyponatremia

hypoparathyroidism

hypoperfusion

hypophosphatemia

hypophyseal-pituitary adrenal axis

hypopiesis
  orthostatic h.

hypoplasia
  mitral valve h.
  h. of right ventricle
  right ventricular h.

hypoplastic
  h. left heart
  h. left heart syndrome
    (HLS)

hypopnea

hypopneic

hyporeninemia

hyporeninemic hypoaldosteronism

hyposphyxia

hypostasis

hypostatic
  h. congestion

hyposystole

hypotension
  acute severe h.
  arterial h.
  chronic idiopathic orthos-
    tatic h.
  orthostatic h.
  postural h.
  vasovagal h.

hypotensive

hypothermia
  h. blanket
  h. cap
  extracorporeal exchange h.
  h. mattress
  topical h.

hypothermic
  h. anesthesia
  h. fibrillating arrest
  h. surgery
  h. technique

hypothesis *pl.* hypotheses
  Gad h.
  leading circle h.
  lipid h.
  Lyon h.
  monoclonal h.
  null h.
  premature ventricular com-
    plex-trigger h.
  response-to-injury h.
  Starling h.
  sulfhydryl depletion h.
  Wu-Hoak h.

hypothyroidism

hypotonia

hypotonicity

hypotonus

hypotony

hypoventilation

hypovenosity

hypovolemia

hypovolemic shock

hypoxemia
  arterial h.
  circulatory h.
  REM sleep-related h.
  rest h.
  h. test

hypoxia
  altitude h.
  anemic h.
  circulatory h.
  hypobaric h.
  hypoxic h.
  ischemic h.
  sleep h.
  stagnant h.

hypoxic
  h. hypoxia
  h. lap swimming
  h. response study

hypoxic *(continued)*
  h. spell
  h. syncope

hypoxidosis

hysteresis
  pacemaker h.
  pacing h.

hysteresis *(continued)*
  protoplasmic h.
  rate h.

hysteric angina

hystericus
  globus h.

hysterosystole

I

I-123
    iodine 123
        I-123 IPPA
        I-123 metaiodobenzyl-
            guanidine
        I-123 MIBG
        I-123 MIBG uptake

I-125
    iodine 125
        I-125 metaiodobenzyl-
            guanidine
        I-125 MIBG

IAB
    intra-aortic balloon
        IAB assist
        IAB catheter
        IAB counterpulsation
        IAB device
        IAB pump

IAIA
    immune adherence immu-
        nosorbent assay

iatrogenic
    i. atrial septal defect
    i. disorder
    i. pneumothorax

I band

ICA
    internal carotid artery

ICD
    implantable cardioverter-
        defibrillator
        Cadence biphasic ICD
        Guardian ICD
        Teletronics Guardian
            ATP II ICD
        Ventritex Cadence ICD
        Vitatron Diamond ICD

ICD-ATP
    implantable cardioverter-
        defibrillator/atrial tachy-
        cardia pacing
        ICD-ATP device

ICHD pacemaker code

ice
    i. slush
    topical i.

iced saline

ice-pick view (on M-mode echo-
    cardiogram)

icing heart

ICS
    intracellular-like, calcium-
        bearing crystalloid solu-
        tion
        ICS cardioplegic solu-
            tion

ictometer

ICTP
    type I collagen telepeptide

ictus
    i. cordis
    i. sanguinis

ICUS
    intracoronary ultrasound

ICXA
    intermediate circumflex ar-
        tery

IDC
    idiopathic dilated cardio-
        myopathy

Ideal cardiac device

idiojunctional rhythm

idionodal
    i. rhythm

idiopathic
    i. arteritis of Takayasu
    i. bradycardia
    i. brown induration
    i. cardiomegaly
    i. cyclic edema
    i. dilated cardiomyopathy
        (IDC)

idiopathic *(continued)*
    i. dilation
    i. hypereosinophilic syn-
        drome
    i. hypertension
    i. hypertrophic subaortic
        stenosis (IHSS)
    i. long Q-T interval syn-
        drome
    i. myocardial hypertrophy
    i. myocarditis
    i. orthostatic hypotension
    i. pericarditis
    i. restrictive cardiomyopa-
        thy
    i. thrombocytopenic pur-
        pura
    i. ventricular fibrillation
    i. ventricular tachycardia

idioventricular
    i. bradycardia
    i. kick
    i. rhythm
    i. tachycardia

IE
    infective endocarditis

IEA
    inferior epigastric artery
        IEA graft

IEL
    internal elastic lamina

IgE
    serum I.

IgE-sensitized cell

IgG avidity test

IHD
    ischemic heart disease

IHSS
    idiopathic hypertrophic
        subaortic stenosis

iliac
    i. artery
    i. artery occlusion

iliac *(continued)*
    i. atherosclerotic occlusive
        disease
    i. fossa
    i. steal
    i. vein
    i. vein thrombosis

iliofemoral

iliopopliteal
    i. bypass

Illumen-8 guiding catheter

IMA
    internal mammary artery
        IMA graft
        IMA pedicle

image
    i. aliasing
    amplitude i.
    i. bundle
    ejection-fraction i.
    ejection shell i.
    equilibrium i.
    end-diastolic i.
    functional i.
    initial i.
    i. intensifier
    paradox i.
    parametric i.
    regional ejection fraction
        (REF1) i.
    phase i.
    phase-encoded velocity i.
    SE i.
    stress washout myocardial
        perfusion i.
    supine rest gated equilibri-
        um i.
    T1 myocardial i.
    T1, T2 weighted i.

Imagecath rapid exchange an-
    gioscope

Image-Measure morphometry
    software

imager
    Hewlett-Packard color
        flow i.

imager *(continued)*
>   Sonos 2000 ultrasound i.

Imager Torque selective catheter

imaging
>   acoustic i.
>   adenosine radionuclide
>   perfusion i.
>   i. agent
>   Aloka color Doppler sys-
>   tem for blood flow i.
>   antifibrin antibody i.
>   antimyosin antibody i.
>   biplane i.
>   blood-pool i.
>   cardiac blood-pool i.
>   i. chain
>   color flow i.
>   color flow Doppler i.
>   continuous-wave Doppler i.
>   digital subtraction i.
>   digital vascular i.
>   dipyridamole-thallium i.
>   direct Fourier transforma-
>   tion i.
>   Doppler color flow i.
>   Doppler tissue i.
>   Doppler transesophageal
>   color flow i.
>   duplex i.
>   echo-planar i.
>   exercise i.
>   four-hour delayed thalli-
>   um i.
>   Fourier two-dimensional i.
>   frequency domain i.
>   functional i.
>   gallium-67 i.
>   gated cardiac blood-pool i.
>   gated sweep magnetic re-
>   sonance i.
>   high-speed volumetric i.
>   hot spot i.
>   indium 111 antimyosin i.
>   indium 111–labeled lym-
>   phocyte i.
>   infarct-avid i.
>   INTEGRIS cardiovascular i.

imaging *(continued)*
>   krypton-81m ventilation i.
>   magnetic resonance i.
>   (MRI)
>   magnetic source i.
>   mask-mode cardiac i.
>   multiple gated equilibrium
>   cardiac blood pool i.
>   myocardial T1 i.
>   myocardial perfusion i.
>   nuclear magnetic resonan-
>   ce i.
>   parametric i.
>   pharmacologic stress per-
>   fusion i.
>   phase i.
>   planar myocardial i.
>   platelet i.
>   postexercise i.
>   PYP i.
>   pyrophosphate i.
>   radioisotope i.
>   radionuclide i.
>   redistribution i.
>   redistribution myocardial i.
>   redistribution thallium
>   201 i.
>   rest myocardial perfusion i.
>   rest-redistribution thallium
>   201 i.
>   rest thallium 201 myocardi-
>   al i.
>   rubidium 82 i.
>   sestamibi i.
>   single-photon emission to-
>   mography (SPET) i.
>   spin-echo i.
>   stress-redistribution-rein-
>   jection thallium-201 i.
>   stress thallium 201 myocar-
>   dial i.
>   stress thallium 201 myocar-
>   dial perfusion i.
>   i. study
>   teboroxime i.
>   technetium (Tc) myocardi-
>   al i.
>   technetium 99m i.
>   technetium 99m MIBI i.

imaging *(continued)*
    technetium 99m pyrophos-
      phate i.
    technetium 99m pyrophos-
      phate myocardial i.
    thallium 201 myocardial i.
    thallium myocardial perfu-
      sion i.
    thallium perfusion i.
    tissue Doppler i.
    transesophageal Doppler
      color flow i.
    velocity-encoded cine-mag-
      netic resonance i.
    video i.
    i. window
    xenon lung ventilation i.

imaging-angioplasty balloon
  catheter

Imatron
    I. C-100 system
    I. C-100 tomographic scan-
      ner
    I. Ultrafast CT scanner

imbalance
    acid-base i.
    electrolyte i.
    protease-antiprotease i.
    sympathovagal i.

IMED
    IMED infusion device
    IMED infusion pump

IMI
    inferior myocardial infarc-
      tion

immune
    i. adherence immunosor-
      bent assay (IAIA)
    i. globulin, intravenous

immune-mediated
    i.-m. disease
    i.-m. membranous nephritis

immunity
    cell-mediated i.

immunoassay
    enzyme i. (EIA)
    nifedipine enzyme i.
    Thrombus Precursor Pro-
      tein i.

immunochemical abnormalities

immunocompetent host

immunocompromised

immunodeficiency
    i. virus

immunofluorescence
    cytometric indirect i.

immunoglobulin
    varicella-zoster i.

immunological theory

immunology

immunometric sandwich
  method

immunonephelometry
    rate i.

immunoperoxidase stain

immunoprecipitin analysis

immunoradiometric assay

immunoseparation

immunostaining technique

immunosuppressant

immunosuppression
    i. therapy

immunotherapy

immunoturbidimetric assay

IMP-Capello arm support

impairment of contractility

impedance
    i. aggregometry
    aortic i.
    arterial i.
    atrial lead i.

impedance *(continued)*
    i. catheter
    lead i.
    i. modulus
    pacemaker i.
    pacemaker lead i.
    i. plethysmography
    pulmonary arterial input i.
    thoracic i.
    i. variables
    vascular i.

implant
    Biocell RTV i.
    bioresorbable i.
    Core-Vent i.
    defibrillator i.

implantable
    i. cardioverter-defibrillator
      (ICD)
    i. cardioverter-defibrillator/
      atrial tachycardia pacing
      (ICD-ATP)
    i. cardioverter electrodes
    i. left ventricular assist sys-
      tem
    i. system

Implantaid Di-Lock cardiac lead
    introducer

implantation
    intrapleural pulse genera-
      tor i.
    i. metastasis
    permanent pacemaker i.
    i. response
    stent i.
    subpectoral pulse genera-
      tor i.

impotence
    vasculogenic i.

Impra
    I. bypass graft
    I. Flex vascular graft
    I. vascular graft
    I. vein graft

Impra-Graft microporous PTFE
    vascular graft

impressio
    i. cardiaca pulmonis

impulse
    afferent i.
    apex i's
    apical i.
    atrial filling i.
    cardiac i.
    cardiac apex i.
    i. conduction
    ectopic i.
    episternal i.
    escape i.
    i. formation
    juxtapical i.
    left parasternal i.
    paradoxic apical i.
    paradoxic rocking i.
    point of maximum i. (PMI)
    i. propagation
    right parasternal i.
    i. summation
    systolic apical i.

impure flutter

IMREG-1

IMT
    intimal-medial thickness

Imulyse t-PA ELISA kit

inaequalis
    pulsus i.

incessant tachycardia

incidence
    peak i.

incident
    vascular i.

incidental murmur

incision
    collar i.
    fish-mouth i.
    flank i.
    infraclavicular i.
    ladder i's
    longitudinal i.

index *(continued)*
 venous filling i.
 volume thickness i.
 wall motion score i.
 Wood units i.
 Woods units i.
 Youden i.

indicator
 i. dilution technique
 i. dilution curve
 i. fractionation principle
 Schneider i.
 xylol pulse i.

indifferent electrode

indirect
 i. diuretic
 i. lead
 i. murmur

indium 111 (^{111}In)
 i. 111 antimyosin antibody
 i. 111 antimyosin imaging
 i. 111–labeled lymphocyte
   imaging
 i. 111 radioisotope
 i. 111 scintigraphy

indium 113m

indocyanine
 i. dilution curve
 i. green
 i. green angiography
 i. green dye
 i. green indicator dilution
   technique
 i. green method

induced pneumothorax

inducibility
 i. basal state
 ventricular tachycardia i.

inducible
 i. arrhythmia
 i. polymorphic ventricular
   tachycardia
 i. sustained orthodromic
   supraventricular tachycardia

induction
 i. of anesthesia, crash
 rapid sequence i.

induration
 idiopathic brown i.

indurative myocarditis

indwelling time

inertia

in extremis

Inf
 infarction

infantile
 i. arteritis
 i. beriberi

infarct
 brain i.
 i. bulging
 cerebral i.
 embolic i.
 i. expansion
 i. extension
 lacunar i.
 pulmonary i.
 red i.
 i. scar
 i. size limitation
 i. thinning
 watershed i.

infarct-avid
 i.-a. hot-spot scintigraphy
 i.-a. imaging
 i.-a. myocardial scintigraphy

infarctectomy

infarction (Inf)
 acute myocardial i. (AMI)
 age indeterminate i.
 age-undetermined myocar-
   dial i.
 anterior myocardial i.
   (AMI)
 anterior wall myocardial i.
 anteroinferior myocardial i.

infarction *(continued)*
    anterolateral myocardial i.
    anteroseptal myocardial i.
    apical myocardial i.
    arrhythmic myocardial i.
    asymptomatic myocardial i.
    atherothrombotic i.
    atrial i.
    atrial myocardial i.
    cardiac i.
    completed myocardial i.
    complicated myocardial i.
    diaphragmatic myocardi-
      al i.
    evolving myocardial i.
    extensive anterior myocar-
      dial i.
    high lateral myocardial i.
    hyperacute myocardial i.
    impending myocardial i.
    inferior myocardial i.
    inferior wall myocardial i.
    inferolateral myocardial i.
    inferoposterolateral my-
      ocardial i.
    ischemic cerebral i.
    lateral myocardial i.
    myocardial i. (MI) i.
    myocardial i. in H-form
    nonarrhythmic myocardi-
      al i.
    nonfatal myocardial i.
    non–Q-wave myocardial i.
    non–ST-segment elevation
      myocardial i.
    nontransmural myocardi-
      al i.
    old myocardial i.
    posterior myocardial i.
    posteroinferior myocardi-
      al i.
    postmyocardial i.
    postmyocardiotomy i.
    Q wave i.
    Q wave myocardial i.
    primary angioplasty in my-
      ocardial i. (PAMI)
    prourokinase in myocardi-
      al i. (PRIMI)

infarction *(continued)*
    recent myocardial i.
    recurrent myocardial i.
    right ventricular i.
    Roesler-Dressler i.
    rule out myocardial i.
      (ROMI)
    septal myocardial i.
    silent myocardial i.
    stuttering myocardial i.
    subacute myocardial i.
    subendocardial i.
    subendocardial myocardi-
      al i.
    thrombolysis and angio-
      plasty in myocardial i.
      (TAMI)
    thrombolysis in myocardi-
      al i. (TIMI)
    through-and-through my-
      ocardial i.
    transmural myocardial i.
    watershed i.

infarct-related vessel

infarctoid cardiopathy

infected
    i. aneurysm
    i. myxoma

infection
    adenoviral type 40/41 i.
    bacterial i.
    community-acquired i.
    endemic fungal i.
    fungal i.
    hospital-acquired i.
    laryngeal i.
    latent i.
    luetic i.
    MAC i.
    MAI i.
    mixed i.
    Mycobacterium avium com-
      plex i.
    Mycobacterium avium intra-
      cellulare i.
    mycotic i.
    nosocomial i.

infection *(continued)*
    opportunistic i.
    rhinocerebral i.
    secondary i.
    spirochetal i.
    staphylococcal i.
    subclinical i.
    syphilitic i.
    systemic i.
    upper respiratory i. (URI)
    viral respiratory i.

infectious
    i. endocarditis
    i. esophagitis
    i. mononucleosis

infective
    i. embolism
    i. endocarditis
    i. pericarditis
    i. thrombosis
    i. thrombus

inferior
    i. epigastric artery (IEA)
    i. mesenteric artery
    i. mesenteric vascular oc-
        clusion
    i. vena cava (IVC)
    i. vena cava occlusion
    i. wall hypokinesis
    i. wall myocardial infarc-
        tion

inferoapical

inferobasal
    i. wall

inferobasilar

inferolateral
    i. myocardial infarction

inferoposterior

inferoposterolateral

infiltrate
    migratory pulmonary i.
    patchy i.
    perivascular eosinophilic
        i's

infiltrate *(continued)*
    strandy i.
    streaky i.

infiltration
    adipose i.
    calcareous i.
    calcium i.
    cellular i.
    fatty i.
    inflammatory i.
    sanguineous i.
    serous i.

infiltrative cardiomyopathy

Infiniti
    I. catheter
    I. catheter introducer sys-
        tem

inflammation
    fibrinous i.

inflammatoria
    dysphagia i.

inflammatory
    i. pericarditis
    i. reaction

inflation
    balloon i.
    i. reflex

inflow
    i. of arterial blood
    i. tract
    i. tract of left ventricle
    turbulent diastolic mitral i.

infra-apical

infra-auricular

infraclavicular
    i. triangle

infracristal

infracubital bypass

infradiaphragmatic portion

infrahisian, infra-Hisian
    i. block

infrahisian *(continued)*
 i. conduction system

infrainguinal

inframalleolar

inframyocardial

infranodal extrasystole

infrapopliteal

infrared
 i.-pulsed laser
 i. thermography

infrarenal abdominal aortic aneurysm

infrequens
 pulsus i.

infundibular
 i. obstruction
 i. resection
 i. septal defect
 i. wedge resection

infundibulectomy
 Brock i.

infundibuloventricular crest

infundibulum *pl.* infundibula
 i. of heart

Infusaid infusion pump

Infus-a-port pump

InfusaSleeve
 Kaplan-Simpson I.
 LocalMed I.

infuser
 Critikon pressure i.

infusion
 volume i.

ingravescent apoplexy

inguinal region

inhibited
 i. pacing

inhibition
 contact i.

inhibition *(continued)*
 leukotriene i.
 potassium i.

inhibitor
 ACE i.
 acyl-CoA:cholesterol acyltransferase i.
 alpha-1 proteinase i.
 angiotensin-converting enzyme i. (ACE)
 beta-lactamase i.
 carbonic anhydrase i.
 cholinesterase i.
 converting enzyme i.
 cyclooxygenase i.
 endopeptidase i.
 HMG-CoA reductase i.
 human menopausal gonad-
  otropic coenzyme A re-
  ductase i.
 hydroxymethylglutaryl coenzyme A reductase i.
 3-hydroxy-3-methylglutaryl
  coenzyme A reductase i.
 lipoprotein-associated coagulation i.
 MAO i.
 mast cell i.
 monoamine oxidase (MAO)
  i.
 mucus i.
 PDI isoenzyme i.
 phosphodiesterase i.
 phosphodiesterase isoen-
  zyme i's
 a_2-plasmin i.
 plasminogen activator i.
 plasminogen activator i.-1
 protease i.
 a_2-proteinase i.
 renin i.
 secretory leukoproteina-
  se i.
 thromboxane synthetase i.

inhomogeneity

injection
 blood patch i.
 bolus i.

injection *(continued)*
- double i.
- dye i.
- hand i.
- heparin i.
- Hep-Lock i.
- intra-arterial i.
- intracutaneous i.
- intradermal i.
- intramuscular i.
- intrathecal i.
- intravascular i.
- intravenous i.
- iodinated I-125 albumin i.
- iodinated I-131 albumin i.
- iron dextran i.
- iron sorbitex i.
- manual i.
- opacifying i.
- i. port
- power i.
- Ringer i.
- Ringer lactated i.
- sclerosing i.
- selective i.
- serial i.
- sodium chloride i.
- straight AP pelvic i.
- vasopressin i.

injector
- flow i.
- Fujinon variceal i.
- Hercules power i.
- Medrad Mark IV angiographic i.
- Medrad power angiographic i.
- modified Mark IV R-wave-triggered power i.
- power i.
- pressure i.
- Viamonte-Hobbs dye i.

injury
- blunt i.
- diastolic current of i.
- electrical i.
- femoral vascular i.
- mesangial immune i.

injury *(continued)*
- myocardial i.
- penetrating i.
- reperfusion i.
- systolic current of i.
- vascular i.

inlet
- thoracic i.

in-memory gating

innervation
- autonomic sensory i.

innocent
- i. heart murmur
- i. murmur of elderly

innominate
- i. aneurysm
- i. artery
- i. artery stenosis
- i. vein

Innovator Holter system

inoblast

inoculation

Inokuchi vascular stapler

inorganic murmur

inosine

inotrope
- negative i.
- positive i.

inotropic
- i. activity of drug
- i. agent
- i. arrhythmia
- i. effect
- i. support
- i. therapy

inotropy

Inoue
- I. balloon catheter
- I. balloon mitral valvotomy

INR
- international normalized ratio

insertion
　　percutaneous catheter i.
　　retrograde catheter i.
　　route of i.
　　wire i.

inspissated

in situ
　　i. s. bypass
　　i. s. grafting

instability
　　catheter i.

instantaneous
　　i. electrical axis
　　i. gradient
　　i. spectral peak velocity
　　i. vector

Insta-Pulse heart rate monitor

InStent CarotidCoil stent

instillation
　　lavage i.

instrument
　　arterial oscillator endarter-
　　　ectomy i.
　　Cooley neonatal i's
　　Diamond-Lite titanium i's
　　KinetiX i's
　　Matsuda titanium surgical
　　　i's
　　NeoKnife electrosurgical i.
　　Neuro-Trace i.
　　OPG-Gee i.
　　Wolvek sternal approxima-
　　　tion fixation i.

instrumentation
　　angiographic i.
　　MIDA CoroNet i.

instrumented

insudate

insufficiency
　　acute coronary i.
　　aortic i.
　　aortic valve i.

insufficiency (continued)
　　arterial i.
　　atrioventricular valve i.
　　cardiac i.
　　cerebrovascular i.
　　congenital pulmonary val-
　　　ve i.
　　coronary i.
　　deep venous i.
　　mitral i.
　　multivalve i.
　　myocardial i.
　　myovascular i.
　　nonrheumatic aortic i.
　　pseudoaortic i.
　　pulmonary i.
　　renal i.
　　respiratory i.
　　rheumatic mitral i.
　　Sternberg myocardial i.
　　tricuspid i.
　　valvular i.
　　velopharyngeal i.
　　venous i.
　　vertebrobasilar arterial i.

insufflation
　　thoracoscopic talc i.

insufflator
　　Venturi i.

Insuflon device

insulin-like growth factor (IGF)

insult
　　cardiac i.
　　vascular i.

Intact xenograft prosthetic
valve

Intec
　　I. AID cardioverter-defibri-
　　　llator generator
　　I. implantable defibrillator

Integra
　　I. catheter
　　I. II balloon

integral
　　i. aortic flow velocity

integral *(continued)*
i. pulmonary flow velocity

integrated
i. bipolar sensing
i. lead system

INTEGRIS
INTEGRIS cardiac imaging
system
INTEGRIS cardiovascular
imaging

IntelliCat pulmonary artery
catheter

intensifier
image i.

intensity
echo i.
i. of heart sounds
spatial i.

intentional transoperative hemodilution

intentionem
per primam i.
per secundam i.

interaction
adhesin-receptor i.
drug i.

interarterial
i. communication
i. septum
i. shunt

interatrial
i. baffle leak
i. conduction delay
i. groove
i. septal defect
i. septum

interauricular

intercadence

intercalary

intercalated

intercapillary

intercapitular

intercarotic

intercarotid

intercellular
i. adhesion molecule-1
(ICAM-1)
i. coupling

intercept angle

interchordal hooding

intercidens
pulsus i.

intercostal
i. artery
i. space

intercurrens
pulsus i.

interdependence
ventricular i.

interdigitating coil stent

interectopic interval

interface
I. arterial blood filter
electrode-skin i.
Monarch Mini Mask nasal i.

interfascicular fibrous tissue

interference
i. beat
dissociation by i.
i. dissociation
electromagnetic i./radiofre-
quency i.

interkinesis

interlaced scanning

intermediary vessel

intermediate
i. artery
i. circumflex artery (ICXA)
i. coronary syndrome
i. heart

intermediate-density lipoprotein

Intermedics
I. Quantum pacemaker
I. RES-Q implantable car-
dioverter-defibrillator
I. Stride pacemaker

intermedius
bronchus i.
ramus i.

intermitotic

intermittence, intermittency

intermittens
dyskinesia i.
pulsus respiratione i.

intermittent
i. claudication
i. coronary sinus occlusion
i. demand ventilation
i. junctional bradycardia
i. pulse
i. sinus arrest

interna
lamina elastica i.

internal
i. adhesive pericarditis
i. carotid artery (ICA)
i. diameter
i. elastic lamina
i. jugular approach for cardiac catheterization
i. jugular vein
i. mammary artery (IMA)
i. mammary artery bypass
i. mammary artery catheter
i. mammary artery graft angiography
i. thoracic artery (ITA)

international
i. normalized ratio (INR)

internodal
i. conduction
i. pathways

internodal (continued)
i. tract
i. tract of Bachman

internum
pericardium i.

interosseous

interphase

interphyletic

interpolated
i. beat
i. extrasystole
i. premature complex

Interpret ultrasound catheter

interquartile range

interrogation
deep Doppler velocity i.
Doppler i.
pacemaker i.
stereoscopic i.

interrupted
i. aortic arch
i. pledgeted suture
i. respiration

interruption
aortic arch i.
azygoportal i.
vena caval i.

intersegmental arteries

Intersept cardiotomy reservoir

Interspec XL ultrasound

interstitium
cardiac i.

intersystolic
i. period

Intertach
I. II pacer
I. 262-12 pacemaker
I. pacemaker

Intertech
I. anesthesia breathing circuit

Intertech *(continued)*
  I. Mapleson D nonrebrea-
    thing circuit
  I. nonrebreathing modified
    Jackson-Rees circuit
  I. Perkin-Elmer gas sam-
    pling line
Intertherapy intravascular ultrasound
interval
  A–A i.
  A_1–A_2 i.
  A–C i.
  Ae–H i.
  A–H i.
  A–N i.
  A_2 incisural i.
  A2 to opening snap i.
  A_2/MVO (aortic valve clo-
    sure/mitral valve open-
    ing) i.
  atrial escape i.
  atriocarotid i.
  atriohisian i.
  atrioventricular (AV) i.
  auriculocarotid i.
  auriculoventricular i.
  AV i.
  AV delay i.
  Bazett corrected QT i.
  B–H i.
  cardioarterial i.
  coupling i.
  critical coupling i.
  electromechanical i.
  escape i.
  f–f i.
  fixed coupling i.
  flutter R i.
  H–Ae i.
  hangout i.
  H_1–H_2 i.
  H–H′ i.
  H′–P i.
  H–Q i.
  H–QRS i.
  H–V i.
  interectopic i.

interval *(continued)*
  isoelectric i.
  isometric i.
  JT i.
  magnet pacing i.
  P–A i.
  P_2–T_0 i.
  pacemaker escape i.
  P–H i.
  postsphygmic i.
  P–P i.
  P–Q i.
  P–R i.
  presphygmic i.
  prolongation of QRS i.
  Q–H i.
  Q–M i.
  Q–R i.
  Q–RB i.
  QRS i.
  QRS–T i.
  Q–S_1 i.
  Q–S_2 i.
  Q–T i.
  Q–Tc i.
  Q–U i.
  Q to first sound i.
  right ventricular systolic ti-
    me i.
  R–P i.
  R–R i.
  R–R′ i.
  RS–T i.
  S_1–S_2 i.
  S_1–S_3 i.
  S_2–OS (second sound to
    opening snap) i.
  sphygmic i.
  S–QRS i.
  ST i.
  systolic time i.
  TP i.
  V–A i.
  V–H i.
interval-strength relation
intervascular
interventional
  i. cardiac catheterization

interventional *(continued)*
  i. echocardiography
  i. study

interventionist

interventricular
  i. foramen
  i. septal defect
  i. septal motion
  i. septal rupture
  i. septal thickness
  i. septum
  i. septum aneurysm
  i. sulcus
  i. veins

intima
  aortic tunica i.
  i.-pia

intimal
  i. dissection
  i. flap
  i. hyperplasia
  i. tear
  i. thickening

intimal-medial thickness

Intimax vascular catheter

intimectomy

intimitis

intolerance
  carbohydrate i.
  exercise i.
  glucose i.

in toto

intra-aortic
  i. balloon (IAB)
  i. balloon assist
  i. balloon catheter
  i. balloon counterpulsation
  i. balloon device
  i. balloon pump

intra-arterial
  i. counterpulsation

intra-atrial
  i. activation sequence
  i. baffle
  i. baffle operation
  i. block
  i. conduction
  i. conduction defect
  i. conduction time
  i. reentry
  i. reentrant tachycardia

intra-auricular

intracardiac
  i. atrial activation sequence
  i. catheter
  i. electrocardiography
  i. electrophysiologic study
  i. electrophysiology
  i. event
  i. lead
  i. mapping
  i. mass
  i. pacing
  i. pressure
  i. pressure curve
  i. pressure in Doppler ech-
    ocardiogram
  i. shunt
  i. sucker
  i. thrombus

Intracath catheter

intracaval
  i. device
  i. endovascular ultrasonog-
    raphy

intracavitary
  i. clot formation
  i. pressure-electrogram dis-
    sociation
  i. pressure gradient

intracellular
  i. calcium concentration
  i. lipid

intracellular-like calcium-bear-
  ing crystalloid solution (ICS)

intracoronary
i. sonicated meglumine
i. thrombolysis balloon valvuloplasty
i. ultrasound

intracorporeal heart

intracranial
i. aneurysm
i. hypertension

intracytoplasmic

IntraDop
Doppler I.

intrahisian, intra-Hisian
i. AV block
i. block
i. delay

intraluminal
i. plaque
i. ultrasound

intramural
i. coronary arteries
i. thrombosis

intramyocardial
i. prearteriolar vessel
i. pressure

intranodal block

Intra-Op autotransfusion system

intraoperative
i. digital subtraction
i. digital subtraction angiography
i. hemodynamics
i. mapping
i. vascular angiography

intrapericardial
i. pressure

intraperitoneal migration of
pacemaker

intraplaque hemorrhage (IPH)

intrapleural implantation of
pulse generator

intraprotoplasmic

intrapulmonary shunting

intraretinal microangiopathy

intrastent
i. recurrent disease
i. restenosis

intrathoracic
i. pressure
i. thyroid

intravascular
i. catheter electrode
i. coagulation
i. foreign body retrieval
i. injection
i. pressure
i. stent
i. thrombus
i. ultrasound
i. ultrasound catheter
i. volume
i. volume status

intravascularly volume de-
pleted

intravenous (IV)
i. angiocardiography
i. digital subtraction angiography
Fungizone i.
immune globulin i.
i. pacing catheter
Saventrine i.

intravenous TKO
to keep open (the vein,
needle, or catheter)

intraventricular
i. aberration
i. block (IVB)
i. block, conduction delay
i. conduction
i. conduction defect

intraventricular *(continued)*
  i. conduction delay (IVCD)
  i. conduction pattern
  i. hemorrhage
  i. pressure
  i. systolic tension

Intrepid balloon catheter

intrinsic sympathomimetic activity

intrinsicoid deflection

introducer
  Angestat hemostasis i.
  Angetear tearaway i.
  aortic assist balloon i.
  Avanti i.
  i. catheter
  Cardak percutaneous catheter i.
  Check-Flo i.
  Davol pacemaker i.
  Desilets i.
  Desilets-Hoffman catheter i.
  electrode i.
  Encapsulon sheath i.
  FasTrac i.
  gum elastic bougie i.
  Hemaquet i.
  Hemaquet catheter i.
  Hemaquet sheath i.
  heparin lock i.
  Implantaid Di-Lock cardiac lead i.
  Littleford-Spector i.
  LPS Peel-Away i.
  Micropuncture Peel-Away i.
  Mullins catheter i.
  Nottingham i.
  peel-away i.
  percutaneous i.
  permanent lead i.
  Razi cannula i.
  i. sheath
  888 i. sheath
  split-sheath i.
  Tuohy-Borst i.
  UMI transseptal Cath-Seal catheter i.

introducer *(continued)*
  USCI i.

intron
  i. 16
  i. A

intubate

intubation

invasive
  i. assessment
  i. cardiologist
  i. pressure measurement

inversion
  T wave i.
  U wave i.
  ventricular i.

inversus
  dextrocardia with situs i.
  levocardia with situs i.
  situs i.

inverted
  i. P wave
  i. T wave
  i. terminal T wave
  i. U wave

in vivo balloon pressure

inward-going rectification

iodine
  i. 123
  i. 123 heptadecanoic acid radioactive tracer
  i. 123 metaiodobenzylguanidine
  i. 123 metaiodobenzylguanidine update
  i. 123 phenylpentadecanoic acid
  i. 125
  i. 125 isotope
  i. 125 radioisotope
  radiolabelled i. i. 131
  i. 131 MIBG scintigraphy

iohexol contrast medium

ion
  calcium i.

ion *(continued)*
    i. channel
    chloride i.
    potassium i.
    i. pump
    sodium i.

Ionescu
    I. method of making a tri-
        leaflet valve
    I. operation
    I. sympathectomy
    I. trileaflet valve
    I.-Shiley bioprosthetic valve
    I.-Shiley bovine pericardial
        valve
    I.-Shiley heart valve
    I.-Shiley low-profile pros-
        thetic valve
    I.-Shiley pericardial patch
    I.-Shiley pericardial valve
    I.-Shiley pericardial xeno-
        graft valve
    I.-Shiley prosthesis
    I.-Shiley standard pericar-
        dial prosthetic valve
    I.-Shiley valve
    I.-Shiley valve prosthesis
    I.-Shiley vascular graft

ionizing radiation

ion-selective electrode

Ionyx lead

iopamidol contrast medium

Iopamiron contrast medium

iothalamate meglumine con-
    trast medium

ioxaglate meglumine contrast
    medium

IPCO-Partridge defibrillator

IPG
    impedance plethysmogra-
        phy

IPLVAS
    implantable left ventricular
        assist system

ipsilateral
    i. nonreversed greater sa-
        phenous vein bypass

IR
    ionizing radiation

Irex Exemplar ultrasound

iridium strand

IRMA
    immunoradiometric assay

iron
    i. chelator
    i. dextran complex
    serum i.
    i. storage disease

irradiation
    total axial node i.
    total lymphoid i.

irregularity
    diffuse i.
    luminal i.
    i. of pulse

irregularly
    i. irregular pulse
    i. irregular rhythm

Irri-Cath suction system

irritability
    myocardial i.
    tactile i.

irritable heart

irritant receptor

Irvine viable organ-tissue trans-
    port system (IVOTTS)

Isambert disease

ischemia
    asymptomatic cardiac i.
    brachiocephalic i.
    cardiac i.
    clandestine myocardial i.
    i. cordis intermittens
    exercise-induced i.

ischemia *(continued)*
  extremity i.
  global myocardial i.
  ischemic i.
  limb i.
  manifest i.
  myocardial i.
  nonlocalized i.
  peri-infarction i.
  regional myocardial i.
  regional transmural i.
  remote i.
  silent i.
  silent myocardial i.
  subendocardial i.
  transient i.
  transient myocardial i.
ischemic-guided medical therapy
ischemic
  i. burden
  i. cardiomyopathy
  persistence of i. changes
  i. contracture of the left
    ventricle
  i. ECG changes
  i. episodes
  i. heart disease (IHD)
  i. heart disease syndrome
  i. hypoxia
  i. mitral regurgitation
  i. myocardium
  i. pericarditis
  i. rest angina
  i. rest pain
  reversible i. changes
  i. segment (on echocardi-
    ogram)
  i. ST segment changes
  i. sudden death
  i. threshold
  i. viable myocardium
  i. zone
ischemically mediated mitral
  regurgitation
ISE
  ion-selective electrode

Iselin forceps
ISH
  isolated septal hypertro-
    phy
isoactin switch
isocapneic condition
isocapnia
isocenter system
isochoric
isocytosis
isodiametric bipolar screw-in
  lead
isodiphasic complex
isoechoic
isoelectric
  i. at J point
  i. interval
  i. line
  i. period
  i. point
  i. ST segment
isoenzyme
  cardiac i.
  CK i.
  CK-MB i.
  CK-MM i.
  CPK i's
  CPK-MB i.
  CPK-MM i.
  LDH_1 i.
  LDH_2 i.
  myocardial muscle creatine
    kinase i. (CK-MB)
isolated
  i. dextrocardia
  i. heat perfusion
  i. heat perfusion of an ex-
    tremity
  i. parietal endocarditis
  i. septal hypertrophy
isomer
  dextro i.

isomer *(continued)*
 levo i.

isomerism

isometric
 i. contraction
 i. contraction period
 i. exercise
 i. exercise test
 i. handgrip
 i. interval
 i. period of cardiac cycle
 i. relaxation period

isomyosin switch

isorhythmic
 i. AV dissociation
 i. dissociation

isotonic
 i. contraction
 i. exercise

isotope
 iodine-125 i.
 radioactive i.
 stable i.

isotypical

isovolumetric
 i. contractility
 i. phase index
 i. relaxation
 i. relaxation period

isovolumic
 i. index
 i. interval
 i. relaxation
 i. relaxation time
 i. systole

Isovue
 I.-330 contrast medium
 I.-370 contrast medium
 I.-M 300 contrast medium

isozyme

isthmectomy

isthmus *pl.* isthmi
 i. of aorta

isthmus *(continued)*
 aortic i.
 Krönig i.
 thyroid i.
 i. of Vieussens

ITA
 internal thoracic artery
 ITA graft

ITC balloon catheter

IVA
 intraoperative vascular angiography

Ivalon
 I. plug
 I. sponge

IVB
 intraventricular block

IVC
 inferior vena cava

IVDSA
 intravenous digital subtraction angiography

Ivemark syndrome

IVOTTS
 Irvine viable organ-tissue transport system

IVOX
 intravascular oxygenator

IVRP
 isovolumetric relaxation period

IVRT
 isovolumic relaxation time

IVT
 idiopathic ventricular tachycardia
  IVT percutaneous catheter introducer sheath

IVUS
 intravascular ultrasound

Ivy bleeding time

J
J-curve
J-exchangewire
J-guidewire
J-junction
J-loop technique
J-loop posterior chamber
lens
J-orthogonal electrode
J-point
J-point electrical axis
J-point treadmill test
J-Rosen guidewire
J-shaped tube
J-tip guidewire
J-wave
J-wire

Jabaley-Stille Supercut scissors

Jaccoud
J. arthritis
J. dissociated fever
J. sign

jacket
Bonchek-Shiley cardiac j.
cardiac cooling j.
cuirass j.
Daily cooling j.
Medtronic cardiac cool-
ing j.

jacket-type chest dressing

Jackman
J. coronary sinus electrode
catheter
J. orthogonal catheter

Jackson
J. bistoury
J. safety triangle
J. sign
J. syndrome
J.-Mosher dilator
J.-Trousseau dilator

Jacobson
J. clamp
J. endarterectomy spatula

Jacobson *(continued)*
J. forceps
J. hemostatic forceps
J. microbulldog clamp
J. modified vessel clamp
J. scissors
J. spatula
J.-Potts clamp
J.-Potts vessel clamp

Jacquet apparatus

Jahnke
J. anastomosis clamp
J.-Barron heart support net

Jako anterior commissure
scope

James
J. accessory tracts
J. atrionodal bypass tract
J. bundle
J. exercise protocol
J. fibers

Jamshidi needle

Janeway
J. lesion in infective endo-
carditis
J. sphygmomanometer

Jannetta aneurysm neck dissector

Jantene operation

Janus syndrome

Janz formula

Jarvik
J. -7 artificial heart
J. -8 artificial heart
J. 7-70 total artificial heart
J.-7 mechanical pump

Jatene
J. arterial switch procedure
J.-Macchi prosthetic valve

Javid
J. carotid artery bypass
clamp

Javid *(continued)*
  J. endarterectomy shunt
  J. internal carotid shunt
  J. shunt

jaw thrust maneuver

jejunal arteries

jelly
  cardiac j.
  electrode j.

jeopardized myocardium

jerky pulse

Jervell and Lange-Nielsen syndrome

jet
  anteriorly-directed j.
  aortic stenosis j.
  Doppler color j.
  j. effect
  mitral regurgitant j.
  mosaic j.
  regurgitant j.
  residual j.
  turbulent j.

Jeune syndrome

Jewel
  J. pacer-cardioverter-defibrillator
  J. PCD

Jinotti closed suctioning system

JL-4 catheter
  Judkins left, 4 cm

Jobst
  J. elastic stockings
  J. extremity pump
  J. pressure garment
  J. VPGS stockings
  J.-Stride support stockings
  J.-Stridette support stockings

Job syndrome

Johnson & Johnson hemopump

Johns Hopkins
  J. H. bulldog clamp
  J. H. coarctation clamp
  J. H. forceps
  J. H. modified Potts clamp
  J. H. occluding forceps
  J. H. thoracic forceps

Jonas modification of Norwood procedure

Jones
  J. criteria for diagnosing acute rheumatic fever
  J. IMA forceps
  J. thoracic forceps

Jonnson maneuver

Jopamiro 370

Jorgenson thoracic scissors

Josephson
  J. quadripolar mapping electrode
  J. quadripolar catheter

Jostra
  J. arterial blood filter
  J. cardiotomy reservoir
  J. catheter

joule (J)

JR-4 catheter
  Judkins right, 4 cm

JR-5 catheter
  Judkins right, 5 cm

JT
  junctional tachycardia
    JT interval

JTc value

Judkins
  J. cardiac catheterization technique
  J. coronary catheter (left/right)
  J. curve LAD catheter
  J. curve LCX catheter
  J. curve STD catheter

Judkins *(continued)*
   J. femoral catheterization
      technique
   J. guiding catheter
   J.-4 guiding catheter
   J. left 4 (JL-4)
   J. left coronary catheter
   J. right coronary catheter
   J. selective coronary arteri-
      ography
   J. technique for coronary
      arteriography
   J. torque control catheter
   J. USCI catheter

Judkins-Sones technique of cardiac catheterization

Juevenelle clamp

jugular
   j. bulb catheter placement
      assessment
   j. embryocardia
   j. notch of sternum
   j. vein
   j. venous arch
   j. venous catechol spillover
   j. venous distention (JVD)
   j. venous pressure (JVP)
   j. venous pulsation
   j. venous pulse tracing

jugulovenous distention (JVD)

Julian thoracic forceps

jump
   j. collaterals
   j. graft

jumping thrombosis

junction
   aortic sinotubular j.
   atrioventricular j.
   AV j.
   cardioesophageal j.
   costochondral j.
   gap j.

junction *(continued)*
   J j.
   loose j.
   QRS–ST j.
   saphenofemoral j.
   sinotubular j.
   ST j.
   sternochondral j.
   tight j.
   tracheoesophageal j.
   triadic j.

junctional
   j. arrhythmia
   j. axis
   j. bigeminy
   j. bradycardia
   j. complex
   j. depression
   j. ectopic tachycardia
   j. escape
   j. escape beat
   j. escape rhythm
   j. extrasystole
   j. pacemaker
   j. reciprocating tachycardia
   j. rhythm
   j. tachycardia

Junod procedure

Jürgensen sign

juvenile
   j. arrhythmia
   j. pattern

juxtacapillary receptor

juxtacardiac
   j. pleural pressure

juxtaductal
   j. coarctation

Juzo
   J. hose
   J. shrinker
   J. stocking for thrombo-
      phlebitis

Juzo *(continued)*
   J. stockings

J-Vac

JVD
     jugular venous distention

JVP
     jugular venous pressure

K
    potassium
K current

kallikrein
    k.-bradykinin system
    k. inactivating units
    k.-kinin system

Kallmann syndrome

Kalos pacemaker

Kaltostat
    K. wound packing dressing
    K. wound packing material

Kangaroo pump

Kantrowitz
    K. hemostatic clamp
    K. pacemaker
    K. thoracic clamp
    K. thoracic forceps
    K. vascular dissecting scis-
       sors
    K. vascular scissors

Kaplan-Meier
    K.-M. event-free survival
       curve
    K.-M. life table
    K.-M. method

Kaplan-Simpson InfusaSleeve

Kaposi
    K. sarcoma
    epicardial K.

Kapp
    K. microarterial clamp
    K.-Beck clamp
    K.-Beck coarctation clamp
    K.-Beck-Thomson clamp

Karell
    K. diet
    K. treatment

Karhunen-Loeve procedure

Karmen units

Karmody venous scissors

Karnofsky rating scale

Karp aortic punch forceps

Karplus sign

Kartagener
    K. syndrome
    K. triad

Kartchner carotid artery clamp

karyapsis

karyenchyma

karyochylema

karyoclasis

karyoclastic

karyocyte

karyogamic

karyogamy

karyogenesis

karyogenic

karyokinesis
    asymmetrical k.
    hyperchromatic k.
    hypochromatic k.

karyokinetic

karyoklasis

karyoklastic

karyolymph

karyolytic

karyomegaly

karyomere

karyometry

karyomitosis

karyomitotic

karyomorphism

karyon

karyoplasm
karyoplasmic
karyoplast
karyoplastin
karyopyknosis
karyopyknotic
karyoreticulum
karyorrhectic
karyorrhexis
karyostasis
karyotheca
karyotin
Kasabach-Merritt syndrome
Kasser-Kennedy method
Kaster mitral valve prosthesis
KATT II Plus intra-aortic balloon pump
Kattus
 K. exercise stress test
 K. treadmill protocol
Katzen
 K. infusion wire
 K. long balloon dilatation catheter
Katz-Wachtle phenomenon
Kawai bioptome
Kawasaki
 K. disease
 K. syndrome
Kawashima intraventricular tunnel
Kay
 K. aortic clamp
 K. balloon
 K. tricuspid valvuloplasty
 K.-Lambert clamp
 K.-Shiley caged-disk valve

Kay (continued)
 K.-Shiley disk prosthetic valve
 K.-Shiley mitral valve
 K.-Shiley valve prosthesis
 K.-Suzuki disk valve prosthesis
 K.-Suzuki valve prosthesis
Kaye-Damus-Stansel operation
KCl
 potassium chloride
kd
 kilodalton
Kearns-Sayre syndrome
Kearns syndrome
keel
 McNaught k.
keeled chest
Keith
 K. bundle
 K. node
 K.-Flack sinoatrial node
 K.-Wagener hypertensive retinopathy classification (I–IV)
 K.-Wagener-Barker (KWB) hypertensive classification
Kellock sign
Kelly
 K. clamp
 K. hemostat
 K.-Murphy hemostatic forceps
 K.-Wick vascular tunneler
Kelvin Sensor pacemaker
Kempner diet
Kendall
 K. compression stockings
 K. Sequential Compression device
Kennedy
 K. area-length method

Kennedy *(continued)*
    K. method for calculating
        ejection fraction

Kensey atherectomy catheter

Kent
    K. bundle
    K. bundle ablation
    bundle of Stanley K.
    K. fibers
    K. pathway
    K. potential
    K.-His bundle

Kerley
    K. A lines
    K. B lines
    K. C lines

Kern technique

Keshan disease

Kety-Schmidt method

KeV
    kiloelectron volt

Key
    ResCue K.

keyhole-limpet hemocyanin

keyhole surgery

kg/m²
    kilogram per meter
        squared

KI antigen

kick
    atrial k.
    idioventricular k.

Kienback phenomenon

Kiethly-DAS series 500 data-ac-
    quisition system

Kifa catheter

Kikuchi disease

Killip
    K. classification of heart
        disease

Killip *(continued)*
    K. wire

Killip-Kimball heart failure clas-
    sification

kilodalton (kd)

kiloelectron volt (keV)

kilogram
    milligrams per k. (mg/kg)
    milliliters per k. (mL/kg)
    k. per meter squared (kg/
        m²)

kilohm

kilopascal (kPA)

kilopond (KP)

kilovolt (kV)

Kimmelstiel-Wilson syndrome

KimRay
    K. Greenfield antiembolus
        filter
    K. Greenfield vena cava fil-
        ter
    K. thermodilution

Kimura cartilage graft

kinase
    creatine k. (CK)
    phosphorylase k.
    protein k.
    serum creatine k.

Kindt carotid artery clamp

kinesin

kinetics
    first-order k.
    zero-order k.

kinetocardiogram

kinetocardiography

kinetoplasm

King
    K. ASD umbrella closure
    K. biopsy method

King *(continued)*
   K. bioptome
   K. cardiac device
   K. double umbrella closure
     system
   K. guiding catheter
   K. of Hearts event recorder
   K. of Hearts Holter monitor
   K. multipurpose catheter
   K. multipurpose coronary
     graft catheter

kinin

kininogen

kinked aorta

kinking
   k. of blood vessel
   k. of graft

kinky-hair disease

kinocentrum

kinocilium

kinosphere

Kinsey
   K. atherectomy
   K. atherectomy catheter
   K. rotation atherectomy ex-
     trusion angioplasty

Kinyoun stain

Kirklin
   K. atrial retractor
   K. fence

Kirstein method

Kirsch reflex

kissing
   k. balloon angioplasty
   k. balloon technique

kit
   BiPort hemostasis intro-
     ducer sheath k.
   Cordis lead conversion k.
   Euro-Collins multiorgan
     perfusion k.

kit *(continued)*
   Fergus percutaneous in-
     troducer k.
   Imulyse t-PA ELISA k.
   neonatal internal jugular
     puncture k.
   No Pour Pak suction cath-
     eter k.
   percutaneous access k.
   percutaneous catheter in-
     troducer k.
   Pro-Vent arterial blood
     gas k.
   Pro-Vent arterial blood
     sampling k.
   Pulsator dry heparin arte-
     rial blood gas k.
   Sub-4 Platinum Plus wire k.
   thermodilution hemostasis
     introducer sheath k.
   TriPort hemostasis intro-
     ducer sheath k.
   UniPort hemostasis intro-
     ducer sheath k.
   Yamasa assay k.

Klebs-Löffler bacillus

Kleihauer-Betke test

Kleihauer test

Klein transseptal introducer
  sheath

Klein-Waardenburg syndrome

Klinefelter syndrome

Klippel-Feil syndrome

Klippel-Trenaunay-Weber syndrome

knife
   A-K diamond k.
   A-OK ShortCut k.
   Bailey-Glover-O'Neill com-
     missurotomy k.
   Bailey-Morse k.
   Bard-Parker k.
   Beaver k.
   Bosher commissurotomy k.
   Brock commissurotomy k.

knife *(continued)*
  commissurotomy k.
  Derra commissurotomy k.
  Gamma k.
  Hufnagel commissuroto-
    my k.
  intimectomy k.
  Koos vessel k.
  Lebsche sternal k.
  Lebsche thoracic k.
  microblade k.
  microvessel k.
  mitral stenosis k.
  Neoflex bendable k.
  Niedner k.
  Nunez-Nunez mitral stenos-
    is k.
  pulmonary valve k.
  Rochester mitral stenos-
    is k.
  roentgen k.
  Sellor k.
  UltraCision ultrasonic k.
  valvotomy k.

knitted
  k. Dacron arterial graft
  k. sewing ring
  k. Teflon prosthesis
  k. vascular prosthesis

knob
  aortic k.

knock
  pericardial k.

knuckle
  aortic k.
  b k.
  cervical aortic k.
  k. sign

Ko-Airan bleeding control procedure

Koate-HP

Koch
  K. sinoatrial node
  triangle of K.
  K. triangle

Kocher-Cushing reflex

Koga treatment

KOH
  potassium hydroxide

Kohn pores

koilocyte

koilocytosis

koilocytotic

Kolff-Jarvik artificial heart

Kolmogorov-Smirnov
  K.-S. Goodness-of-fit test
  K.-S. procedure

Kommerell diverticulum

Konigsberg catheter

Konno
  K. biopsy method
  K. bioptome

Kono
  K. operation
  K. patch enlargement of as-
    cending aorta

Kontron
  K. balloon
  K. balloon catheter
  K. intra-aortic balloon

Korányi
  K. auscultation
  K. percussion
  K. sign

Korotkoff
  K. method
  K. phase (I–V)
  K. sound
  K. test

Kostmann syndrome

Kotonkan virus

K-37 pediatric arterial blood filter

Krasky retractor

Krayenbuehl vessel hook

Krebs
  K. cycle
  K. solution
  K.-Henseleit buffer
  K.-Henseleit solution

Krehl
  tendon of K.

Kreiselman unit

Kreysig sign

kringle

Krishaber disease

Kronecker aneurysm needle

Krönig
  K. area
  K. fields
  K. isthmus
  K. percussion
  K. steps

Krovetz-Gessner equation

Kruskal-Wallis test

k-space segmentation

K-sponge

Kugel
  K. anastomosis
  K. artery

Kugel *(continued)*
  K. collaterals

Kuhn
  K. mask
  K. tube

Kulchitsky cell

Kurten vein stripper

Kussmaul
  K. breathing
  K. paradoxical pulse
  K. respirations
  K. sign
  K.-Kien respiration
  K.-Maier disease

kV
  kilovolt
    kV fluoroscopy

Kveim
  K. antigen skin test
  K. reaction

KWB
    Keith-Wagener-Barker
      KWB classification

Kwelcof

kymogram

kymograph

kymography

kymoscope

kyphoscoliosis

L
    L-transposition of great arteries

LA
    left atrium

LAA
    left atrial appendage
    LAA thrombi

La:Ao
    left atrial to aortic
    L. ratio

LABA
    laser-assisted balloon angioplasty

labeled FFA scintigraphy

labile
    l. blood pressure
    l. hypertension
    l. pulse

LaBorde method

lacertus
    l. cordis

LACI
    lipoprotein-associated coagulation inhibitor

lactamase
    beta l.

lactate
    amrinone l.
    l. dehydrogenase (LDH)
    l. extraction
    milrinone l.
    Ringer's l.
    l. threshold

lactea
    macula l.

lactic
    l. acid
    l. acid dehydrogenase
    l. acidosis
    l. dehydrogenase (LDH)

lacunar
    l. angina
    l. infarct
    l. infarction
    l. stroke

LAD
    left anterior descending artery
        LAD saphenous vein
            graft angioplasty
    left axis deviation

ladder
    l. diagram
    l. incisions

laddergram

LAE
    left atrial enlargement

Laënnec
    L. catarrh
    L. cirrhosis
    L. pearls
    L. sign

Lagrangian
    L. definition
    L. strain

LAH
    left anterior hemiblock
    left atrial hypertrophy

Lahey
    L. arterial forceps
    L. hemostatic forceps
    L. lock arterial forceps
    L. thoracic clamp
    L. thoracic forceps

laid-back
    l.-b. balloon occlusion aortography
    l.-b. view

LAIS laser

laiteuses
    taches l.

lake
 venous l's

Lam procedure

LAMA
 laser-assisted microanastomosis

Lambda pacemaker

Lambert
 L. aortic clamp
 canals of L.
 L.-Kay vascular clamp

Lambl excrescences

lamella
 annulate lamellae

lamellipodia

lamellipodium

lamin

lamina *pl.* laminae
 elastic l.
 external elastic l.
 internal elastic l.
 l. elastica interna
 l. fibrosa
 fibrous nuclear l.
 nuclear l.
 l. parietalis pericardii ser-
 osi
 l. visceralis pericardii ser-
 osi

laminar blood flow

laminated
 l. clot
 l. thrombus

laminin

lamp
 Wood l.

Lancisi sign

Landolfi sign

Landry-Guillain-Barré syndrome

Landry Vein Light Venoscope

Lange calipers

Lange-Nielsen syndrome

Langendorff
 L. apparatus
 L. heart preparation

Langer axillary arch

Langerhans giant cells

Langevin updating procedure

Langhans cells

Lanz low-pressure cuff endotracheal tube

Laplace law

Laplacian mapping

lapping murmur

Lap Sac

Large vena caval clamp

large-bore
 l.-b. catheter
 l.-b. needle

large-vessel disease

laser
 l. ablation
 alexandrite l.
 l. angioplasty
 ArF excimer l.
 argon l.
 argon-krypton l.
 argon pulsed-dye l.
 argon-pumped tunable
 dye l.
 atheroablation l.
 l.-balloon angioplasty
 balloon-center argon l.
 carbon dioxide (CO_2) l.
 continuous-wave pulsed l.
 cool-tip l.
 coumarin pulsed-dye l.
 dye l.
 ELCA l.

laser *(continued)*
  l. endarterectomy
  erbium:YAG l.
  excimer cool l.
  excimer gas l.
  l. firing
  flashlamp-pulsed Nd:YAG l.
  fluorescence-guided
    smart l.
  free-beam l.
  helium-cadmium diagnos-
    tic l.
  helium-neon l.
  HF infrared l.
  high-energy l.
  holmium l.
  Ho:YAG l.
  infrared-pulsed l.
  krypton l.
  LAIS l.
  long-pulsed alexandrite l.
  long-pulsed ruby l.
  low-energy l.
  Lumonics YAG l.
  MCM smart l.
  microsecond pulsed flash-
    lamp pumped dye l.
  mid-infrared pulsed l.
  Nd:YAG l.
  neodymium:yttrium-alumi-
    num-garnet l.
  l. photoablation
  l. photocoagulation
  pulsed angio l.
  pulsed dye l.
  Q-switched alexandrite l.
  Q-switched Nd:YAG l.
  l. recanalization
  rotational ablation l.
  ruby l.
  Septranetics l.
  spectroscopy-directed l.
  Surgica K6 l.
  Surgilase 150 l.
  THC:YAG l.
  ultraviolet l.
  XeCl excimer l.
  xenon chloride excimer l.
  YAG l.

laser-assisted
  l.-a. balloon angioplasty
  l.-a. microanastomosis

Laserdish
  L. electrode
  L. pacing lead

Laserflow blood perfusion monitor

LaserHarmonic laser

laser-induced
  l.-i. arterial fluorescence
  l.-i. thrombosis

Laserpor pacing lead

Laserprobe catheter

Laserprobe-Hatle equation

Lasertek YAG laser

late
  l. apical systolic murmur
  l. apnea
  l. cyanosis
  l. death
  l. deceleration
  l. diastole
  l. diastolic murmur
  l. potential activity
  l. proarrhythmic effect
  l. reperfusion
  l. systole

latent pacemaker

late-peaking systolic murmur

lateral
  l. myocardial infarction
  l. sac
  l. thrombus
  l. wall

Laubry-Soulle syndrome

Laurell method

Laurence-Moon-Bardet-Biedl
  syndrome

Lautier test

lavage
  bronchoalveolar l.
  continuous pericardial l.
  pericardial l.

law
  all-or-none l.
  Bowditch l.
  Du Bois-Reymond l.
  Einthoven l.
  l. of the heart
  Hooke l.
  Laplace l.
  Louis l.
  Marey l.
  Ohm l.
  Poiseuille l.
  Starling l.
  Sutton l.
  Torricelli l.

laxa
  cutis l.

layer
  adventitial l.
  fascial l.
  half-value l.
  hypertrophic smooth mus-
    cle l.
  parietal l. of pericardium
  parietal l. of serous pericar-
    dium
  subendocardial l.
  subendothelial l.
  subepicardial l.
  visceral l. of pericardium
  visceral l. of serous peri-
    cardium

LBBB
  left bundle branch block

LCA
  left coronary artery

LCX
  left circumflex coronary ar-
    tery

LDH
  lactic dehydrogenase

LDL
  low-density lipoprotein

lead
  l. I
  l. II
  l. III
  ABC l's
  Accufix bipolar l.
  Accufix pacemaker l.
  active fixation l.
  anterior precordial l.
  anterolateral l.
  atrial l.
  atrial J l.
  augmented unipolar limb l.
  aVF l.
  aVL l.
  aVR l.
  barbed epicardial pacing l.
  bifurcated J-shaped tined
    atrial pacing and defibril-
    lation l.
  bipolar l.
  bipolar limb l.
  bipolar precordial l.
  Cadence TVL nonthoraco-
    tomy l.
  capped l.
  CapSure cardiac pacing l.
  CB l.
  CCS endocardial pacing l.
  CF l.
  cobra-head epicardial l.
  Cordis Ancar pacing l's
  CPI endocardial defibrilla-
    tion/rate-sensing/pacing l.
  CPI Endotak SQ electrode l.
  CPI porous tined-tip bipo-
    lar pacing l.
  CPI Sentra endocardial l.
  CPI Sweet Tip l.
  CR l.
  direct l.
  Einthoven l.
  Ela ventricular pacing l.
  electrocardiographic l's
  Elema l's
  Encor pacing l.

lead *(continued)*
 endocardial balloon l.
 Endotak C tripolar pacing/
  sensing/defibrillation l.
 Endotak C tripolar transvenous l.
 epicardial pacemaker l.
 esophageal l.
 Frank XYZ orthogonal l.
 Golum EKG l.
 Heartwire l.
 Hombach placement of l's
 l. impedance
 indirect l.
 inferior precordial l.
 inferolateral l.
 intracardiac l.
 Ionyx l.
 isodiametric bipolar screw-
  in l.
 Laserdish pacing l.
 lateral precordial l.
 Lewis l.
 limb l.
 Mason-Likar placement of
  EKG l's
 Medtronic l's
 monitor l's
 myocardial l.
 Myopore l.
 negative sensing rate l.
 Nehb D l.
 nonintegrated transvenous
  defibrillation l.
 nonintegrated tripolar l.
 Oscor atrial l.
 Oscor pacing l's
 Osykpa atrial l.
 pacemaker l.
 pacing l.
 passive fixation l.
 permanent cardiac pa-
  cing l.
 Permathane l.
 l. placement
 positive sensing rate l.
 Precept l.
 precordial l.
 l. reversal

lead *(continued)*
 reversed arm l's
 scalar l's
 screw-in l.
 screw-on epicardial l.
 screw-tipped l.
 segmented ring tripolar l.
 semidirect l.
 single-pass l.
 standard l's
 standard limb l.
 Stela electrode l.
 steroid-eluting pacemaker l.
 Sweet Tip l.
 l. system
 Target Tip l.
 Telectronics l's
 temporary pacemaker l.
 temporary pervenous l.
 three-turn epicardial l.
 l. threshold
 Transvene-RV l.
 transvenous defibrillator l.
 transvenous ventricular
  sensing l.
 tripolar l.
 two-turn epicardial l.
 Unipass endocardial pa-
  cing l.
 unipolar limb l's
 unipolar precordial l.
 V_1 to V_6 l's
 Viatron l's
 V-Pace transluminal pa-
  cing l.
 Wilson l.
 XYZ Frank l.

3-lead electrocardiogram

12-lead electrocardiogram

leaflet
 anterior mitral l.
 anterior tricuspid l.
 aortic valve l.
 arching of mitral valve l.
 ballooning of mitral valve l.
 bowing of mitral valve l.
 calcified l.
 cleft l.

leaflet *(continued)*
    degenerated l.
    doming of l's
    doughnut-shaped prolapsing l.
    flail mitral l.
    fluttering of valvular l.
    fused l.
    hammocking of l.
    incompetent l.
    mitral valve l.
    l. motion
    myxomatous valve l.
    nodularity of l.
    noncoronary l.
    paradoxical motion of l.
    posterior l.
    posterior mitral l. (PML)
    posterior tricuspid l.
    l. prolapse
    prolapsed l.
    redundant l.
    retracted l.
    l. retractor
    sail-like anterior l.
    thickened l.
    l. thickening
    l. tip
    tricuspid valve l.
    l. vegetation

leak
    baffle l.
    interatrial baffle l.
    paraprosthetic l.
    paravalvular l.
    perivalvular l.

leaky valve

Leather
    L. valve cutter
    L. venous valvulotome
    L.-Karmody in-situ valve scissors

Lebsche
    L. forceps
    L. shears
    L. sternal knife
    L. sternal punch

Lebsche *(continued)*
    L. sternal shears
    L. thoracic knife

lecithin

lecithin-cholesterol acyltransferase

lecithin/sphingomyelin

Lecompte maneuver

Lectron II electrode gel

Lee
    L. bronchus clamp
    L. delicate hemostatic forceps
    L. microvascular clamp
    L.-White method

Lees
    L. arterial forceps
    L. vascular clamp

left
    l. anterior descending artery (LAD)
    l. anterior fascicular block
    l. anterior hemiblock (LAH)
    l. anterior oblique (LAO)
    l. aortic angiography
    l. atrial angiography
    l. atrial to aortic (La:Ao)
    l. atrial appendage (LAA)
    l. atrial dimension
    l. atrial emptying index
    l. atrial enlargement (LAE)
    l. atrial hypertension
    l. atrial myxoma
    l. atrial pressure
    l. atrium (LA)
    l. atrium to distal arterial aortic bypass
    l. axis deviation (LAD)
    l. border of cardiac dullness
    l. bundle branch block (LBBB)
    l. circumflex coronary artery
    l. common carotid artery

left *(continued)*
l. coronary artery (LCA)
l. dominant coronary circulation
l. fifth intercostal space
l. heart
l. heart bypass
l. heart catheterization
l. iliac system
l. inferior pulmonary vein
l. intercostal space
l. internal jugular vein
l. internal mammary artery
(LIMA)
l. Judkins catheter
l. lateral projection
l. main coronary artery
(LMCA)
l. main coronary artery disease
l. main coronary stenosis
l. main disease
l. middle hemiblock
l. posterior hemiblock
l. septal hemiblock
l. sternal border
l. subclavian artery
l. ventricle (LV)
l. ventricular aneurysm
l. ventricular angiography
l. ventricular apex
l. ventricular assist device
(LVAD)
l. ventricular assist system
l. ventricular bypass pump
l. ventricular chamber compliance
l. ventricular clamp catheter
l. ventricular contactility
l. ventricular dam
l. ventricular diastolic
phase index
l. ventricular diastolic pressure
l. ventricular diastolic relaxation
l. ventricular dysfunction
(LVD)

left *(continued)*
l. ventricular ejection fraction (LVEF)
l. ventricular ejection time
l. ventricular end-diastolic
dimension
l. ventricular end-diastolic
pressure
l. ventricular end-diastolic
volume
l. ventricular end-systolic
dimention
l. ventricular end-systolic
stress
l. ventricular end-systolic
volume
l. ventricular failure
l. ventricular filling pressure
l. ventricular forces
l. ventricular function
l. ventricular hypertrophy
(LVH)
l. ventricular inflow tract
obstruction
l. ventricular internal diastolic diameter
l. ventricular internal diastolic dimension
l. ventricular-l. atrial crossover dynamics
l. ventricular mass
l. ventricular muscle compliance
l. ventricular myxoma
l. ventricular outflow tract
l. ventricular outflow tract
velocity
l. ventricular output
l. ventricular power
l. ventricular pressure-volume curve
l. ventricular puncture
l. ventricular-right atrial
communication murmur
l. ventricular regional wall
motion
l. ventricular segmental
contraction

left (continued)
l. ventricular stroke volume
l. ventricular sump catheter
l. ventricular systolic performance
l. ventricular systolic pressure
l. ventricular systolic pump
function
l. ventricular tension
l. ventricular wall
l. ventricular wall motion
abnormality
l. ventricular wall stress
l. ventriculography

left-sided heart failure

left-to-right shunt

leg
l. fatigue
milk l.
l. pain at rest
white l.

Legend pacemaker

legionellosis

Legionnaire
L. disease
L. pneumonia

Legroux remission

Lehman
L. cardiac device
L. catheter
L. ventriculography cathe-
ter

leiomyoma pl. leiomyomata

leiomyomatosis of heart

leiomyosarcoma

Leios pacemaker

leishmaniasis

Leitner syndrome

Lejeune thoracic forceps

Leksell
L. cardiovascular rongeur
L.-Stille thoracic-cardiovas-
cular rongeur

Leland-Jones
L.-J. forceps
L.-J. peripheral vascular
clamp
L.-J. vascular clamp

Lemakalim

Lemmon
L. intimal dissector
L. rib spreader
L. self-retaining sternal re-
tractor
L. sternal approximator
L. sternal elevator
L. sternal spreader

Lenègre
L. disease
L. syndrome

length
antegrade block cycle l.
atrial-paced cycle l.
basic cycle l.
basic drive cycle l.
block cycle l.
chordal l.
cycle l.
drive cycle l.
flutter cycle l.
paced cycle l.
pacing cycle l.
sinus cycle l.
tachycardiac cycle l.
ventricular tachycardia cycle l.
wave l.

length-active tension curve

length-dependent activation

length-resting tension relation

length-tension relation

Lennarson suction tube

lensed fiber-tip laser delivery
　catheter

lenta
　　endocarditis l.

lentiginosis
　　cardiomyopathic l.

lentis
　　ectopia l.

Lenz syndrome

Leocor hemoperfusion system

lepocyte

lepromin test

leptochromatic

leptonema

leptoscope

leptotene

Leptos pacemaker

leptospirosis

Leredde syndrome

Leriche
　　L. hemostatic forceps
　　L. operation
　　L. syndrome

Lerman-Means scratch

lesion
　　aorto-ostial l.
　　atherosclerotic l.
　　bifurcation l.
　　bird's nest l.
　　Blumenthal l.
　　Bracht-Wachter l.
　　braid-like l.
　　branch l.
　　calcified l.
　　cavitary l.
　　coin l.
　　concentric l.
　　coronary artery l.

lesion (continued)
　　critical l.
　　culprit l.
　　dendritic l.
　　de novo l.
　　dilatable l.
　　discrete coronary l.
　　eccentric l.
　　enhancing l.
　　fibrocalcific l.
　　fibromusculoelastic l.
　　flow-limiting l.
　　Ghon primary l.
　　hemodynamically signifi-
　　　cant l.
　　high-grade l.
　　honeycomb l.
　　Janeway l.
　　jet l.
　　Libman-Sacks l.
　　Lohlein-Baehr l.
　　long l.
　　macrovascular coronary l.
　　monotypic l.
　　nonbacterial thrombotic
　　　endocardial l.
　　occlusive l.
　　onion scale l.
　　ostial l.
　　partial l.
　　plexiform l.
　　polypoidal l.
　　regurgitant l.
　　restenosis l.
　　satellite l.
　　space-occupying l.
　　stenotic l.
　　synchronous airway l's
　　tandem l.
　　target l.
　　vegetative l.
　　wire-loop l.

lesser resection

lethal arrhythmia

Letterer-Siwe disease

leucine

leucovorin

leukocidin

leukocyte
l.-poor red blood cells

leukocytoblastic vasculitis

leukocytoclastic angiitis

leukocytosis
transient l.

LeukoNet Filter

Leukos pacemaker

Leukotrap red cell storage system

leukotriene
l. B4
l. C
l. E
l. inhibition

Lev
L. classification of complete AV block
L. disease
L. syndrome

LeVeen
L. endarterectomy
L. peritoneovenous shunt
L. plaque-cracker
L. valve

level
air-fluid l.
blood oxygen l.
digoxin l.
ELF l's
isoelectric l.
multiple shunt l's
myofibrillar calcium l.
peak and trough l's
predose l.
reflecting l.
sarcolemmal l.
serum renin l.
triglyceride l.

level (continued)
trough l.
trough-and-peak l's

Levenberg-Marquardt algorithm

Levin catheter

Levine
L. gradation of cardiac murmurs (grades 1–6)
L. sign
L.-Harvey classification of heart murmur

Levinson-Durbin recursion

Levinthal-Coles-Lillie (LCL) (LCL)

levoatriocardinal vein

levocardia
isolated l.
l. malposition
mixed l.
l. with situs inversus

levocardiogram

levo isomer

levophase of angiogram

levoisomerism

levo-transposed position

levotransposition of great arteries (L-transposition)

levoversion

Lewis
L. index
L. lead
L. lines
L. thoracotomy
L. upper limb cardiovascular disease
L.-Pickering test
L.-Tanner procedure

Lewy
L. chest holder
L.-Rubin needle

Leycom volume conductance
    catheter

LFT
    liver function test

LIAF
    laser-induced arterial fluo-
        rescence

Libman
    L.-Sacks disease
    L.-Sacks endocarditis
    L.-Sacks lesion
    L.-Sacks syndrome

Liddle aorta clamp

Liebermann-Burchard test

Liebermeister rule

Lifeline electrode

Lifepak
    L. 7 monitor-defibrillator

Lifesaver disposable resuscita-
    tor bag

Lifescan

Lifestream coronary dilation
    catheter

lifestyle
    sedentary l.

lift
    aneurysmal l.
    late systolic parasternal l.
    left ventricular l.
    parasternal systolic l.
    pulmonary artery l.
    right ventricular l.
    substernal l.
    sustained right ventricu-
        lar l.

ligament
    Bérard l.
    l. of Botallo
    conus l.
    Cooper l.
    l. of left vena cava

ligament (continued)
    l's of Luschka
    Marshall l.
    pericardiosternal l.
    sternopericardiac l's

ligamentum pl. ligamenta
    l. arteriosum
    l. sternopericardiaca
    l. teres cardiopexy
    l. venae cavae sinistrae

ligand
    macromolecular l.

ligate

ligation
    Bardenheurer l.
    l. of bleeders
    l. clip
    Desault l.
    patent ductus arteriosus l.
    l. of perforators
    proximal l.
    variceal l.
    varicose vein stripping
        and l.
    l. of vessels

ligature
    l.-carrying aneurysm for-
        ceps
    pursestring l.
    silk l.
    Stannius l.
    wire l.
    Woodbridge l.

light
    l. chain
    l. microscope
    l. pen
    l. pen-determined ejection
        fraction

lightwire

Ligniere test

Lilienthal
    L. incision
    L. rib guillotine
    L. rib spreader

Lilienthal *(continued)*
    L.-Sauerbruch retractor
    L.-Sauerbruch rib spreader

Lillehei
    L. pacemaker
    L. valve
    L. valve forceps
    L. valve-grasping forceps
    L. valve prosthesis
    L.-Cruz-Kaseter prosthesis
    L.-Kaster aortic valve pros-
        thesis
    L.-Kaster cardiac valve
        prosthesis
    L.-Kaster mitral valve pros-
        thesis
    L.-Kaster pivoting-disk
        prosthetic valve

LIMA
    left internal mammary ar-
        tery
    LIMA graft

limb
    anacrotic l.
    ascending l.
    l. of bifurcation graft
    catacrotic l.
    descending l.
    Gore-Tex l.
    l. ischemia
    l. lead
    l. salvage
    thoracic l.

limb-girdle muscular dystrophy

limbus *pl.* limbi
    l. fossae ovalis
    l. of Vieussens

lime
    bruit de l.

limit
    Hayflick l.
    Nyquist l.

Lincoln scissors

Lincoln-Metzenbaum scissors

Lindbergh pump

Lindesmith operation

line
    A l. (arterial line)
    anterior axillary l.
    aortic l.
    arterial mean l.
    Cantlie l.
    central venous l.
    central venous pressure
        (CVP) l.
    commissural l.
    Conradi l.
    Correra l.
    Eberth l's
    indwelling l.
    Intertech Perkin-Elmer gas
        sampling l.
    isoelectric l.
    Kerley A, B, C l's
    Lewis l.
    Linton l.
    M l.
    midaxillary l.
    midclavicular l. (MCL)
    radial arterial l.
    suture l.
    tram l's
    Z l.
    Zahn l's

linea alba

lineage
    cell l.

linear
    l. echodensity
    l. phonocardiograph
    l. regression

linearity
    amplitude l.
    count-rate l.

lingular artery

linin

linoleic acid

Linton
    L. elastic stockings
    L. flap
    L. line
    L. radical vein ligation
    L. vein stripper

Linx
    L. exchange guide wire
    L. extension wire
    L.-EZ cardiac device
    L. guide wire extension
    L. guide wire extension cardiac device

Liotta
    L.-BioImplant prosthetic valve
    L. total artificial heart

lipase
    diacylglycerol l.
    hepatic l.
    lipoprotein l.

lipedema

lipemia retinalis

lipid
    l. accumulation
    endogenous l.
    exogenous l.
    extracellular l.
    l. fractionation
    l. hypothesis
    intracellular l.
    l. panel
    l. peroxidation product
    renomedullary l.
    sarcolemma l.
    l. solubility

lipid-A

lipodosis *pl.* lipidoses

lipid-rich plaque

lipocardiac

lipodystrophy
    intestinal l.

lipofuscinosis
    neuronal ceroid l.

lipogenic theory of atherosclerosis

lipohyalinosis

lipoid pneumonia

lipoparticle

lipoperoxide

lipophanerosis

lipophilicity

lipopolysaccharidase

lipopolysaccharide

lipoprotein
    alpha l.
    beta l.
    high density l. (HDL)
    intermediate-density l.
    l. lipase
    low-density l. (LDL)
    plasma l.
    pre-beta l.
    triglyceride-rich l's
    very-low-density l. (VLDL)

lipoprotein-associated coagulation inhibitor

lipoproteinemia

liposarcoma

Liposorber LA-15 system

lipothymia

lipoxygenase

5-lipoxygenase

Lissajou loop

Liston-Stille forceps

Liteguard mini-defibrillator

lith-II pacemaker

lithium
    l. battery

lithium *(continued)*
l. pacemaker
l. -powered pacemaker

Litten
L. diaphragm sign
L. phenomenon

Little disease

Littleford-Spector introducer

Littman
L. Class II pediatric stethoscope
L. defibrillation pad

littoral

Litwak
L. cannula
L. left atrial-aortic bypass
L. mitral valve scissors
L. scissors
L. utility scissors

livedo
l. reticularis
l. vasculitis

liver
cardiac l.
cirrhosis of l.
l. function test
l. palm

livida
asphyxia l.

livid cyanosis

Livierato
L. reflex
L. sign
L. test

LIZ-88 ablation unit

L-looping of the ventricle

LMCA
left main coronary artery

LMWH
low-molecular-weight heparin

load
electronic pacemaker l.
exercise l.
heat l.
peak work l.

loading
l. dose
glycogen l.
methionine l.
relaxation l.
saline l.
volume l.

localized
l. lesion
l. plaque formation
l. signs of weakness
l. tenderness

LocalMed
L. catheter infusion sleeve
L. InfusaSleeve

lock
heparin l.

Löffler (Loeffler)
L. basillus
L. disease
L. endocarditis
L. parietal fibroplastic endocarditis
L. syndrome

Lohlein-Baehr lesion

Lombardi sign

lone atrial fibrillation

long
l. ACE fixed-wire balloon catheter
l. axial oblique view
l. axis
l. lesion
l. pulse
l. Q–T syndrome
l. Q–TU syndrome
l. segment narrowing
L. Skinny over-the-wire balloon catheter

long-acting nitrate

long-axis
l.-a. parasternal view
l.-a. view

Longdwel Teflon catheter

longitudinal
l. arteriography
l. dissociation
l. midline incision
l. narrowing

Longmire
L. anastomosis
L. valvotomy
L. valvulotome
L.-Mueller curved valvulotome

loop
atrial vector l.
bulboventricular l.
Cannon endarterectomy l.
capillary l's
cine l.
D l.
l. diuresis
l. diuretic
elliptical l.
endarterectomy l.
flow-volume l.
Gerdy interatrial l.
Gerdy interauricular l.
Gerdy intra-auricular l.
guide wire l.
heart l.
Henle l.
L l.
Lissajou l.
maxi-vessel l's
memory l.
P l.
pressure-volume l's
QRS l.
reentrant l.
rubber vessel l.
sewing ring l.
Silastic l.
T l.

loop (continued)
U l.
Uresil radiopaque silicone band vessel l's
U-shaped catheter l.
vector l.
ventricular l.
ventricular pressure-volume l.
vessel l.

loose junction

Lo-Por
L. arterial prosthesis
L. vascular graft prosthesis

Lo-Profile
L. II balloon catheter
L. steerable dilatation catheter

Lortat-Jacob approach

loss
l. of capture
l. of sensing

Louis
sternal angle of L.

Love-Gruenwald forceps

Loven reflex

low
l. amplitude P wave
l. energy direct current
l. flow rate
l. grade
L. Profile Port vascular access
l. septal atrium

low-compliance
l.-c. balloon
l.-c. perfusion system

low-density lipoprotein (LDL)

Löwenberg cuff sign

low-energy
l.-e. laser

low-energy *(continued)*
l.-e. synchronized cardioversion

Lower rings

Lower-Shumway cardiac transplant

lower
l. body negative pressure
l. extremity bypass graft
l. extremity noninvasive
l. nodal extrasystole
l. nodal rhythm

low-fat diet

low-frequency murmur

low-methioine diet

low-molecular-weight
l.-m.-w. dextran
l.-m.-w. heparin

Lown
L. arrhythmia
L. cardioverter
L. class 4a or b ventricular
ectopic beats
L. classification
L. modified grading system
L. technique
L. and Woolf method
L.-Edmark waveform
L.-Ganong-Levine variant
syndrome

low-osmolality contract material

low-output heart failure

low-pitched murmur

low-pressure tamponade

low-salt (low-sodium)
l.-s. diet
l.-s. syndrome

low-speed rotation angioplasty
catheter

LPL
lipoprotein lipase

LPS Peel-Away introducer

LQTS
long Q–T syndrome

L/S
lecithin/sphingomyelin

L-transposition
levotransposition

LT V-105 implantable cardioverter-defibrillator

lubb

lubb-dupp

lubricity

Lucas-Championnière disease

Lucchese mitral valve dilator

lucency

lucent defect

Luciana-Wenckebach atrioventricular block

lucigenin

lucocorticosteroid

Ludwig
L. angina
L. angle

Luer-Lok
L. connector
L. needle
L. port
L. syringe

luetic
l. aneurysm
l. aortitis
l. disease

Luke procedure

Lukens
L. retractor
L. thymus retractor

Lumaguide infusion catheter

Lumelec pacing catheter

lumen *pl.* lumina
  aortic l.
  l. of artery
  double l.
  l. finder
  single l.
  ThruLumen l.
  l. of vein
  vessel l.

luminal
  l. defect
  l. diameter
  l. encroachment
  l. irregularity
  l. narrowing
  l. stenosis

luminescence

Lumonics YAG laser

lung
  cardiac l.

lunula *pl.* lunulae
  l. of aortic valve
  l. of valves of pulmonary
    trunk
  l. valvularum semilunarium
    valvae aortae
  l. valvularum semilunarium
    valvae trunci pulmonalis
  l. of cusps of aortic valve
  l. of pulmonary valves
  l. of cusps of pulmonary
    valve

lupoid

lupus
  l. anticoagulant
  l. erythematosus (LE)
  l. pernio

lupus-associated valve disease

Lurselle

lusitrophy

lusitropic
  l. abnormality

lusitropy

lusoria
  dysphagia l.

Lutembacher
  L. complex
  L. disease
  L. syndrome

Lutz-Splendore-Almeida disease

Luxtec fiberoptic system

luxus heart

LV
  left ventricle
    LV function
    LV wall motion

LVAD
  left ventricular assist de-
    vice
      HeartMate LVAD
      Novacor LVAD
      vented-electric
        HeartMate LVAD

LVAS
  left ventricular assist sys-
    tem

LVD
  left ventricular dysfunction

LVEDD
  left ventricular end-dia-
    stolic dimension

LVEDP
  left ventricular end-dia-
    stolic pressure

LVEF
  left ventricular ejection
    fraction

LVESD
  left ventricular end-systolic
    dimension

LVET
  left ventricular ejection
    time

LVH
     left ventricular hypertro-
          phy
LVOT
     left ventricular outflow
          tract
LW
     lateral wall
Lyme
     L. borreliosis
     L. disease
     L. titer
lymphadenitis
lymphadenopathy
     hilar l.
lymphangiectasis
     chronic pulmonary cystic l.
lymphangioendothelioma
lymphangioma
Lymphapress compression
     therapy
lymphatic
     l. channel
     l. edema
     obtuse marginal l.
     subclavian l.
lymphedema
lymph node
lymphocyte
     l. immune globulin
lymphokines
lymphoma
     African Burkitt l.

lymphoma *(continued)*
     B cell l.
     Burkitt l.
     Kiel classification of l.
     noncleaved cell l.
     non-Hodgkin l.
     pulmonary l.
lymphomatoid granulomatosis
lymphoplasm
lymphosarcoma
lymphotoxin
Lyo-Ject
Lyon hypothesis
Lyon-Horgan procedure
lyophilize
lyophilized powder
lysate
lyse
lysine
lysine-acetylsalicylate
lysis
     clot l.
     l. time
lysosomal
     l. enzyme
     l. hydrolases
lysosome
     primary l.
     secondary l.
lysosomal enzyme
lys-plasminogen
     recombinant l.

M
  M gate
  M lignocaine
  M lines
  M-mode
  M pattern on right atrial
    wave form
  M protein

M_1
  mitral first sound

M_2
  mitral second sound

M1
  marginal branch #1

m7E3 Rab

mA
  milliampere

MABP
  mean arterial blood pressure

MAC
  mitral annular calcification

McArdle
  M. disease
  M. syndrome

MacCallum patch

McCort sign

McDowall reflex

Macewen sign

McGinn-White sign

McGoon
  M. coronary perfusion
    catheter
  M. guidelines
  M. technique

Machado-Guerreiro test

McHenry treadmill exercise
  protocol

machine
  Aloka echocardiograph m.
  Apogee CX 100 Interspect
    ultrasound m.
  Bird m.
  Burdick EKG m.
  bypass m.
  Cobe-Stockert heart-lung m.
  Corometrics-Aloka echocar-
    diograph m.
  Crafoord-Senning heart-
    lung m.
  General Electric Pass-C
    echocardiograph m.
  G5 massage and percus-
    sion m.
  heart-lung m.
  Mayo-Gibbon heart-lung m.
  Respironics CPAP m.
  Respitrace m.
  Toshiba electrocardi-
    ograph m.

machinery murmur

MacIntosh
  M. blade anesthesia
  M. laryngoscopy

McIntosh double-lumen catheter

Mackenzie polygraph

Mackler tube

Macleod syndrome

McNaught keel

McNealy
  M.-Glassman-Mixter forceps
  M.-Glassman-Mixter liga-
    ture-carrying aneurysm
    forceps

McNemar test

McPheeters treatment

macroangiopathy
  coronary m.

macrocardia

macroglobulin
alpha-2 m.

macroglobulinemia
Waldenström m.

macrolide
m. antibiotic
m. antimicrobial

macromolecular ligand

macronucleus

macrophage
foamy m.
hemosiderin-laden m.

macroreentrant
m. atrial tachycardia
m. circuit

macroshock

macrosteatosis

macrovascular coronary lesion

macula *pl.* maculae
m. albida
m. lactea
m. tendinea

Maestro implantable cardiac
pacemaker

Magellan monitor

Magic Torque guide wire

Magnascanner
Picker M.

magnesium
m. oxide
m. sulfate
m. sulfate heptahydrate

magnet
Equen m.
m. application over pulse
generator
m. pacing interval

magnet *(continued)*
m. rate
m. wire

magnetic
m. moment
m. relaxation time
m. resonance angiography
(MRA)
m. resonance flowmetry
m. resonance imaging
(MRI)
m. resonance signal
m. resonance spectroscopy
m. source imaging

magnetocardiogram

magnetocardiograph (MCG)

magnetocardiography (MCG)

magnification
loupe m.

magnitude
average pulse m.
peak m.

Magnum guide wire

Magnum-Meier system

Magovern
M. ball-valve mallet
M. ball-valve prosthesis
M.-Cromie ball-cage pros-
thetic valve
M.-Cromie valve prosthesis

Mag-Ox 400

Mahaim
M. bundle
M. fibers
M.-type tachycardia

Mahalanobis distance

Mahler sign

mahogany flush

Maigret-50

main
  m. bundle
  m. pulmonary artery
  m. renal vein
  m. stem bronchus

mainstem coronary artery

Makin murmur

malabsorption

maladie
  m. de Roger

malaise

malformation
  angiographically occult in-
    tracranial vascular m.
  arteriovenous m. (AVM)
  atrioventricular m.
  congenital m.
  coronary artery m.
  Mondini pulmonary arter-
    iovenous m.
  neural crest m.
  pulmonary arterioven-
    ous m.
  Uhl m.

malfunction
  pacemaker m.

malignant
  m. beat
  m. endocarditis
  m. hypertension
  m. ventricular arrhythmia
  m. ventricular tachycardia

Mallinckrodt
  M. angiographic catheter
  M. radioimmunoassay

Mallory
  M. RM-1 cell pacemaker
  M. stain
  M.-Weiss syndrome
  M.-Weiss tear

malnutrition
  alcoholic m.

malnutrition *(continued)*
  myocardial m.
  protein-calorie m.

malposition
  crisscross heart m.
  double-outlet left ventri-
    cle m.
  double-outlet right ventri-
    cle m.
  m. of great arteries
  levocardia m.
  mesocardia m.
  single ventricle m.

maltase deficiency

malum
  m. cordis

mammary
  m. artery
  m. artery graft
  m. souffle murmur
  m. souffle sound

mammary-coronary tissue forceps

mandrel, mandril
  m. graft

maneuver
  Addison m.
  Adson m.
  Catell m.
  cold pressor testing m.
  costoclavicular m.
  Ejrup m.
  Heimlich m.
  hemodynamic m.
  Hillis-Müller m.
  hyperabduction m.
  hyperventilation m.
  jaw thrust m.
  Jonnson m.
  Lecompte m.
  Mattox m.
  Mueller m.
  Osler m.
  Rivero-Carvallo m.

maneuver *(continued)*
  Sellick m.
  Valsalva m.

manifest
  m. ischemia
  Morse m.
  m. vector

manipulation
  catheter m.

Mann-Whitney test

manner
  Creech m.
  DeBakey-Creech m.

Mannkopf sign

manofluorography

manometer
  Dinamap ultrasound blood
    pressure m.
  Hürthle m.
  Riva-Rocci m.
  strain gauge m.

manometer-tipped catheter

Mansfield
  M. Atri-Pace 1 catheter
  M. balloon
  M. balloon dilatation cathe-
    ter
  M. bioptome
  M. orthogonal electrode
    catheter
  M. Polaris electrode
  M. Scientific dilatation bal-
    loon catheter
  M.-Webster catheter

Mantel
  M.-Haenszel statistic
  M.-Haenszel test

Mantoux test

manual edge detection

manubrium

MAO
  monoamine oxidase
    MAO inhibitor (MAOI)

MAP
  mean arterial pressure
  monophasic action poten-
    tial

map
  polar coordinate m.

MAPD
  monophasic action poten-
    tial duration

maple bark disease

Mapper hemostasis EP mapping
  sheath

mapping
  activation-sequence m.
  atrial activation m.
  body surface Laplacian m.
  bull's-eye polar coordina-
    te m.
  cardiac m.
  catheter m.
  color-coded flow m.
  digital phase m.
  Doppler color flow m.
  electrophysiologic (EP) m.
  endocardial catheter m.
  endocardial m. of ventricu-
    lar tachycardia
  epicardial m.
  flow m.
  ice m.
  intracardiac m.
  intramural m.
  intraoperative m.
  Laplacian m.
  pace-m.
  precordial m.
  pulsed-wave Doppler m.
  retrograde atrial activa-
    tion m.
  sinus rhythm m.
  spectral temporal m.

mapping *(continued)*
    spectral turbulence m.
    tachycardia pathway m.
    ventricular m.

mapping/ablation catheter

marantic
    m. endocarditis
    m. thrombosis
    m. thrombus

marasmic
    m. thrombosis
    m. thrombus

marasmus

Marathon guiding catheter

Marbach-Weil technique

Marey law

Marfan syndrome

margin
    costal m.
    m. of heart, acute
    m. of heart, left
    m. of heart, obtuse
    m. of heart, right
    rib m.

marginal
    m. arteries of Drummond
    m. artery of colon
    m. branch
    m. circumflex artery
    obtuse m.

margo
    m. dexter cordis

Marie
    Marie syndrome
    Marie-Bamberger syn-
        drome

Marion-Clatworthy side-to-end
    vena caval shunt

mark
    alignment m.

mark *(continued)*
    strawberry m.

Mark VII cooling vest

marker
    m. catheter
    m. channel
    gold m.
    lead-letter m.
    vein graft m.

marking
    perihilar m's
    vascular m's

Marquette
    M. Case-12 electrocardio-
        graphic system
    M. Case-12 exercise system
    M. 3-channel laser Holter
    M. electrocardiograph
    M. 8000 Holter monitor
    M. Holter recorder
    M. Responder 1500 multi-
        functional defibrillator
    M. Series 8000 Holter ana-
        lyzer
    M. treadmill

Marriott method

Marshall
    M. fold
    M. ligament
    M. oblique vein

marsupialization

Martorell syndrome

Mary Allen Engle ventricle

masked hypertension

mask-mode
    m.-m. cardiac imaging
    m.-m. node subtraction

Mason
    M. vascular clamp
    M.-Likar 12-lead EKG sys-
        tem

Mason *(continued)*
  M.-Likar limb lead modifica-
    tion
  M.-Likar placement of EKG
    leads

mass
  achromatic m.
  cardiac m.
  echodense m.
  echogenic m.
  fibrillar m. of Flemming
  fungating m.
  intracardiac m.
  intracavity m.
  intraventricular m.
  left ventricular m.
  myocardial m.
  pulsatile abdominal m.
  right ventricular m.

massage
  cardiac m.
  carotid sinus m.
  closed chest cardiac m.
  direct cardiac m.
  external cardiac m.
  heart m.
  open chest cardiac m.
  vapor m.

Massier solution

massive
  m. bleeding
  m. collapse
  m. heart attack
  m. hemorrhage
  m. involvement

Masson
  M. bodies
  M. trichrome stain

MAST
  military anti-shock trousers
  MAST pants
  MAST suit

mast
  m. cell
  m. cell inhibitor

Master
  M. exercise stress test
  M. Flow Pumpette
  SpaceLabs Event M.
  M. two-step exercise test

mastocytosis syndrome

Masy angioscope

MAT
  multifocal atrial tachycar-
    dia

Matas
  M. aneurysmectomy
  M. aneurysmoplasty
  M. operation
  M. test

match defect

matching
  afterload m.

material
  Biobrane/HF graft m.
  Biograft bovine hetero-
    graft m.
  Carbo-Seal graft m.
  Cellolite m.
  contrast m.
  embolized foreign m.
  fibrinohematic m.
  Haynes 25 m.
  Hexabrix contrast m.
  Kaltostat wound packing m.
  Kifa catheter m.
  low-osmolality contract m.
  MycroMesh graft m.
  Myoview contrast m.
  nonionic contrast m.
  PermaMesh m.
  Soludrast contrast m.
  Stellite ring m.
  Zenotech graft m.

matrix
  cytoplasmic m.
  extracellular m.
  m. mode
  mitochondrial m.

matrix *(continued)*
  myocardial collagen m.

Matson
  M. rib elevator
  M. rib spreader
  M. rib stripper
  M.-Alexander rib elevator
  M.-Alexander rib stripper

Matsuda titanium surgical instruments

Mattox
  M. aorta clamp
  M. maneuver

mattress
  apnea alarm m.
  eggcrate m.
  hypothermia m.
  m. sutures

maturation
  affinity m.

Maugeri syndrome

Mavik

Maxilith pacemaker

maximal
  m. velocity

maximum
  m. predicted heart rate (MPHR)
  m. ventricular elastance
  m. walking time

maxi-vessel loops

Maxon suture

May-Grünwald-Giemsa stain

Mayo
  M. cannula
  M. exercise treadmill protocol
  M. hemostat
  M. vein stripper
  M. vessel clamp
  M.-Gibbon heart-lung machine

Mayo *(continued)*
  M.-Péan forceps

maze procedure

MB
  myocardial band
  myocardial bridging
    MB enzymes of CPK
    MB fraction
    MB isoenzyme of CK (CK-MB)

MCI
  mean cardiac index

MCL
  midclavicular line

MCM smart laser

MCV
  mean corpuscular volume

M/D 4 defibrillator system

Meadows syndrome

Meadox
  M. bifurcated graft
  M. Dardik biograft
  M. graft
  M. graft sizer
  M. ICP monitor
  M. Microvel double-velour knitted Dacron arterial graft
  M. Teflon felt pledget
  M. vascular graft
  M. woven velour prosthesis
  M.-Cooley woven low-porosity prosthesis

mean
  arterial m.
  m. aortic pressure
  m. arterial blood pressure
  m. arterial pressure (MAP)
  m. cardiac vector
  m. circulation time
  m. corpuscular volume (MCV)
  m. diastolic left ventricular pressure

mean *(continued)*
    m. electrical axis
    m. mitral valve gradient
    m. normalized systolic
      ejection rate
    m. pulmonary artery pres-
      sure
    m. pulmonary artery wedge
      pressure
    m. QRS axis
    m. systolic left ventricular
      pressure
    m. vectors

Means-Lernan mediastinal
  crunch

measurement
    blood flow m.
    cardiac output m.
    coronary blood flow m.
    Doppler m.
    hemodynamic m.
    invasive pressure m.
    physiologic m.
    PR-AC m.
    pressure m.
    Reid index m.
    thermodilution m.
    transstenotic pressure gra-
      dient m.
    venous flow m.

mechanical
    m. alternation
    m. alternation of heart
    m. cough
    m. heart
    m. valve
    m. ventilation

mechanics
    fluid m.

mechanism
    m. of action
    compensatory m.
    coronary steal m.
    deglutition m.
    escape m.
    Frank-Starling m.
    gating m.

mechanism *(continued)*
    Laplace m.
    leading circle m.
    peeling-back m.
    pinchcock m.
    reentrant m.
    reserve m.
    sensing m.
    sinus m.
    Starling m.
    steal m.
    wave-speed m.

mechanocardiography

mechanoelectrical feedback

mechanoreceptor

mechanoreflex

Medcor pacemaker

MedGraphics
    M. Cardio O2 system
    M. CPX/D metabolic cart

media
    aortic tunica m.
    arterial m.

medial
    m. incision
    m. tear

median
    m. antebrachial vein
    m. artery
    m. basilic vein
    m. cephalic vein
    m. sternotomy
    m. cubital vein
    m. sacral artery
    m. sternotomy incision
    m. survival time

medianus
    ramus m.

mediastinal
    m. amyloidosis
    m. cannula
    m. cavity
    m. crunch
    m. drain

mediastinal *(continued)*
    m. flutter
    m. node biopsy
    m. shadow
    m. shift
    m. space
    m. sump filter
    m. thickening
    m. wedge
    m. widened

mediastinitis
    descending necrotizing m.
    fibrous m.

mediastinopericarditis
    adhesive m.

mediastinoscope
    Carlens fiberoptic m.
    Goldberg-MPC m.

mediastinoscopy
    Chamberlain m.

mediastinotomy

mediastinum

mediator
    vasoactive m.

Medicon
    M. rib retractor
    M. rib spreader
    M. wire-twister forceps

Mediflex-Bookler device

Medi-graft vascular prosthesis

Medigraphics 2000 analyzer

MEDILOG 4000 ambulatory ECG
    recorder

medionecrosis
    m. of aorta
    m. aortae idiopathica cystica

Medi-Quet tourniquet

Medi-Strumpf stockings

Meditape

Medi-Tech
    M. balloon catheter
    M. catheter system
    M. guide wire
    M. multipurpose basket
    M. steerable catheter

Mediterranean anemia

medium
    Adenoscan contrast m.
    m. chain triglycerides
    Conray contrast m.
    contrast m.
    Eagle m.
    iothalamate meglumine
        contrast m.
    ioxaglate meglumine contrast m.
    Isovue contrast m.
    Joklik m.
    metrizamide contrast m.
    nonionic contrast m.
    Obturay contrast m.
    polygelin colloid contrast m.
    SHU-454 contrast m.

Medi vascular stockings

Medivent
    M. self-expanding coronary
        stent
    M. vascular stent

Medlar bodies

Medrad angiographic injector

Medtel pacemaker

Medtronic
    M. Activitrax rate-responsive unipolar ventricular
        pacemaker
    M. aortic punch
    M. automated coagulation
        timer
    M. balloon catheter
    M. cardiac cooling jacket
    M. Chardack pacemaker
    M. corkscrew electrode
        pacemaker

Medtronic *(continued)*
    M. Cyberlith pacemaker
    M. defibrillator implant
       support device
    M. demand pulse generator
    M. Elite DDDR pacemaker
    M. Elite II pacemaker
    M. external cardioverter-
       defibrillator
    M. External Tachyarrhyth-
       mia Control Device
    M. Intact valve
    M. Interactive Tachycardia
       Terminating system
    M. interventional vascular
       stent
    M. Jewell 7219D and C de-
       vice
    M. Kappa 400 pacemaker
    M. leads
    M. PCD implantable cardio-
       verter-defibrillator
    M. prosthetic valve
    M. Pulsor Intrasound pain
       reliever
    M. radiofrequency receiver
    M. RF 5998 pacemaker
    M. SPO pacemaker
    M. SP 502 pacemaker
    M. Symbios pacemaker
    M. SynchroMed implanta-
       ble pump
    M. Thera "I-series" cardiac
       pacemaker
    M. Transvene electrode
    M. Transvene endocardial
       lead system
    M.-Hall device
    M.-Hall heart valve
    M.-Hall monocuspid tilting-
       disk valve
    M.-Hall prosthetic heart
       valve
    M.-Hall tilting-disk valve
       prosthesis
    M.-Hancock device
    M.-Hancock valve
megacardia

megaelectron volt (MeV)

megahertz (MHz)

megaloblastic anemia

megalocardia

Meier-Magnum system

Meigs' capillaries

meiogenic

meiosis

meiotic

melena

melioidosis

Meltzer
    M. method
    M. sign

Melzack-Wall gate theory

membranacea
    angina m.
    pars m.

membranaceous

membrane
    antibasement m.
    basement m.
    Bichat m.
    cell m.
    m. channel
    chromatic m.
    cuprophane m.
    cytoplasmic m.
    m. current
    Debove m.
    elastic m.
    excitable m.
    fenestrated m.
    Gore-Tex surgical m.
    Henle elastic m.
    Henle fenestrated m.
    nuclear m.
    m. oxygenator
    plasma m.
    pleuropericardial m.

membrane *(continued)*
  polyacrylonitrile m.
  m. potential
  Preclude pericardial m.
  m. rupture
  sarcolemmal m.
  serous m's
  supramitral m.
  syncytiovascular m.
  unit m.
  Wachendorf m.
  m.-stabilizing activity

membranous
  m. septum
  m. ventricular septal defect
  m. wall

membranolysis

memory
  cardiac m.
  m. catheter
  m. loop

MemoryTrace
  M. AT
  M. AT ambulatory cardiac
    monitor

mendelian disorder

Mendelson syndrome

Menière syndrome

meningococcal
  m. pericarditis

meningococcemia

meningococcus

meningoencephalitis

mEq
  milliequivalent

mercury-in-rubber strain gauge
  plethysmograph

mercury-in-Silastic strain gauge
  for blood flow determination

mercury 195m

Merendino technique

meridian
  m. echocardiogram
  m. echocardiography

meridional wall stress

merodiastolic

meromyosin

meropenem

merosystolic

merotomy

Merilene braided nonabsorbable suture

mesangial
  m. cell
  m. immune injury

mesaortitis

mesarteritis
  Mönckeberg m.

mesenchymal
  m.-derived tumor
  m. intimal cell

mesenteric
  m. angiography
  m. arteritis
  m. artery
  m. artery occlusion
  m. bypass graft
  m. inferior artery
  m. ischemia
  m. infarction
  m. superior artery
  m. superior vein
  m. thrombosis
  m. vascular occlusion

mesh
  m. stent
  m. wrapping of aortic aneu-
    rysm

meso-aortitis
  m. syphilitica

mesocardia
  m. malposition

mesocardium
    arterial m.
    dorsal m.
    lateral m.
    venous m.
    ventral m.

mesocaval
    m. anastomosis
    m. shunt

mesoderm
    precardiac m.

mesodermal tumor

mesodiastolic

mesophlebitis

mesosystolic

mesothelioma of atrioventricular node

messenger
    m. ribonucleic acid
      (mRNA)
    second m.

Mester test

MET
    metabolic equivalents of
      task

Meta
    M. II pacemaker
    M. MV pacemaker
    M. rate-responsive pacemaker

metabolator
    Sanborn m.

metabolic
    m. acidosis
    m. alkalosis
    m. cart
    m. equivalents of task
      (MET) (METs)
    m. parameter determination
    m. rate meter
    m. vasodilatory capacity

metabolism
    aerobic m.
    anaerobic m.
    arachidonate m.
    glucose m.
    myocardial m.

metabolite
    arachidonic acid m's
    prostacyclin m.

metaboreceptor

metacholin

metakinesis

metal
    m. electrode
    heavy m.
    m. sewing ring
    trace m.

metallic
    m. clicks
    m. echo
    m. tinkle

metaphase

metaplasia
    goblet cell m.

metaplastic mucus-secreting cell

metarteriole

metasynapsis

metasyndesis

metazoal myocarditis

met-enkephalin

methicillin-sensitive right-sided endocarditis

method
    Abell-Kendall m.
    Anel m.
    Antyllus m.
    Ashby m.
    atrial extrastimulus m.
    Brasdor m.

method *(continued)*
    Carrel m.
    catheter introduction m.
    dye-dilution m.
    Eggleston m.
    Fick m.
    Gärtner m.
    Gräupner m.
    indicator dilution m.
    Ionescu m.
    Jaboulay m.
    Korotkoff m.
    Langendorff m.
    Lee-White m.
    Lown and Woolf m.
    Moore m.
    Orsi-Grocco m.
    Pachon m.
    Purmann m.
    Scarpa m.
    Theden m.
    thermodilution m.
    Wardrop m.
    Welcker m.
    Westergren m.

Metras catheter

Metrix atrial defibrillation system

metrizamide
    m. contrast medium

metrocyte

Metzenbaum scissors

MeV
    megaelectron volt

Mewissen infusion catheter

Meyer
    M. olive-tipped vein stripper
    M. spiral vein stripper

Meyerding retractor

MGA
    malposition of great arteries

Mgb
    myoglobulin

MHz
    megahertz

MI
    mitral incompetence
    mitral insufficiency
    myocardial infarction
    myocardial ischemia

Michel aortic clamp

Micro
    M. Minix pacemaker
    M. SI Holter system
    M. stent

microalbuminuria

microanastomosis
    m. approximator
    m. clip
    m. clip approximator
    laser-assisted m.

microaneurysm
    Charcot-Bouchard m.

microangiopathic
    m. anemia

microangiopathy
    coronary m.
    thrombotic m.

microangioscopy

microarterial
    m. clamp
    m. clamp applier

microatheroma

microballoon
    m. probe
    Rand m.

microbubble

microbulldog clamp

microcalcification

microcardia

microcatheter
    Terumo SP hydrophilic-
        polymer-coated m.
    Tracker m.

microcavitation

microcentrum

microcirculation

microcirculatory

microelectrode

microembolic disease

microembolism

microembolization

microembolus

microfibrillar collagen hemostat

microfilament

microfilaria

microfilter

microfluorometry

Micro-Guide catheter

microhemagglutination *Trepo-
    nema pallidum* (MHA-TP)

microinvasive

Microjet Quark portable pump

microjoule

Microknit
    M. arterial prosthesis
    M. patch graft
    M. vascular graft prosthe-
        sis

Micro-Line artery forceps

Microlith
    M. pacemaker pulse gener-
        ator
    M. P pacemaker

micromanometer
    m. catheter

micromanometer *(continued)*
    m.-tip catheter

micromanometry

micron needle

micronucleus

microorganism

microparticle

microphage
    fat-laden m's

microphone
    cardiac catheter-m.

micropinocytosis

Micropuncture Peel-Away intro-
    ducer

microreentry

Microsampler device

microscope
    acoustic m.
    capillary m.
    darkfield m.
    electron m.
    light m.
    scanning electron m.

microscopic polyangiitis

microsecond pulsed flashlamp
    pumped dye laser

microshock

Microsoftrac catheter

microsomal

microsome

microsphere
    albumin m.
    magnetic m.
    m. perfusion scintigraphy
    polystyrene latex m's
    radiolabeled m.
    Ultrasound Contrast M.

microsphygmia

microsphygmy

microsphyxia

Micross
    M. dilatation catheter
    M. SL balloon

microsteatosis

Microsulfon

Microthin P2 pacemaker

microtome
    Cryo-Cut m.
    Stadie-Riggs m.

Micro-Tracer
    M.-T. portable ECG (EKG)

microthrombosis

microthrombus

microtubule

microvascular
    m. abnormalities
    m. angina
    m. clamp
    m. clamp-applying forceps
    m. forceps
    m. free flap
    m. modified Alm retractor
    m. needle holder

microvasculature

microvasculopathy

Microvasive sclerotherapy needle

microvessel

microvoltometer

Microvel double velour graft

midaxillary line

midbody

MID-CAB
    minimally invasive direct
        coronary artery bypass

midclavicular line (MCL)

mid-diastolic
    m. murmur
    m. rumble

middle
    m. cardiac cervical nerve
    m. cardiac vein
    m. cerebral artery (MCA)
    m. colic artery
    m. colic vein
    m. collateral artery
    m. genicular artery
    m. meningeal artery
    m. meningeal vein
    m. rectal artery
    m. rectal vein
    m. suprarenal artery
    m. temporal artery
    m. temporal vein
    m. thyroid vein
    m. vesical artery

mid-infrared pulsed laser

midline
    m. shift
    m. sternum-splitting incision

midnodal
    m. extrasystole
    m. rhythm

midodrine

midsagittal plane

midsystole

midsystolic
    m. buckling
    m. click
    m. closure of aortic valve
    m. dip
    m. murmur
    m. notching

migrating
    m. pacemaker
    m. phlebitis

Mikity-Wilson disease

Mikros pacemaker

Mikro-tip
    M. angiocatheter
    M. micromanometer-tipped
        catheter
    M. transducer

Milano
    apolipoprotein A-I M.
    apolipoprotein B M.
    apolipoprotein D M.
    apolipoprotein E M.

Miles vena cava clip

miliary
    m. embolism

military anti-shock trousers
    (MAST)

Millar
    M. catheter-tipped trans-
        ducer
    M. Doppler catheter
    M. micromanometer cathe-
        ter
    M. Mikro-Tip catheter pres-
        sure transducer
    M. MPC-500 catheter
    M. pigtail angiographic
        catheter

mille-feuilles effect

Miller
    M. elastic stain
    M. Fisher variant
    M. septostomy catheter
    M.-Dieker syndrome
    M.-Senn double-ended re-
        tractor
    M.-Senn retractor

mill-house murmur

milliampere (mA)

milliequivalent (mEq)

millijoule (mJ)

Milliknit
    M. arterial prosthesis
    M. Dacron prosthesis

Milliknit *(continued)*
    M. vascular graft prosthe-
        sis

milliliter (mL)

millimeters of mercury (mm
    Hg)

millimole (mmol)

Millipore filter

millisecond (msec)

milliunit (mU)

millivolt (mV)

Mills
    M. arteriotomy scissors
    M. cautery
    M. coronary endarterec-
        tomy set
    M. coronary endarterec-
        tomy spatula
    M. microvascular needle
        holder
    M. operative peripheral an-
        gioplasty catheter
    M. rib spreader
    M. valvulotome

mill-wheel murmur

Miltex rib spreader

Milton disease

mineralocorticoid-induced hy-
    pertension

Mingograf
    M. 62 6-channel electrocar-
        diograph
    M. 82 recorder

miniballoon

Minibird II

mini-defibrillator

Minilith pacemaker

minimal
    m. leak technique
    m. luminal diameter

Mini-Motionlogger Actigraph

minimum
    m. bactericidal concentra-
        tion
    m. inhibitory concentration

Mini-Profile dilatation catheter

Minix pacemaker

Minnesota
    M. classification of EKG
    M. code
    M. criteria for high R waves

minor
    pectoralis m.

Minuet DDD pacemaker

minute
    beats per m. (bpm)
    m. output
    m. volume

miocardia

miosis

miotic

Mirage over-the-wire balloon
    catheter

mirror-image
    m.-i. dextrocardia
    m.-i. brachiocephalic
        branching

Mirsky
    formula of M.
    M. thick wall model

missed beat

mitapsis

mitochondrial
    m. calcium deposition
    m. cardiomyopathy
    m. enzymes
    m. function

mitochondrion *pl.* mitochondria

mitogen

mitogenesia

mitogenesis

mitogenetic

mitogenic

mitokinetic

mitome

mitoplasm

mitoschisis

mitosis *pl.* mitoses
    heterotypic m.
    homeotypic m.
    multicentric m.
    pathologic m.
    pluripolar m.

mitosome

mitotic

mitral
    m. annular calcification
    m. annuloplasty
    m. annulus
    m. atresia
    m. balloon commissurot-
        omy
    m. balloon valvotomy
    m. buttonhole
    m. click
    m. E to F slope
    m. facies
    m. first sound (M_1)
    m. forceps
    m. funnel
    m. incompetence
    m. insufficiency
    m. knife
    m. opening snap
    m. prolapse murmur
    m. prosthesis
    m. regurgitant jet
    m. regurgitation (MR)
    m. restenosis
    m. second sound (M_2)
    m. stenosis (MS)
    m. stenosis murmur
    m. stenosis knife

mitral *(continued)*
  m. tap
  m. valve (MV)
  m. valve aneurysm
  m. valve annulus
  m. valve area (MVA)
  m. valve billowing
  m. valve closure index
  m. valve commissurotomy
  m. valve dilator
  m. valve echocardiography
  m. valve endocarditis
  m. valve fusion
  m. valve gradient
  m. valve hypoplasia
  m. valve leaflet
  m. valve leaflet tip
  m. valve parachute defor-
    mity
  m. valve prolapse (MVP)
  m. valve prolapse syn-
    drome
  m. valve prosthesis
  m. valve regurgitation
  m. valve replacement
  m. valve retractor
  m. valve ring
  m. valve septal separation
  m. valve spreader
  m. valve stenosis
  m. valve valvotomy
  m. valve valvulotomy
  m. valvulitis
  m. valvuloplasty

mitrale
  P m.

mitralis
  facies m.

mitralism

mitralization

mitral-septal apposition

mitroarterial

Mitroflow pericardial prosthetic
  valve

Mitrothin P2 pacemaker

Mitsubishi
  M. angioscope
  M. angioscopic catheter

mixed
  m. aneurysm
  m. angina
  m. beat
  m.-cholesterol gallstone
  m. levocardia
  m. thrombus
  m. venous blood

Mixter
  M. forceps
  M. hemostat
  M. right angle clamp
  M. thoracic clamp
  M. ventricular needle

mJ
  millijoule

mL
  milliliter

M-line protein

MM band

mm Hg
  millimeters of mercury

M-mode
  motion mode
    M-m. Doppler
    M-m. echocardiogra-
      phy
    M-m. recording
    M-m. transducer

mobile
  carina sharp and m.
  cor m.

Mobin-Uddin
  M.-U. filter
  M.-U. umbrella filter
  M.-U. vena cava filter

Mobitz
  M. heart block
  M. I AV heart block
  M. I second-degree block

Mobitz *(continued)*
    M. II AV heart block
    M. II second-degree block

modafinil

modality
    pacing m.
    therapeutic m.

mode
    A-m.
    m. abandonment
    atrial burst m.
    atrial triggered and ventricular inhibited m.
    atrioventricular dual-demand m.
    B-m.
    bipolar pacing m.
    DDD m.
    demand pacemaker m.
    dual-demand pacing m.
    DVI m.
    fixed-rate m.
    gated list m.
    histogram m.
    inhibited m.
    M-m.
    matrix m.
    motion m. (M-mode)
    pacing m.
    passive m.
    rate-responsive m.
    sequential m.
    stimulation m.
    m. switching
    synchronous pacemaker m.
    triggered pacing m.
    underdrive m.
    unipolar pacing m.
    VVI m.

model
    Cox stepwise regression m.
    figure-of-eight m.
    fluid mosaic m.
    Hodgkin-Huxley m.
    leading circle m.
    Mirsky thick wall m.
    ring m.

model *(continued)*
    Torricelli m.

moderator band

modified
    m. brachial technique
    m. Bruce protocol
    m. Ellestad protocol
    m. Mark IV R-wave-Triggered power injector
    m. multifactorial index of cardiac risk
    m. Seldinger technique

modification
    Mason-Likar limb lead m.

modulation
    autonomic m.
    brightness m.

modulus
    impedance m.

molecule
    adhesion m's
    cell adhesion m's

Molina needle catheter

mollis
    pulsus m.

moment
    magnetic m.

monad

Monark bicycle ergometer

monaster

Mönckeberg
    M. arrhythmia
    M. arteriosclerosis
    M. degeneration
    M. sclerosis

Mondor
    M. disease
    M. syndrome

monitor
    Accucap CO_2/O_2 m.
    Accucom cardiac output m.

monitor *(continued)*
    Accutorr A1 blood pressure m.
    Accutracker II ambulatory blood pressure m.
    Acuson V5M transesophageal echocardiographic m.
    ambulatory Holter m.
    Arrhythmia Net arrhythmia m.
    automatic oscillometric blood pressure m.
    bedside m.
    Biotrack coagulation m.
    blood perfusion m.
    cardiac m.
    cardiac apnea m.
    CardioDiary heart m.
    Colin ambulatory BP m.
    continuous Holter m.
    Dinamap blood pressure m.
    Dopplette m.
    Doppler-Cavin m.
    Doppler fetal heart m.
    Electrodyne cardiac m.
    event m.
    Finapres blood pressure m.
    HeartCard m.
    HemoTec activated clotting time m.
    Holter m.
    Insta-Pulse heart rate m.
    King of Hearts Holter m.
    Lifepak 7 m./defibrillator
    Magellan m.
    Marquette 8000 Holter m.
    MemoryTrace AT ambulatory cardiac m.
    Ohmeda 6200 O2 m.
    Omega 5600 noninvasive blood pressure m.
    Pressurometer blood pressure m.
    SpaceLabs Holter m.
    telemetry m.
    VEST ambulatory ventricular function m.

monitoring
    24-hour ambulatory blood pressure m.
    ambulatory Holter m.
    bedside m.
    hemodynamic m.
    m. line
    pulse oximetry m.
    transtelephonic arrhythmia m.

Moniz carotid siphon

Monneret pulse

monoballoon

monocardiogram

monoclonal
    m. antibody 3G4
    m. antimyosin antibody
    m. hypothesis
    m. theory of atherogenesis

monocrotic
    m. pulse

monocrotism

monocyte

monofilament
    m. absorbable suture
    m. polypropylene suture

monofoil catheter

monoform tachycardia

monolayer

monometer-tipped catheter

monomorphic
    m. ventricular tachycardia

mononuclear

mononucleate

monophasic
    m. action potential (MAP)
    m. action potential duration
    m. complex

monophasic *(continued)*
   m. contour of QRS complex

monopolar temporary electrode

Monorail
   M. angioplasty catheter
   M. Speedy balloon

Monostrut
   M. Björk-Shiley valve
   M. cardiac valve prosthesis

monotherapy

Monro
   foramen of M.

Montgomery
   M. Safe-T-Tube
   M. speaking valve

Moore procedure

morbid obesity

morcellation

Moretz clip

Morgagni
   M. disease
   foramen of M.
   M. sinus
   M.-Adams-Stokes syndrome

moriens
   ultimum m.

morphologic

morphology
   QRS m.

morphoplasm

Morquio
   M. syndrome
   M.-Brailsford disease

Morris
   M. aortic clamp
   M. cannula
   M. mitral valve spreader
   M. Silastic thoracic drain
   M. thoracic catheter

Morse
   M. backward-cutting aortic
     scissors
   M. modified Finochietto re-
     tractor
   M. scissors
   M. sternal spreader
   M. valve retractor

MOS
   mitral opening snap

Mosaic cardiac bioprosthesis

mosaic
   m. jet
   m.-jet signals
   m. perfusion

Moschcowitz
   M. disease
   M. test

mosquito
   m. clamp
   m. forceps
   m. hemostat
   m. hemostatic forceps

motion
   anterior wall m.
   apical wall m.
   atrioventricular junction m.
   brisk wall m.
   cusp m.
   diastolic m.
   m. display echo
   dyskinetic wall m.
   hypokinetic wall m.
   inferior wall m.
   interventricular septal m.
   leaflet m.
   left ventricular regional
     wall m.
   m. mode (M-mode)
   paradoxic wall m.
   paradoxical leaflet m.
   paradoxic septal m.
   posterior wall m.
   posterolateral wall m.
   precordial m.
   regional wall m.

motion *(continued)*
    segmental wall m.
    septal wall m.
    systolic anterior m.
    ventricular wall m.
    wall m.
    whorl m.

motoricity

mottling of extremities

Moulaert
    muscle of M.

moulin
    bruit de la roué de m.

Mounier-Kuhn syndrome

Mount-Mayfield forceps

mountain sickness

mousetail pulse

movable
    m. core straight safety wire
        guide
    m. heart
    m. pulse

Movat
    M. pentachromic
    M. stain

movement
    air m.
    ameboid m.
    circus m.
    precordial m.

moyamoya cerebrovascular disease

Moynahan syndrome

MPA
    main pulmonary artery

MPHR
    maximum predicted heart
        rate

M-protein serotype

MR
    mitral reflux

MR *(continued)*
    mitral regurgitation

MRA
    magnetic resonance angiography

MRF
    mitral regurgitant flow

MRI
    magnetic resonance imaging
        cine gradient-echo MRI
        FLASH MRI
        gd-DTPA-enhanced
            MRI
        GRASS MRI
        spin-echo MRI
        ThromboScan MRI

MS
    mitral stenosis
    MS Classique balloon dilatation catheter

MS-3
    Miniscope MS-3

MS-857

m/sec
    meters per second

msec
    millisecond

M-shaped pattern of mitral
    valve

MSOF
    multisystem organ failure

MTC catheter

M-type alpha-1 antitrypsin

mU
    milliunit
    Much granules

Mueller
    M. maneuver
    M. sign

muffled heart sounds

MUGA
  multiple gated acquisition
    MUGA cardiac blood
      pool scan
    MUGA exercise stress
      test
    MUGA scan

Muller
  M. banding
  M. test

Müller
  M. catheter guide
  M. maneuver
  M. sign
  M. vena cava clamp

Mullins
  M. blade and balloon sep-
    tostomy
  M. blade technique
  M. cardiac device
  M. catheter introducer
  M. dilator
  M. modification of trans-
    septal catheterization
  M. sheath/dilator
  M. sheath system
  M. transseptal atrial sep-
    tostomy
  M. transseptal catheter
  M. transseptal catheteriza-
    tion sheath

multi-access catheter (MAC)

Multicor
  M. II cardiac pacemaker
  M. Gamma pacemaker

multicrystal gamma camera

multiflanged Portnoy catheter

Multiflex catheter

multifocal
  m. atrial tachycardia
    (MAT)
  m. contractions
  m. heartbeats

multifocal (continued)
  m. premature ventricular
    contractions

multiform
  m. premature ventricular
    complex
  m. tachycardia

multigated angiography

Multileaf Collimator device

multilinear regression analysis

Multi Link stent

Multilith pacemaker

Multi-Med triple-lumen infusion
  catheter

multimer assay

multinucleate

multiple
  m. embolism
  m. gated acquisition
    (MUGA)
  m. lentigines syndrome
  m. lipoprotein-type hyper-
    lipidemia
  m. regression
  m. shunt levels
  m. system atrophy

multiple-balloon valvuloplasty

multiple-parameter telemetry

multiplex
  m. catheter
  mononeuritis m.

multipolar
  m. catheter
  m. catheter electrode

multiprogrammable
  m. pacemaker
  m. pulse generator

multipurpose catheter

multisensor catheter

Multistage Maximal Effort exercise stress test

multisystem organ failure (MSOF)

multivalve insufficiency

multivalvular
   m. disease
   m. disease murmur

multivessel
   m. coronary artery obstruction
   m. disease

multiwire gamma camera

mural
   m. aneurysm
   m. endocarditis
   m. thrombosis
   m. thrombus

Murat sign

Murgo pressure contours

mu rhythm

murmur
   accidental m.
   amphoric m.
   anemic m.
   aneurysmal m.
   aortic m.
   aortic diastolic m.
   aortic insufficiency m.
   aortic-left ventricular tunnel m.
   aortic-mitral combined disease m.
   aortic regurgitation m.
   aortic stenosis m.
   apex m.
   apical m.
   apical diastolic m.
   apical mid-diastolic m.
   apical systolic m.
   arterial m.
   m. at the apex and left sternal border
   atriosystolic m.

murmur *(continued)*
   atrioventricular flow rumbling m.
   attrition m.
   Austin Flint m.
   basal diastolic m.
   bellows m.
   blood m.
   blowing m.
   blubbery diastolic m.
   brain m.
   Bright m.
   bronchial collateral artery m.
   Cabot-Locke m.
   carcinoid m.
   cardiac m.
   cardiopulmonary m.
   cardiorespiratory m.
   Carey Coombs m.
   carotid artery m.
   click m.
   coarse m.
   Cole-Cecil m.
   congenital m.
   continuous m.
   cooing m.
   cooing-dove m.
   Coombs m.
   crescendo m.
   crescendo-decrescendo m.
   Cruveilhier-Baumgarten m.
   decrescendo m.
   deglutition m.
   diamond ejection m.
   diamond-shaped m.
   diastolic m.
   diastolic flow m.
   diffusely radiating m.
   diminuendo m.
   direct m.
   Docke m.
   Duroziez m.
   dynamic m.
   early diastolic m.
   early-peaking systolic m.
   early systolic m.
   ejection m.

murmur *(continued)*
    end-diastolic m.
    endocardial m.
    end-systolic m.
    Eustace Smith m.
    exit block m.
    exocardial m.
    expiratory m.
    extracardiac m.
    Fisher m.
    Flint m.
    Fräntzel m.
    friction m.
    functional m.
    Gallavardin m.
    Gibson m.
    goose-honk m.
    grade 1 through 6 m.
    Graham Steell m.
    groaning m.
    Hamman m.
    harsh m.
    heart m.
    hemic m.
    high-frequency m.
    high-pitched m.
    Hodgkin-Key m.
    holodiastolic m.
    holosystolic m.
    honking m.
    hourglass m.
    humming m.
    humming-top m.
    incidental m.
    indirect m.
    innocent m.
    inorganic m.
    inspiratory m.
    lapping m.
    late apical systolic m.
    late diastolic m.
    late-peaking systolic m.
    late systolic m.
    left ventricular-right atrial
      communication m.
    Levine Harvey gradation 1
      through 6 cardiac m's
    loud m.

murmur *(continued)*
    low-frequency m.
    low-pitched m.
    machinery m.
    Makin m.
    mammary souffle m.
    mid-diastolic m.
    midsystolic m.
    mid-to-late diastolic m.
    mill-house m.
    mill-wheel m.
    mitral m.
    mitral prolapse m.
    mitral regurgitation m.
    mitral stenosis m.
    multivalvular m.
    muscular m.
    musical m.
    noninvasive m.
    nun's venous hum m.
    obstructive m.
    organic m.
    outflow m.
    pansystolic m.
    Parrot m.
    patent ductus arteriosus m.
    pathologic m.
    pericardial m.
    physiologic m.
    pleuropericardial m.
    physiologic m.
    prediastolic m.
    presystolic m.
    presystolic crescendo m.
    primary pulmonary hyper-
      tension m.
    protodiastolic m.
    pulmonary outflow m.
    pulmonary valve flow m.
    pulmonic m.
    m. radiating to apex of
      heart
    m. radiating to axilla
    m. radiating to neck
    m. radiating to sternal bor-
      der
    rasping m.
    reduplication m.

murmur *(continued)*
    regurgitant m.
    respiratory m.
    Roger m.
    rumbling m.
    rumbling diastolic m.
    scratchy m.
    seagull m.
    seesaw m.
    soft m.
    Steell m.
    stenosal m.
    Still m.
    subclavian m.
    subclavicular m.
    systolic m.
    systolic apical m.
    systolic ejection m. (SEM)
    systolic regurgitant m.
    to-and-fro m.
    transmitted m.
    Traube m.
    tricuspid m.
    vascular m.
    venous m.
    vesicular m.
    water-wheel m.
    whooping m.

Murphy
    M. method
    M. percussion

muscle
    anterior papillary m.
    cardiac m.
    Chassaignac axillary m.
    latissimus dorsi m.
    m. of Moulaert
    Oehl m.
    papillary m.
    papillary m. of conus arteriosus
    papillary m. of left ventricle, anterior
    papillary m. of left ventricle, posterior
    papillary m. of right ventricle, anterior

muscle *(continued)*
    papillary m. of right ventricle, posterior
    papillary m's of right ventricle, septal
    pectinate m's of left atrium
    pectinate m's of right atrium
    posterior papillary m.
    rectus abdominis m.
    m. relaxant
    ribbon m's
    skeletal m.
    strap m's
    m. sympathetic nerve activity (MSNA)
    venous smooth m.

muscular
    m. bridging
    m. incompetence
    m. murmur
    m. subaortic stenosis
    m. venous pump

musculus
    musculi papillares
    m. papillaris anterior ventriculi dextri
    m. papillaris anterior ventriculi sinistri
    m. papillaris posterior ventriculi dextri
    m. papillaris posterior ventriculi sinistri
    musculi pectinati atrii dextri
    musculi pectinati atrii sinistri

mush
    m. clamp
    m. heart

musical
    m. bruit
    m. murmur

Musset sign

Mustard
    M. atrial baffle

Mustard *(continued)*
    M. atrial baffle repair
    M. intra-atrial operation
    M. operation
    M. procedure for transposition of great vessels

mute
    m. reflexes
    m. toe signs

MV
    mechanical ventilation
    mitral valve

mV
    millivolt

MVA
    malignant ventricular arrhythmia
    mitral valve area

MVE-50 implantable myocardial electrode

MVG
    mitral valve gradient

MVP
    mitral valve prolapse
    MVP catheter

MVR
    mitral valve replacement

MycoAKT latex bead agglutination test

mycobacteria

mycobacterial

mycotic
    m. aortic aneurysm
    m. aortography
    m. endocarditis
    m. infection

MycroMesh graft material

mydriatic

myectomy
    septal m.

myeloma

myelonecrosis

myelosuppression

Myers vein stripper

Mylar catheter

myocardial
    m. abscess
    m. anoxia
    m. band (MB)
    m. band enzymes of CPK (CPK-MB)
    m. bed
    m. blood flow
    m. blush
    m. bridging
    m. clamp
    m. cold-spot perfusion scintigraphy
    m. collagen matrix
    m. concussion
    m. conduction defect
    m. contractility
    m. contrast appearance time
    m. contrast echocardiography
    m. contusion
    m. depolarization
    m. depressant factor
    m. depressant substance
    m. depression
    m. dilator
    m. disease
    m. edema
    m. failure
    m. fiber shortening
    m. fibrosis
    m. function
    m. hamartoma
    m. hibernation
    m. hypertrophy
    m. hypothermia
    m. infarction (MI)
    m. infundibular stenosis
    m. injury
    m. insufficiency
    m. ischemia

myocardial *(continued)*
  m. ischemic syndrome
  m. jeopardy
  m. jeopardy index
  m. lactate extraction
  m. lead
  m. malnutrition
  m. mass
  m. metabolism
  m. muscle creatine kinase
    isoenzyme (CK-MB)
  m. necrosis
  m. oxygen consumption
  m. oxygen demand
  m. oxygen supply
  m. perforation
  m. perfusion
  m. perfusion imaging
  m. perfusion scintigraphy
  m. perfusion study
  m. protection
  m. reserve
  m. revascularization
  m. rigor mortis
  m. rupture
  m. salvage
  m. scar
  m. sparing
  m. stiffness
  m. straining
  m. stunning
  m. tension
  m. tissue
  m. uptake of thallium
  m. viability

myocardiectomy

myocardiograph

myocardiopathy
  alcoholic m.
  chagasic m.
  idiopathic m.

myocardiorrhaphy

myocarditic

myocarditis
  acute bacterial m.

myocarditis *(continued)*
  acute isolated m.
  antidepressant induced m.
  bacterial m.
  carbon monoxide-indu-
    ced m.
  Candida m.
  cardiac sarcoidosis m.
  chronic m.
  clostridial m.
  cocaine-induced m.
  coxsackievirus m.
  cryptococcal m.
  diphtheritic m.
  echovirus m.
  eosinophilic m.
  fibrous m.
  Fiedler m.
  fragmentation m.
  fungal m.
  giant cell m.
  granulomatous m.
  heat stroke-induced m.
  helminthic m.
  Histoplasma m.
  hypersensitivity m.
  idiopathic m.
  indurative m.
  infectious m.
  interstitial m.
  lymphocytic m.
  metazoal m.
  neutrophilic m.
  penicillin-induced m.
  parenchymatous m.
  peripartum m.
  protozoal m.
  rheumatic m.
  rickettsial m.
  m. scarlatinosa
  spirochetal m.
  subepicardial m.
  syphilitic m.
  toxic m.
  tuberculoid m.
  tuberculous m.
  viral m.

myocardium
  dysfunctional m.

myocardium *(continued)*
  fragmentation of m.
  hibernating m.
  ischemic m.
  jeopardized m.
  postischemic m.
  senescent m.
  stunned m.
  underperfused m.

myocardiotomy

myocardosis
  Reisman m.

myocyte
  Anichkov (Anitschkow) m.
  m. de-energization
  m. hypertrophy
  m. magnesium stores
  m. metabolic activity
  m. necrosis

myocytolysis
  coagulative m.
  focal m. of heart
  m. of heart

myoendocarditis

myofascial

myofibril

myofibrillar
  m. ATPase
  m. calcium level

myofibroblast

myofibrosis
  m. cordis

myofilament
  m. calcium responsiveness
  m. contractile activity

myogenic theory

myoglobin
  m. assay

myoglobulin (Mgb)

myoglobulinuria

myointimal plaque

myolysis
  cardiotoxic m.

myomalacia cordis

myopathia cordis

myopathy
  mitochondrial myolysis m.

myopericarditis

myopleuropericarditis

Myopore lead

myosin
  cardiac m.
  m. heavy chain
  m. light chain

myosin-specific antibody

myositis

myotomy
  septal m.

myotomy-myectomy-septal re-section

Myoview contrast material

Myowire II cardiac electrode

myurus
  pulsus m.

myxedema
  pericardial effusion in m.

myxedematous

myxoma *pl.* myxomata
  atrial m.
  cardiac m.
  familial m.
  vascular m.
  ventricular m.

myxomatous
  m. change
  m. degeneration of valve
  m. proliferation
  m. valve leaflet

N
N cell
N region

N-13
nitrogen 13
N-13 ammonia
N-13 ammonia uptake

N_2
nitrogen

Nachlas tube

nadir of QRS complex

Nagle exercise stress test

nail
n. bed
cyanosis of n. beds
n. pulse
n.-to-n. bed angle

Nakayama
N. anastomosis apparatus
N. microvascular stapler

Namic
N. angiographic syringe
N. catheter

Nanos 01 pacemaker

napkin-ring
n.-r. calcification
n.-r. defect
n.-r. stenosis

narrow-complex tachycardia

narrowed pulse pressure

narrowing
arterial n.
atherosclerotic n.
diffuse n.
eccentric n.
focal n.
high-grade n.
luminal n.
residual luminal n.
subcritical n.

Nathan
N. pacemaker
N. test

native
n. coarctation
n. coronary anatomy
n. valve
n. ventricle
n. vessel

natriuresis

natriuretic
n. hormone
n. peptide

Naughton
N. graded exercise stress
test
N. treadmill protocol
N.-Blake treadmill protocol

Nauheim
N. bath
N. treatment

Navier-Stokes equation

NBIH cardiac device

NBTE
nonbacterial thrombotic
endocarditis

NCEP
National Cholesterol Edu-
cation Program

Nd:YAG laser

nebenkern

neck
n. of the aneurysm
distended n. veins
flat n. veins
fullness of n. veins

necrocytosis

necrocytotoxin

necrosis *pl.* necroses
arteriolar n.

necrosis *(continued)*
  avascular n.
  coagulation n.
  contraction band n.
  cystic medial n.
  digital n.
  dirty n.
  embolic n.
  Erdheim cystic medial n.
  n. factor
  fibrinoid n.
  medial n.
  myocardial n.
  myocyte n.
  renal cortical n.
  tissue n.
  tubular n.

necrotisans
  phlebitis nodularis n.

necrotizing
  n. angiitis
  n. arterial disease
  n. arteriolitis
  n. vasculitis

needle
  Abrams n.
  Adson n.
  Aldrete n.
  AMC n.
  Amplatz angiography n.
  aneurysm n.
  aortic root perfusion n.
  aortic vent n.
  aortogram n.
  argon n.
  Arrow-Fischell EVAN n.
  arterial blood n.
  arterial n.
  arteriogram n.
  n. aspirate
  aspirating n.
  Atraloc n.
  Becton-Dickinson Teflon-
    sheathed n.
  Bengash n.
  beveled thin-walled n.
  Brockenbrough n.
  Brughleman n.

needle *(continued)*
  butterfly n.
  cardioplegic n.
  Cardiopoint cardiac sur-
    gery n.
  Cooley aortic vent n.
  Cournand n.
  Cournand-Grino angiogra-
    phy n.
  Cournand-Potts n.
  Crown n.
  Curry n.
  Cushing n.
  cutting n.
  DeBakey n.
  Deschamps' n.
  DLP cardioplegic n.
  Dos Santos n.
  ergonomic vascular ac-
    cess n. (EVAN)
  Ethalloy n.
  eyeless n.
  Fergie n.
  Ferguson n.
  Flynt n.
  front wall n.
  Harken heart n.
  n. holder
  Hustead n.
  Jamshidi n.
  Karras angiography n.
  Kronecker n.
  large-bore slotted aspira-
    ting n.
  Lewy-Rubin n.
  ligature n.
  Luer-Lok n.
  Menghini n.
  metal n.
  micron n.
  Microvasive sclerothera-
    py n.
  Nordenstrom Rotex II biop-
    sy n.
  olive-tipped n.
  Parhad-Poppen n.
  PercuCut biopsy n.
  percutaneous cutting n.
  pericardiocentesis n.

needle *(continued)*
    pilot n.
    Potts n.
    Potts-Cournand n.
    Ranfac n.
    Rashkind septostomy n.
    Retter n.
    Riley n.
    root n.
    Rochester n.
    Ross n.
    Rotex biopsy n.
    Sanders-Brown-Shaw n.
    Seldinger n.
    Seraflo A-V fistula n. set
    Sheldon-Spatz n.
    slotted n.
    Smiley-Williams n.
    standard n.
    steel-winged butterfly n.
    sternal puncture n.
    Stifcore aspiration n.
    swaged-on n.
    Terumo AV fistula n.
    THI n.
    thin-walled n.
    thoracentesis n.
    transseptal n.
    Tuohy n.
    Tru-Cut biopsy n.
    UMI n.
    Venflon n.
    venipuncture n.
    venting aortic Bengash n.
    Vim-Silverman n.
    Wasserman n.
    Wood n.

needle holder
    Baum-Metzenbaum sternal
        n. h.
    Berry sternal n. h.
    cardiovascular n. h.
    intracardiac n. h.
    Jarit sternal n. h.
    microvascular n. h.
    Mills microvascular n. h.
    Potts-Smith n. h.
    prosthetic valve n. h.

needle holder *(continued)*
    Stille-French cardiovascular
        n. h.
    vascular n. h.
    Vital-Cooley intracardiac
        n. h.
    Vital-Cooley microvascular
        n. h.
    Vital-DeBakey cardiovascu-
        lar n. h.
    Vital-Mills vascular n. h.
    Vital-Ryder microvascular
        n. h.

needlepoint electrocautery

Needle-Pro needle protection
    device

Neff percutaneous access set

negative deflection on EKG

Negri bodies

Nehb D lead

Nellcor Symphony N-3100 non-
    invasive blood pressure mon-
    itor

Nelson
    N. thoracic scissors
    N. thoracic trocar

nemaline myopathy

neodymium:yttrium-aluminum-
    garnet laser (Nd:YAG laser)

Neoflex bendable knife

neointima

neointimal
    n. hyperplastic response
    n. proliferation
    n. tear

NeoKnife electrosurgical in-
    struction

neolumen

neoplasia

neoplasm
    extrathoracic n.

neoplastic
n. disease
n. pericarditis

Neo-Sert umbilical vessel catheter insertion set

Neos M pacemaker

neovascularization

nephropathic cardiomyopathy

nephropathy
hypertensive n.

nephrosclerosis

nephrotoxicity

Nernst equation

nerve
accelerator n's
n. action potential
aortic n.
n. block anesthesia
cardiac sensory n.
carotid sinus n.
Cyon n.
depressor n.
eleventh cranial n.
n. of Hering
hypoglossal n.
n. of Kuntz
laryngeal n.
Ludwig n.
parasympathetic n.
phrenic n.
sensory n.
sympathetic n.
thoracic n.
vagus n.
vasoconstrictor n.
vasodilator n.
vasomotor n.

nest
bird's n.
n. of veins

Nestor guiding catheter

net
chromidial n.

net (continued)
Arrhythmia N.
Jahnke-Barron heart support n.

network
acromial n.
arterial n.
arterial n., cutaneous
arterial n., subpapillary
arterial n. of dermis
articular n. of elbow
articular n. of knee
calcaneal n.
carpal n., dorsal
cell n.
Chiari n.
fibrillar collagen n.
interstitial and perivascular collagen n.
malleolar n., lateral
malleolar n., medial
patellar n.
Purkinje n.
subendocardial terminal n.
subpapillary n.
vascular n., articular
venous n.
venous n., plantar
venous n., plantar cutaneous
venous n. of foot, dorsal
venous n. of hand, dorsal

Neubauer artery

neuf
bruit de cuir n.

neural
n. crest malformation
n. crest migration

neuralgia
glossopharyngeal n.
red n.

neurocardiac

neurocardiogenic syncope

neurocirculatory asthenia

neurofibroma

neurofibromatosis

neurogenic

neurohormonal function

neurohormone

neuromediated syncope

neuromuscular hypertension

neuromyopathic disorder

neuronal ceroid lipofuscinosis

neuropathy
    angiopathic n.
    peripheral n.
    vasculitic n.

neuropeptide

neurosis *pl.* neuroses
    cardiac n.

neurosyphilis

neuroticism

neurotoxic effect

neurotransmitter substance

neurovascular bundle

neuroxanthoendothelioma

neutropenic angina

neutrophil
    n. elastase
    segmented n's

neutrophilia

Neville stent

nevus *pl.* nevi
    n. araneus
    strawberry n.
    vascular n.
    n. vascularis
    n. vasculosus

New Orleans endarterectomy
    stripper

New Weavenit Dacron prosthesis

New York Heart Association
    classification of heart disease
    (I–IV)

Newman-Keuls test

Newton
    N. guide wire
    N. law of motion and variables

n-3 fatty acid

n-6 fatty acid

NH
    NH region
    NH region of AV node

NHLBI
    National Heart, Lung, and
    Blood Institute

Nichol clamp

NiCad
    nickel-cadmium

Nickerson-Kveim test

nicking
    arteriovenous n.

Nicks procedure

Nicoladoni-Branham sign

nidus

Niedner
    N. anastomosis clamp
    N. commissurotomy knife
    N. dissecting forceps
    N. valvulotome

Niemann-Pick disease

nigra
    cardiopathia n.

NIH
    National Institutes of
    Health
        NIH cardiomarker
        catheter
        NIH catheter

NIH *(continued)*
    NIH left ventriculography catheter
    NIH marking catheter
    NIH mitral valve forceps
    NIH mitral valve-grasping forceps

Nikaidoh translocation

Nikaidoh-Bex technique

Nimbus Hemopump cardiac assist device

NI-NR
    no infection-no rejection

nipple
    aortic n.
    blind n.

NIPS
    noninvasive programmed stimulation

nitinol
    n. guide wire
    n. mesh stent
    n. stent
    n. thermal memory stent

nitrate

nitric oxide

nitrogen
    blood urea n. (BUN)
    n. curve
    n. mustard

nitroglycerin (NTG)
    n. drip
    sublingual n.
    topical n.
    transdermal n.
    n. transdermal patch
    transmucosal n.

nitrovasodilator

NK cells

NMR
    nuclear magnetic resonance

NO
    nitric oxide

Nobis aortic occluder

nocardiosis

nociceptive threshold

nocturnal
    n. angina
    n. dyspnea

nod
    bishop's n.

nodal
    n. arrhythmia
    n. artery
    n. beat
    n. bigeminy
    n. bradycardia
    n. escape
    n. escape rhythm
    n. extrasystole
    n. paroxysmal tachycardia
    n. premature contraction
    n. reentrant tachycardia
    n. rhythm
    n. tachycardia
    n. tissue

node
    aortic window n.
    Aschoff n.
    Aschoff-Tawara n.
    atrioventricular n.
    AV n.
    axillary lymph n.
    Cruveilhier n's
    Delphian n.
    Flack n.
    Fraenkel n's
    Heberden n's
    His-Tawara n.
    Keith n.
    Keith-Flack n.

node *(continued)*
    Koch sinoatrial n.
    lymph n.
    mediastinal lymph n.
    NH region of AV n.
    Osler n.
    paratracheal lymph n's
    pericardial lymph n.
    perihilar lymph n's
    pretracheal lymph n's
    n. of Ranvier
    SA (sinoatrial) n.
    sentinel n.
    shotty n's
    singer's n.
    sinoatrial n.
    sinus n.
    supraclavicular lymph n.
    Tawara atrioventricular n.
    teacher's n.

nodo-Hisian bypass tract

nodosa
    arteritis n.
    periarteritis n.
    polyarteritis n.

nodose arteriosclerosis

nodosum
    erythema n.

nodoventricular
    n. fiber
    n. pathway
    n. tachycardia
    n. tract

nodularity of valve leaflet

nodule
    Albini n.
    aortic valve n.
    Arantius n.
    Aschoff n.
    Bianchi n.
    Cruveilhier n.
    Kerckring n.
    Morgagni n.
    ossific n.

nodule *(continued)*
    n. of pulmonary valve
    n. of semilunar valves
    n. of valves of pulmonary
      trunk

nodulus
    noduli valvularum semilu-
      narium valvae aortae
    noduli valvularum semilu-
      narium valvae trunci pul-
      monalis

nodus
    n. atrioventricularis
    n. sinuatrialis

noisy chest

no-leak technique

nomotopic stimulus

nonacute total occlusion

nonbacterial
    n. thrombotic endocardial
      lesion
    n. thrombotic endocarditis
    n. verrucous endocarditis

noncalcified valve

noncardiac
    n. angiography
    n. surgery
    n. syncope

noncaseating

noncavitary

noncompensatory pause

noncompetitive pacemaker
    atrial demand n. p.
    atrial synchronous n. p.
    atrial triggered n. p.
    demand ventricular n. p.
    ventricular synchronous
      n. p.
    ventricular triggered n. p.

noncoronary
    n. cusp

noncoronary *(continued)*
  n. sinus

noncrushing vascular clamp

non-disjunction

nondominant vessel

nonejection systolic click

nonesterified fatty acid (NEFA)

noneverting suture

nonexertional angina

nonflotation catheter

non–flow-directed catheter

nonhemodynamic effect

non-Hodgkin lymphoma

nonimmunocompromised host

nonintegrated
  n. transvenous defibrilla-
    tion lead
  n. tripolar lead

noninvasive
  n. assessment
  n. continuous cardiac out-
    put monitor
  n. evaluation
  n. pacemaker programming
  n. temporary pacemaker
  n. technique
  n. testing

nonionic
  n. contract material
  n. contrast medium

nonischemic dilated cardiomyopathy

nonnecrotizing angiitis

non-nucleated

nonocclusive
  n. mesenteric ischemia
  n. mesenteric thrombosis

nonoperative closure

nonparoxysmal atrioventricular
  junctional tachycardia

nonpenetrating rupture

nonpharmacologic

nonphasic sinus arrhythmia

nonpitting edema

nonpressor doses

non-Q-wave myocardial infarction

nonreset nodus sinuatrialis

nonselective
  n. beta blocker
  n. coronary angiography

non-sensing
  atrial n.-s.

nonspecific
  n. ST segment changes
  n. ST–T wave changes
  n. T wave abnormality
  n. T wave aberration
  n. T wave changes

nonsteroidal anti-inflammatory
  drug (NSAID)

nonsustained ventricular tachycardia

nonthoracotomy
  n. defibrillation lead sys-
    tem
  n. lead implantable cardio-
    verter-defibrillator
  n. system antitachycardia
    device

nonthrombogenic

nontransmural myocardial infarction

nontraumatic cardiac tamponade

nontraumatizing
  n. forceps

nonuniform rotational defect

Noon AV fistula clamp

Noonan syndrome

No Pour Pak suction catheter
    kit

NoProfile
    N. balloon
    N. balloon catheter

no-reflow phenomenon

Nordenstrom biopsy needle

normal
    n. electrical axis
    n. intravascular pressure
    n. S_1 and S_2
    n. sinus rhythm (NSR)

normalization of inverted T
    waves

normocapnia

normokinesia

normolipidemic

normomagnesemia

normonatremic

normotensive

normothermic cardioplegia

normovolemia

Norton flow-directed Swan-Ganz
    thermodilution catheter

Norwood
    Fontan modification of N.
        procedure
    Gill-Jonas modification of
        N. procedure
    Jonas modification of N.
        procedure
    N. operation for hypoplas-
        tic left-sided heart
    Sade modification of N.
        procedure

Norwood (continued)
    N. univentricular heart pro-
        cedure

NOS
    not otherwise specified

nosocomial
    n. endocarditis
    n. infection

notch
    anacrotic n.
    aortic n.
    atrial n.
    cardiac n.
    n. of cardiac apex
    dicrotic n.
    Sibson n.
    sternal n.
    suprasternal n.

notched P wave

notching
    midsystolic n.
    n. of pulmonic valve
    rib n.

notha
    angina n.

Nottingham introducer

Nova
    N. II pacemaker
    N. MR pacemaker

Novacor
    N. DIASYS cardiac device
    N. LVAD (left ventricular
        assist device)

Novofil suture

Novoste catheter

NoxBOX monitor

NSR
    normal sinus rhythm

NSVT
    nonsustained ventricular
        tachycardia

NTMI
  nontransmural myocardial
    infarction
nuclear
  n. magnetic resonance
    (NMR)
  n. magnetic resonance im-
    aging (NMRI)
  n. pacemaker
  n. scanner
nucleated
nuclei
nucleiform
nucleochylema
nucleochyme
nucleocytoplasmic
nucleofugal
nucleohyaloplasm
nucleoid
nucleolar
nucleoli
nucleoliform
nucleolin
nucleolinus
nucleoloid
nucleololus
nucleolonema
nucleoloneme
nucleolonucleus
nucleolus
  secondary n.
nucleolymph
nucleopetal
nucleophilic
nucleoplasm

nucleoreticulum
nucleospindle
nucleotoxin
nucleus
  cell n.
  cellular n.
  compact n.
  daughter n.
  diploid n.
  free n.
  gonad n.
  haploid n.
  polymorphic n.
  reproductive n.
  vesicular n.
null
  n. hypothesis
  n. point
number
  Reynolds n.
  Strouhal n.
Numed intracoronary Doppler
  catheter
nummular aortitis
Nunez-Nunez knife
nun's venous hum murmur
Nurolon suture
nutrient cardioplegia
Nyboer esophageal electrode
Nycore
  N. angiography catheter
  N. cardiac device
  N. pigtail catheter
NYHA
  New York Heart Associa-
    tion
      NYHA classification of
        angina
      NYHA classification of
        congestive heart fail-
        ure

O
O antigen
O point of cardiac apex
pulse

OA
occipital artery

obesity
exogenous o.
morbid o.

obesity-hypoventilation syndrome

oblique
left anterior o.
right anterior o.
o. sinus of pericardium

obliterans
arteriosclerosis o.
arteritis o.
endarteritis o.
pericarditis o.
phlebitis o.
thromboangiitis o.

obliterating
o. pericarditis
o. phlebitis

obliterative
o. cardiomyopathy
o. vascular disease

obstruction
aortic outflow o.
aortoiliac o.
congenital left-sided outflow o.
coronary artery o.
cowl-shaped o.
dynamic intracavitary o.
fixed coronary o.
infundibular o.
left ventricular inflow
tract o.
left ventricular outflow
tract o.
microvascular o.

obstruction *(continued)*
multivessel coronary artery o.
pulmonary outflow o.
pulmonary vascular o.
right ventricular inflow o.
right ventricular outflow o.
shunt o.
subvalvular diffuse o.
vena cava o.
ventricular inflow tract o.
ventricular outflow tract o.

obstructive
o. hypertrophic cardiomyopathy
o. mitral valve murmur
o. murmur
o. thrombus

obturating embolus

obturator
double-catheterizing
sheath and o.
Fitch o.
Hemaflex PTCA sheath
with o.
Hemaquet PTCA sheath
with o.

Obturay contract medium

obtuse
o. marginal (OM)
o. marginal artery (OMA)
o. marginal artery branch
(OMB)
o. marginal lymphatic

occluder
air clamp inflatable vessel
o. clamp
aorta o.
Bard Clamshell septal o.
Brockenbrough curved-
tip o.
catheter tip o.
Clamshell septal o.
Flo-Rester vascular o.
Heifitz carotid o.

occluder *(continued)*
    Heishima balloon o.
    Hunter detachable bal-
        loon o.
    Hunter-Sessions balloon o.
    Nobis aortic o.
    radiolucent o.
    tilting-disk o.

occluding thrombus

occlusion
    angioplasty-related ves-
        sel o.
    aortoiliac o.
    balloon o.
    branch retinal vein o.
    branch vessel o.
    complete o.
    coronary o.
    embolic o.
    femoral artery o.
    femoral vein o.
    femoropopliteal o.
    graft o.
    iliac artery o.
    inferior mesenteric vascu-
        lar o.
    inferior vena cava o.
    intermittent coronary sin-
        us o.
    mesenteric artery o.
    mesenteric vascular o.
    nonacute total o.
    popliteal-femoral o.
    pressure-controlled inter-
        mittent coronary o.
    recurrent mesenteric vas-
        cular o.
    side branch o.
    subtotal o.
    superior mesenteric vascu-
        lar o.
    temporary unilateral pul-
        monary artery o.
    thrombotic o.
    total o.
    venous mesenteric vascu-
        lar o.

occlusive
    o. disease
    o. thromboaortopathy
    o. thrombus

occult
    o. blood loss
    o. infection
    o. pericardial constriction
    o. pericarditis

ochronosis

Ochsner
    O. aortic clamp
    O. arterial clamp
    O. arterial forceps
    O. retractor
    O. thoracic clamp
    O. thoracic trocar
    O. vascular retractor
    O.-Dixon arterial forceps
    O.-Mahorner echocardi-
        ogram
    O.-Mahorner test

octapolar
    o. catheter
    o. lead

oculocardiac reflex

oculomucocutaneous syndrome

oculopharyngeal reflex

oculoplethysmography

oculopneumoplethysmography

oculovagal reflex

ODAM defibrillator

Oehler symptoms

Oertel treatment

office
    o. angina
    o. hypertension

Ogata method

OHD
    organic heart disease

Ohm
    O.'s law

ohm

Ohmeda
    O. 6200 CO_2 monitor
    O. thoracic suction regula-
        tor

ohmic heating

ohmmeter

Öhnell
    X wave of Ö.

OHT
    orthotopic heart transplant

oil
    canola o.
    o. embolism
    fish o.
    MCT o.
    rapeseed o.

Olbert
    O. balloon
    O. balloon catheter

oligemia

oligemic
    o. shock

oligonucleotides

oliguria

Oliver-Rosalki method

olive-tipped needle

Olivre sign

Olympix II PTCA dilatation
    catheter

Olympus angioscope

OM
    obtuse marginal
        OM-1
        OM-2

OMA
    obtuse marginal artery

OMB
    obtuse marginal branch

Omega
    O. 5600 noninvasive blood
        pressure monitor
    O.-NV balloon

omega-3 unsaturated fatty acids

omentopexy

Omni
    O. SST balloon
    O. tract retractor system
    O.-Atricor pacemaker

Omnicarbon
    O. heart valve prosthesis
    O. prosthetic heart valve

Omnicor
    O. pacemaker
    O. Programmer

Omni-Ectocor pacemaker

Omniflex
    O. balloon
    O. balloon catheter

Omni-Orthocor pacemaker

Omnipaque contrast medium

OmniPlane TEE

Omniscience
    O. cardiac valve prosthesis
    O. single leaflet cardiac
        valve prosthesis
    O. tilting-disk valve
    O. tilting-disk valve pros-
        thesis
    O. valve device

Omni-Stanicor pacemaker

Omni-Theta pacemaker

Omni-Ventricor pacemaker

omphalitis

omphalocele

omphalomesenteric
    o. duct
    o. veins
    o. vessels

omphalophlebitis

oncotic pressure

one-block claudication

one-flight exertional dyspnea

one-hole angiographic catheter

O'Neill cardiac clamp

one-ventricle heart

onion scale lesion

onychogram

onychograph

oocyte
    Xenopus o's

OPCAB
    off-pump coronary artery
        bypass

open
    o. chest cardiac massage
    o. heart surgery

Open-Cath
    Abbokinase O.-C.

opening
    o. amplitude of valve
    aortic o.
    atrioventricular o., left
    atrioventricular o., right
    o. of coronary artery
    o. of coronary sinus
    o. of inferior vena cava
    o. pressure
    o. of pulmonary trunk
    o. of pulmonary veins
    o. snap
    o. of superior vena cava
    valvular o.

operation
    ablation of bundle of His o.
    aneurysmectomy o.
    annuloplasty o.
    aortic root replacement o.
    aortic valve repair o.
    aortic valve replacement o.
    aortic valvuloplasty o.
    aortofemoral bypass o.
    aortopulmonary window o.
    arterial switch o.
    arteriotomy o.
    atrial baffle o.
    Babcock o.
    balloon atrial septosto-
        my o.
    balloon mitral valvuloplas-
        ty o.
    balloon valvuloplasty o.
    banding of pulmonary ar-
        tery o.
    Beck I, II o.
    Bentall inclusion techni-
        que o.
    Berger o.
    blade and balloon atrial
        septostomy o.
    Blalock-Hanlon o.
    Blalock-Taussig o.
    Brauer o.
    Brock o.
    Brockenbrough commissu-
        rotomy o.
    Carpentier annuloplasty o.
    Carpentier tricuspid valvu-
        loplasty o.
    catheter balloon valvulo-
        plasty o.
    coarctectomy o.
    commissurotomy o.
    Cooley anastomosis o.
    cryosurgical interruption of
        AV node o.
    Damus-Kaye-Stansel o.
    Delorme o.
    De Vega annuloplasty o.
    division of accessory bun-
        dle of Kent o.

operation *(continued)*

    electrode catheter ablation o.

    encircling endocardial ventriculotomy o.

    endocardial to epicardial resection o.

    femorodistal bypass o.

    femoropopliteal bypass o.

    Fontan-Kreutzer repair o.

    Fontan tricuspid atresia o.

    Freund o.

    Glenn o.

    Harrington o.

    Heller-Belsey o.

    Heller-Nissen o.

    Hufnagel o.

    Hunter o.

    inferior vena cava interruption o.

    infundibular resection o.

    intra-arterial baffle o.

    Jantene o.

    Kay tricuspid valvuloplasty o.

    Kaye-Damus-Stansel o.

    Kono o.

    laser recanalization o.

    Leriche o.

    Lindesmith o.

    Lower-Shumway heart transplant o.

    Lyon-Horgan o.

    Matas o.

    Mayo o.

    medial sternotomy o.

    mitral valve replacement o.

    Moore o.

    Müller-Dammann pulmonary artery banding o.

    Mullins blade and balloon septostomy o.

    Mullins transseptal atrial septostomy o.

    Mustard transposition of great arteries o.

    Norwood hypoplastic left-sided heart o.

operation *(continued)*

    Norwood univentricular heart o.

    open heart o.

    open mitral commissurotomy o.

    orthotopic cardiac transplant o.

    Park blade and balloon atrial septostomy o.

    patent ductus arteriosus (PDA) ligation o.

    percutaneous aortic valvuloplasty o.

    percutaneous mitral balloon valvotomy o.

    percutaneous transluminal balloon dilatation o.

    pericardiectomy o.

    peripheral artery bypass o.

    peripheral laser angioplasty o.

    phlebectomy o.

    plication repair of flail leaflet o.

    Potts o.

    Potts-Smith-Gibson o.

    profundaplasty o.

    pulmonary artery banding o.

    Rashkind-Miller atrial septostomy o.

    Rastelli o.

    redirection of inferior vena cava o.

    regional cardiac sympathectomy o.

    Sade modification of Norwood o.

    Scarpa o.

    second-look o.

    Senning o.

    septostomy o.

    Simpson atherectomy o.

    Sucquet-Hoyer anastomosis o.

    switch o.

    thromboendarterectomy o.

operation *(continued)*
    transcatheter closure of
        atrial septal defect o.
    Trendelenburg o.
    triangular resection of leaf-
        let o.
    tricuspid valve annuloplas-
        ty o.
    transmural resection o.
    valvotomy o.
    valvuloplasty o.
    valvulotomy o.
    vein stripping o.
    ventriculorrhaphy o.
    ventriculotomy o.
    Vineberg o.
    Waterston o.
    wrapping of abdominal aor-
        tic aneurysm o.

OPG
    oculoplethysmography
        OPG-Gee instrument

Opitz syndrome

opportunistic
    o. infection

oppositipolar

Opta 5 catheter

Opticath oximeter catheter

Optichin disc test

Opti-Flex

Optima
    O. MP pacemaker
    O. MPI Series III pacemaker
    O. MPI Series III pulse gen-
        erator
    O. SPT pacemaker

Optiray
    O. 320
    O. contrast

Optiscope
    O. angioscope
    O. catheter

Optison echocardiography
    opacification agent

OptiView digital system

Opus
    O. cardiac troponin I assay

Oracle
    O. Focus PTCA catheter
    O. Micro intravascular ul-
        trasound catheter
    O. Micro Plus
    O. Micro Plus PTCA cathe-
        ter

Oregon
    O. prosthesis
    O. tunneler

Oreopoulos-Zellerman catheter

organ
    cell o.
    Golgi tendon o's
    o's of Zuckerkandl

organic
    o. murmur
    o. phosphorus

organism
    Cox o.
    encapsulated o.
    gram-negative o.
    gram-positive o.

organized thrombus

organizer
    nucleolar o.
    nucleolus o.
    procentriole o.

oriental hemoptysis

orifice
    aortic o.
    atrioventricular o.
    cardiac o.
    o. of coronary sinus
    double coronary o.
    effective regurgitant o.
    flow across o.
    o. of inferior vena cava
    mitral o.
    narrowed o.

orifice *(continued)*
    pulmonary o.
    o. of pulmonary trunk
    o. of superior vena cava
    tricuspid o.
    valvular o.

orificial
    o. stenosis

origin
    anomalous o.

Orion
    O. balloon
    O. pacemaker

Orlowski stent

Ornish diet

Orsi-Grocco method

ORT
    orthodromic reciprocating
    tachycardia

orthoarteriotomy

orthocardiac reflex

Orthocor II pacemaker

orthodromic
    o. AV reentrant tachycardia
    o. circus movement tachy-
    cardia
    o. reciprocating tachycar-
    dia (ORT)

orthogonal
    o. electrocardiogram
    o. lead arrangement on
    EKG
    o. plane
    o. view

orthograde conduction

orthopercussion

orthopnea
    three-pillow o.
    two-pillow o.

orthopneic

orthostasis

orthostatic
    o. blood pressure
    o. dyspnea
    o. hypopiesis
    o. hypotension
    o. syncope
    o. tachycardia

orthotopic
    o. biventricular artificial
    heart
    o. cardiac transplant
    o. heart transplant
    o. univentricular artificial
    heart

Osborne wave

oscillating
    o. saw
    o. sternotomy saw

oscillation
    high-frequency o.

oscillator

oscillometer

oscillometrics

oscillometry

oscilloscope
    Tektronix digital o.

Oscor
    O. active fixation leads
    O. pacing leads
    O. pacemaker

OSF
    outlet strut fracture

O'Shaughnessy
    O. artery forceps
    O. clamp

Osler
    O. node
    O. sign
    O. triad
    O.-Weber-Rendu disease
    O.-Weber-Rendu syndrome

osmolality

osmolarity

osmometer

osmoregulation

osmoregulatory

osmotaxis

osmotic
  o. diuretic
  o. pressure

osteoarthritis

osteochondroma

osteogenesis imperfecta

osteomyelitis of sternum

osteosarcoma of heart

ostium *pl.* ostia
  o. aortae
  o. arteriosum cordis
  o. atrioventriculare dextrum
  o. atrioventriculare sinistrum
  o. cardiacum
  o. primum
  o. primum defect
  o. secundum
  o. secundum defect
  o. sinus coronarii
  sinusoidal o.
  o. trunci pulmonalis
  o. venae cavae inferioris
  o. venae cavae superioris
  o. venarum pulmonalium
  o. venosum cordis

Osypka
  O. atrial lead
  O. Cereblate electrode

Ototemp 3000 thermometer

ototoxicity

OTW
  over-the-wire
  OTW perfusion catheter

ouabain

outflow
  o. anastomosis
  o. tract

output
  cardiac o.
  Dow method for cardiac o.
  Fick method for cardiac o.
  Gorlin method for cardiac o.
  left ventricular o.
  pacemaker o.
  pulmonic o.
  stroke o.
  thermodilution cardiac o.
  ventricular o.
  work o. of the heart

ovale
  foramen o.
  patent foramen o.

oval foramen

ovalis
  annulus o.
  fossa o.

overdilation

overdrive
  o. pacing
  o. suppression

overflow wave

Overholt
  O. elevator
  O. thoracic forceps
  O.-Geissendörfer arterial forceps
  O.-Geissendörfer dissection forceps

overload
  circulatory o.
  diastolic o.
  pressure o.
  right ventricular o.
  systolic ventricular o.
  volume o.

override
   aortic o.

oversampling

oversensing
   afterpotential o.
   o. pacemaker

oversewing

over-the-wire (OTW)
   o.-t.-w. balloon dilatation
      system
   Buchbinder Thruflex
      o.-t.-w.
   o.-t.-w. probe
   o.-t.-w. PTCA balloon cathe-
      ter

Owens
   O. balloon
   O. balloon catheter
   O. Lo-Profile dilatation
      catheter

Owren
   O. disease
   O. factor V deficiency

Oxford
   O. Medilog frequency-mod-
      ulated recorder
   O. technique

ox heart

oxide
   endothelium-derived ni-
      tric o.
   magnesium o.
   nitric o.
   nitrous o.

oxidized
   o. cellulose

oximeter
   American Optical o.
   Armstrong hand-held
      pulse o.
   CO-o.
   Criticare pulse o.

oximeter *(continued)*
   Datascope pulse o.
   ear o.
   intracardiac o.
   Nellcor N series pulse o.
   Novametrix pulse o.
   Ohmeda pulse o.
   Oxypleth pulse o.
   OxyTemp hand-held
      pulse o.
   Oxytrak pulse o.
   pulse o.
   SpaceLabs pulse o.

oximetric catheter

oximetry
   CO-o.

oxygenator
   Bentley o.
   bubble o.
   Capiox-E bypass system o.
   Cobe Optima hollow-fiber
      membrane o.
   DeBakey heart pump o.
   disk o.
   extracorporeal mem-
      brane o.
   extracorporeal pump o.
   intravascular o. (IVOX)
   Lilliput o.
   Maxima Plus plasma resis-
      tant fiber o.
   membrane o.
   Monolyth o.
   plasma-resistant fiber o.
   pump o.
   Sarns membrane o.
   Shiley o.

oxygen
   o.-binding capacity
   o.-carrying capacity
   o.-diffusing capacity

oxyhemoglobin
   o. dissociation curve

oxytropism

ozonophore

P
P cell
P congenitale
P loop
P mitrale
P pulmonale syndrome
P pulmonary in leads II, III, aVF
P synchronous pacing
P terminal force
P vector

P_2
pulmonic heart sound
pulmonary valve closure

P24
P24 antigen
P24 antigen test

PA
pulmonary artery
PA banding
PA diastolic pressure
PA filling pressure
PA interval
PA pressure
PA systolic pressure
PA Watch position-monitoring catheter

P&A
percussion and auscultation

pAAT
plasma alpha$_1$-antitrypsin

PAB
premature atrial beat

PAC
premature atrial contraction

Paceart complete pacemaker patient testing system

paced
p. cycle length
p. impulse
p. rhythm

paced *(continued)*
p. ventricular evoked response

Pacejector

pacemaker
AAI p.
AAIR p.
AAT p.
Accufix p.
Acculith p.
Activitrax single-chamber responsive p.
Activitrax variable-rate p.
activity-sensing p.
AEC p.
Aequitron p.
AFP II p.
AICD p.
AICD-B p.
AICD-BR p.
Alcatel p.
American Optical Cardio-Care p.
American Optical R-inhibited p.
Amtech-Killeen p.
antitachycardia p. (ATP)
AOO p.
Arco atomic p.
Arco lithium p.
p. artifact
artificial p.
Arzco p.
Astra p.
ASVIP p.
asynchronous p.
asynchronous atrial p.
asynthronous mode p.
asynchronous ventricular p.
atrial asynchronous p.
atrial demand inhibited p.
atrial demand noncompetitive p.
atrial demand triggered p.
atrial synchronous p.

pacemaker *(continued)*

- atrial synchronous non-competitive p.
- atrial synchronous ventricular inhibited p.
- atrial tracking p.
- atrial triggered noncompetitive p.
- atrial triggered ventricular inhibited p.
- Atricor Cordis p.
- atrioventricular junctional p.
- atrioventricular (AV) sequential p.
- Aurora dual-chamber p.
- Autima II dual-chamber p.
- automatic p.
- p. AV disable mechanism
- Avius sequential p.
- AV sequential demand p.
- AV synchronous p.
- Axios 04 p.
- Basix p.
- p. battery status
- Betacel-Biotronik p.
- bifocal demand DVI p.
- Biorate p.
- Biotronik demand p.
- bipolar p.
- breathing p.
- burst p.
- Byrel SX p.
- Byrel-SX/Versatrax p.
- p. capture
- cardiac p.
- Cardio-Control p.
- Cardio-Pace Medical Dura-pulse p.
- p. catheter
- Chardack-Greatbatch p.
- Chardack Medtronic p.
- Chorus DDD p.
- Chorus dual-chamber p.
- Chorus RM rate-responsive dual-chamber p.
- Chronocor IV external p.
- Chronos p.

pacemaker *(continued)*

- Circadia dual-chamber rate-adaptive p.
- Classix p.
- p. code system
- Comand P5 p.
- committed mode p.
- Cooke p.
- Coratomic R-wave inhibited p.
- Cordis Atricor p.
- Cordis Chronocor IV p.
- Cordis Ectocor p.
- Cordis fixed-rate p.
- Cordis Gemini cardiac p.
- Cordis Multicor p.
- Cordis Omni Stanicor Theta transvenous p.
- Cordis Sequicor cardiac p.
- Cordis Stanicor unipolar ventricular p.
- Cordis Synchrocor p.
- Cordis Ventricor p.
- Cosmos 283 DDD p.
- Cosmos II DDD p.
- Cosmos pulse-generator p.
- CPI Astra p.
- CPI DDD p.
- CPI Maxilith p.
- CPI Microthin DI, DII lithium-powered programmable p.
- CPI Minilith p.
- CPI Ultra II p.
- CPI Vista-T p.
- crosstalk p.
- Cyberlith demand p.
- Cybertach automatic-burst atrial p.
- Cybertach 60 bipolar p.
- Daig ESI-II or DSI-III screw-in lead p.
- Dart p.
- Dash single-chamber rate-adaptic p.
- DDD p.
- DDDR p.
- DDI p.
- Delta TRS p.

pacemaker *(continued)*
    demand p.
    demand ventricular non-
      competitive p.
    Devices, Ltd. P.
    Dialog p.
    Diplos M 05 p.
    Dromos p.
    dual-chamber p.
    dual-demand p.
    Durapulse p.
    DVI p.
    ECT p.
    Ectocor p.
    ectopic p.
    ectopic atrial p.
    Ela Chorus DDD p.
    Elecath p.
    electric cardiac p.
    p. electrodes
    electronic p.
    Electrodyne p.
    Elema p.
    Elema-Schonander p.
    Elevath p.
    Elgiloy p.
    Elgiloy lead-tip p.
    Elite p.
    Encor p.
    endocardial p.
    end-of-life p.
    Enertrax p.
    epicardial p.
    Ergos O_2 dual-chamber
      rate-responsive p.
    erratic p. capture
    escape p.
    p. escape interval
    external p.
    externally controlled nonin-
      vasive programmed sti-
      mulation p.
    external transthoracic p.
    p. failure
    fixed-rate p.
    fully automatic p.
    Galaxy p.
    GE p.
    Gemini DDD p.

pacemaker *(continued)*
    Gen2 p.
    p. generator pouch
    Genisis dual-chamber p.
    Guardian p.
    Hancock bipolar balloon p.
    heart p.
    hermetically-sealed p.
    p. hysteresis
    implantable p.
    implanted p.
    p. impedance
    Intermedics lithium-power-
      ed p.
    Intermedics Quantum uni-
      polar p.
    Intermedics Stride p.
    Intermedics Thinlith II p.
    internal p.
    Intertach p.
    isotopic pulse generator p.
    junctional p.
    Kalos p.
    Kantrowitz p.
    Kelvin Sensor p.
    lack of p. capture
    Lambda Omni Stanicor p.
    latent p.
    Laurens-Alcatel nuclear
      powered p.
    p. lead fracture
    p. leads
    Legend p.
    Leukos p.
    lithium-powered p.
    Maestro implantable car-
      diac p.
    p. malfunction
    Malith p.
    Mallor p.
    Mallory RM-1 cell p.
    malsensing p.
    Maxilith p.
    Medcor p.
    p.-mediated tachycardia
    Medtel p.
    Medtronic Activitrax rate-
      responsive unipolar ven-
      tricular p.

pacemaker *(continued)*
  Medtronic-Alcatel p.
  Medtronic bipolar p.
  Medtronic-Byrel-SX p.
  Medtronic Chardack p.
  Medtronic corkscrew elec-
    trode p.
  Medtronic demand p.
  Medtronic Elite DDDR p.
  Medtronic Elite II p.
  Medtronic Pacette p.
  Medtronic RF 5998 p.
  Medtronic SP 502 p.
  Medtronic SPO p.
  Medtronic Symbios p.
  Medtronic temporary p.
  Medtronic Thera "I-series"
    cardiac p.
  Medtronic-Zyrel p.
  mercury cell-powered p.
  Meta II p.
  Meta MV p.
  Meta rate-responsive p.
  Microlith P p.
  Micro Minix p.
  Microthin P p.
  migrating p.
  Mikros p.
  Minilith p.
  Minix p.
  Minuet DDD p.
  Multicor Gamma p.
  Multicor II cardiac p.
  Multilith p.
  multiprogrammable p.
  Nanos 01 p.
  Nathan p.
  natural p.
  Neos M p.
  Nomos multiprogrammable
    R-wave inhibited de-
    mand p.
  noncompetitive p.
  noninvasive temporary p.
  Nova II p.
  Nova MR p.
  nuclear-powered p.
  Omni-Atricor p.
  Omnicor p.

pacemaker *(continued)*
  Omni-Ectocor p.
  Omni-Orthocor p.
  Omni-Stanicor p.
  Omni-Theta p.
  Omni-Ventricor p.
  Optima MP p.
  Optima MPI Series III p.
  Optima SPT p.
  Opus p.
  Orion p.
  Orthocor II p.
  Oscor p.
  p. output
  oversensing p.
  Pacesetter p.
  Pacesetter Synchrony p.
  Pacette p.
  Paragon p.
  Paragon II p.
  PASAR tachycardia rever-
    sion p.
  Pasys p.
  PDx pacing and diagnos-
    tic p.
  permanent p.
  permanent myocardial p.
  permanent rate-respon-
    sive p.
  permanent transvenous p.
  permanent ventricular p.
  Permathane Pacesetter
    lead p.
  pervenous p.
  phantom p.
  Phoenix single-chamber p.
  Phoenix 2 p.
  Phymos 3D p.
  physiologic p.
  Pinnacle p.
  p. pocket
  PolyFlex implantable pac-
    ing lead p.
  PolyFlex lead p.
  p. potential
  Precept DR p.
  Prima p.
  Prism p.
  Prism-CL p.

pacemaker *(continued)*
    Programalith p.
    Programalith AV p.
    Programalith II p.
    Programalith III p.
    programmable p.
    Programmer III p.
    Prolith p.
    Prolog p.
    Pulsar NI implantable p.
    P-wave-triggered ventricu-
      lar p.
    Q-T interval sensing p.
    Quantum p.
    radiofrequency p.
    rate-modulated p.
    rate-responsive p.
    Reflex p.
    refractory period of elec-
      tronic p.
    Relay cardiac p.
    rescuing p.
    respiratory-dependent p.
    reversion p.
    RS4 p.
    R-synchronous VVT p.
    runaway p.
    screw-in lead p.
    secondary p.
    Seecor p.
    p. sensitivity
    Sensolog III p.
    sensor-based single-cham-
      ber p.
    Sensor Kelvin p.
    Sequicor II, III p.
    Shaldach electrode p.
    Shaldach p.
    shifting p.
    Siemens-Elema p.
    Siemens-Pacesetter p.
    single-chamber p.
    single-pass p.
    sinus p.
    sinus node p.
    Sohes p.
    Solar p.
    Solis p.
    Solus p.

pacemaker *(continued)*
    Sorin p.
    p. sound
    Spectraflex p.
    Spectrax bipolar p.
    Spectrax programmable
      Medtronic p.
    Spectrax SX, SX-HT, SXT,
      VL, VM, VS p.
    p. spike
    standby p.
    Stanicor p.
    Stanicor Gamma p.
    Stanicor Lambda de-
      mand p.
    Starr-Edwards hermetically
      sealed p.
    Stride cardiac p.
    subsidiary atrial p.
    Swing DR1 DDDR p.
    Symbios p.
    synchronous p.
    synchronous burst p.
    synchronous mode p.
    Synchrony I, II p.
    p. syndrome
    Synergyst DDD p.
    Synergyst II p.
    Syticon 5950 bipolar de-
      mand p.
    tachycardia-terminating p.
    Tachylog p.
    Telectronics p.
    temperature-sensing p.
    temporary p.
    temporary transvenous p.
    Thera-SR p.
    Thermos p.
    Thinlith II p.
    p. threshold
    tined lead p.
    transcutaneous p.
    transpericardial p.
    transthoracic p.
    transvenous p.
    transvenous ventricular de-
      mand p.
    Trios M p.
    Triumph VR p.

pacemaker *(continued)*
  p. undersensing
  Ultra p.
  Unilith p.
  unipolar p.
  unipolar atrial p.
  unipolar atrioventricular p.
  unipolar sequential p.
  Unity-C cardiac p.
  Unity VDDR p.
  USCI Vario permanent p.
  universal p.
  variable rate p.
  VAT p.
  VDD p.
  Ventak AICD p.
  Ventak ECD P.
  Ventricor p.
  ventricular p.
  ventricular asynchronous p.
  ventricular demand inhibited p.
  ventricular demand triggered p.
  ventricular suppressed p.
  ventricular synchronous noncompetitive p.
  ventricular triggered p.
  ventricular triggered noncompetitive p.
  Versatrax cardiac p.
  Versatrax II p.
  Vicor p.
  Vista 4, T, TRS p.
  Vitatrax II p.
  Vitatron p.
  VOO p.
  VVD mode p.
  VVI p.
  VVIR p.
  VVT p.
  wandering atrial p.
  Xyrel p.
  Zitron p.
  Zoll NTP noninvasive p.
Paceport catheter
pacemapping

pacer
  Intertach II p.
  PolySafe p.
Pacer-Tracer
Pacesetter
  P. cardiac pacemaker
  P. programmable pulse generator
  P. Synchrony pacemaker
pace-terminable
pace-terminate
Pacewedge dual-pressure bipolar pacing catheter
Pachon
  P. method
  P. test
pachynema
pachytene
pacing
  AAI p.
  AAI-RR p.
  AAT p.
  antitachycardia p.
  AOO p.
  asynchronous p.
  asynchronous atrioventricular sequential p.
  atrial p.
  atrial overdrive p.
  atrial train p.
  autodecremental p.
  AV sequential p.
  backup bradycardia p.
  bipolar p.
  burst atrial p.
  burst overdrive p.
  cardiac p.
  p. catheter
  p. code
  committed p.
  competitive p.
  continuous p.
  coronary sinus p.
  coupled p.

pacing *(continued)*
    p. cycle length
    DDD p.
    DDDR p.
    DDI p.
    DDIR p.
    decremental atrial p.
    demand p.
    diaphragmatic p.
    dual-chamber p.
    DVI p.
    endocardial p.
    epicardial p.
    esophageal p.
    external p.
    fixed rate p.
    p. hysteresis
    implantable cardioverter-defibrillator/atrial tachycardia p. (ICD-ATP)
    p. impulse
    incremental atrial p.
    incremental ventricular p.
    p.-induced angina
    p.-induced termination of arrhythmia
    inhibited p.
    intracardiac p.
    p. modalities
    noncommitted p.
    overdrive p.
    pacemaker burst p.
    paired p.
    permanent p.
    physiologic p.
    P triggered ventricular p.
    ramp p.
    rapid atrial p.
    rapid-burst p.
    rapid ventricular p.
    rate-adaptive p.
    rate-responsive p.
    sequential p.
    single chamber p.
    p. stimulus
    synchronous p.
    p. system analyzer
    temporary p.
    p. threshold

pacing *(continued)*
    trains of ventricular p.
    transatrial p.
    transcutaneous p.
    transesophageal p.
    transesophageal atrial p.
    transesophageal echocardiography with p.
    transthoracic p.
    transvenous p.
    triggered p.
    ultrafast train p.
    ultrarapid p.
    underdrive p.
    unipolar p.
    VAT p.
    VDD p.
    ventricular p.
    ventricular demand p.
    ventricular overdrive p.
    ventricular triggered p.
    vibration based p.
    VOO p.
    VVI p.
    VVIR p.
    VVI-RR p.
    VVI/VVIR p.
    VVT p.
    p. wire
    p. wire fracture

pack-year smoking history

pack-years of cigarette smoking

P-A conduction time

PAD
    peripheral artery disease
    pulsatile assist device

pad
    defibrillator p.
    disposable electrode p.
    electrode p.
    Littman defibrillation p.
    pericardial fat p.
    p. sign of aortic insufficiency

paddle
    anteroposterior p's

paddle *(continued)*
    cardioversion p's
    defibrillation p's
    defibrillator p's
    electrode p's

PAF
    paroxysmal atrial fibrillation

Page episodic hypertension

Paget disease

Paget-Schröetter venous thrombosis

Paget-von Schrötter syndrome

PAH
    pulmonary artery hypertension

PAI
    plasminogen activator inhibitor

PAI-1
    plasminogen activator inhibitor-1

pain
    anginal p.
    atypical chest p.
    burning p.
    calf p.
    crushing chest p.
    dream p.
    dull p.
    exertional chest p.
    focal p.
    p.-free walking time
    functional p.
    ischemic rest p.
    phantom p.
    pinching chest p.
    postprandial p.
    precordial chest p.
    pressure chest p.
    psychogenic p.
    radiating chest p.
    referred cardiac p.
    rest p.
    retrosternal chest p.

pain *(continued)*
    squeezing chest p.
    staccato p.
    suffocating chest p.

P–A interval

paired
    p. beats
    p. electrical stimulation
    p. *t* test

pairing
    somatic p.

pale
    p. hypertension
    p. thrombus

palisading
    p. histiocytes

palliation

palliative surgery

pallor

palm
    liver p.
    tripe p.

Palma operation

palmar
    p. arch
    p. erythema
    p. xanthoma

palmare
    xanthoma striatum p.

Palmaz
    P. arterial stent
    P. balloon-expandable iliac stent
    P. vascular stent
    P.- Schatz balloon-expandable stent
    P.- Schatz coronary stent
    P.- Schatz Crown balloon-expandable stent

palmic

palmitate
    C-11 p.

palmitate *(continued)*
    clofazimine p.
    colfosceril p.

palmitic acid

palmitocylcarnitine

palmodic

palmoscopy

palmus *pl.* palmi

palpitatio cordis

palpitation
    bimanual precordial p.
    flip-flop p's
    fluttering p's
    paroxysmal p's
    premonitory p's

palsy
    ischemic p.

PAM2 monitor

PAM3 monitor

pamoate

panangiitis
    diffuse necrotizing p.

panarteritis
    p. nodosa

pancarditis

panchamber enlargement

Pancoast syndrome

panconduction defect

pandiastolic

panel
    lipid p.
    South Florida RAST p.
    thyroid p.

pang
    breast p.

panhyperemia

panniculitis

panophthalmitis

pansystolic
    p. flow
    p. murmur

pantaloon
    p. embolism

pantothenate synthetase

pants
    MAST p.

pantyhose
    Glattelast compression p.

panzerherz

PAP
    pulmonary artery pressure

papain

Papercuff

papillary
    p. fibroelastoma
    p. muscle dysfunction
    p. muscle rupture

papilledema

papillitis

papillotome
    Wilson-Cook p.

papulosis
    atrophic p.

para-aortic

paracentesis
    p. cordis
    p. pericardii
    p. thoracis

paracardiac

parachromatin

parachute
    p. deformity
    p. mitral valve

paracorporeal heart

paradox
  calcium p.
  French p.
  p. image
  oxygen p.
  thoracoabdominal p.

paradoxic, paradoxical
  p. embolization
  p. embolus
  p. motion
  p. pulse
  p. respiration
  p. rocking impulse
  p. septal motion
  p. split of S_2
  p. wall motion

paradoxically split S_2 sound

paradoxus
  p. parvus et tardus
  pulsus p.

Paragon II pacemaker

paralinin

parallel shunt

parallel-loop electrode

paralysis
  ischemic p.
  periodic p.
  phrenic nerve p.
  tick p.
  vasomotor p.
  Volkmann ischemic p.

paralytica
  dysphagia p.

paralytic chest

paralyticus
  p. thorax

paramagnetic

paramedian

parameter
  clinical p's

parameter *(continued)*
  physiologic p's
  systemic hemodynamic p's

parametric
  p. image
  p. imaging

paramitome

paraneoplastic process

paranuclear

paranucleolus

paranucleus

paraortic

paraplane echocardiography

paraplasm

paraplasmic

paraplastin

paraprosthetic leakage

pararrhythmia

parasagittal plane

paraseptal motion

parasitic cardiomyopathy

parasoma

parasternal
  p. examination
  p. heave
  p. long-axis view
  p. long-axis view echocardi-
    ogram
  p. short-axis view
  p. short-axis view echocar-
    diogram
  p. systolic lift
  p. systolic thrill
  p. view of the heart

parasympathetic
  p. function
  p. nerve fibers
  p. nervous system

parasympathomimetic

parasynapsis

parasyndesis

parasystole
    atrial p.
    junctional p.
    pure p.
    ventricular p.

parasystolic
    p. beat
    p. ventricular tachycardia

paravalvular

paravenous

parchemin
    bruit de p.

parchment heart

parenchyma

parenchymal
    p. amyloidosis
    p. fibrosis

parenchymatous
    p. myocarditis

Parhad-Poppen needle

Parham bands

paries
    p. caroticus cavi tympani

parietal
    p. endocarditis
    p. pericardiectomy
    p. pericardium
    p. thrombus

parieto-occipital artery

Park
    P. aneurysm
    P. blade and balloon atrial
        septostomy
    P. blade septostomy cathe-
        ter

paroxysmal
    p. atrial fibrillation (PAF)

paroxysmal *(continued)*
    p. atrial tachycardia (PAT)
    p. burst
    p. cough
    p. junctional tachycardia
    p. nocturnal dyspnea
        (PND)
    p. nocturnal hemoglobinu-
        ria
    p. nodal tachycardia
    p. palpitation
    p. reentrant supraventricu-
        lar tachycardia
    p. sinus tachycardia
    p. supraventricular ar-
        rhythmia
    p. supraventricular tachy-
        cardia
    p. ventricular tachycardia

Parrot
    P. murmur

parrot
    p. fever

pars
    p. amorpha
    p. corticalis arteriae cere-
        bri mediae
    p. corticalis arteriae cere-
        bri posterioris
    p. fibrosa
    p. granulosa
    p. infrasegmentalis
    p. membranacea septi
        atriorum
    p. membranacea septi in-
        terventricularis
    p. muscularis septi inter-
        ventricularis
    p. terminalis arteriae cere-
        bri mediae
    p. terminalis arteriae cere-
        bri posterioris
    p. atlantis arteriae verte-
        bralis

Parsonnet
    P. aortic clamp
    P. coronary probe

Parsonnet *(continued)*
    P. dilator
    P. epicardial retractor
    P. pulse generator pouch

part
    basal p. of left pulmonary
      artery
    basal p. of right pulmonary
      artery
    cervical p. of vertebral ar-
      tery
    first p. of vertebral artery
    fourth p. of vertebral ar-
      tery
    horizontal p. of middle ce-
      rebral artery
    second p. of vertebral ar-
      tery
    sphenoid p. of middle cere-
      bral artery
    third p. of vertebral artery

partial
    p. anomalous pulmonary
      venous connection
    p. anomalous pulmonary
      venous return
    p. atrioventricular canal
    p. encircling endocardial
      ventriculotomy
    p. heart block
    p.-occlusion clamp
    p.-occlusion forceps
    p.-occlusion inferior vena
      cava clip
    p. thromboplastin time
      (PTT)

particle
    Amberlite p's
    attraction p.
    Dane p's
    elementary p's of mito-
      chondria

partitioning
    left atrial particle p.

parvus
    p. alternans
    p. et tardus pulsus

parvus *(continued)*
    pulsus p.

Parzen window

PASAR tachycardia reversion
    pacemaker

P.A.S. Port
    P.A.S. P. catheter
    P.A.S. P. Fluoro-Free cathe-
      ter
    P.A.S. P. Fluoro-Free pe-
      ripheral access system

passage
    adiabatic fast p.

passer

passive
    p. clot
    p. edema
    p. hyperemia
    p. interval
    p. mode
    p. smoking

Pasys pacemaker

PAT
    paroxysmal atrial tachycar-
      dia

patch
    p. angioplasty
    autologous pericardial p.
    cardiac p.
    Carrel p.
    p. closure of septal defect
    Dacron intracardiac p.
    Dacron onlay p.-graft
    Dacron Sauvage p.
    defibrillation p.
    Edwards p.
    epicardial p.
    epicardial defibrillator p.
    Gore-Tex cardiovascular p.
    Gore-Tex soft-tissue p.
    p.-graft angioplasty
    p.-graft aortoplasty
    Ionescu-Shiley pericar-
      dial p.
    MacCallum p.

patch *(continued)*
    nitroglycerin transdermal p.
    outflow cardiac p.
    pericardial p.
    Peyer p.
    polypropylene intracardiac p.
    Silastic p.
    soldier's p.
    Teflon felt p.
    Teflon intracardiac p.
    transannular p.

patchplasty
    profunda Dacron p.

Patella disease

patency
    catheter p.
    coronary bypass graft p.
    epicardial vessel p.
    probe p. of foramen ovale
    p. of vein graft

patent
    p. ductus arteriosus (PDA)
    p. ductus arteriosus ligation
    p. ductus arteriosus murmur
    p. ductus arteriosus umbrella
    p. foramen ovale
    p. graft

Pathfinder catheter

pathogenesis

pathogenicity

pathologic murmur

pathology
    coexistent p.

pathophysiology

pathostimulation

pathway
    accessory p.

pathway *(continued)*
    accessory conducting p.
    antegrade internodal p.
    anterior internodal p.
    atrio-His p.
    atrioventricular p.
    AV nodal p.
    Bachmann p.
    circus p.
    concealed accessory p.
    conduction p.
    internodal p.
    Kent p.
    metabolic p.
    multiple accessory p.
    paraseptal accessory p.
    posterior septal p.
    reentrant p.
    retrograde p.
    scavenger cell p.
    selective past p.
    septal p.
    shunt p.
    slow AV node p.
    Thorel p.
    Wenckebach p.

patient-controlled analgesic

Patil stereotactic system

pattern
    A fib (atrial fibrillation) p.
    bigeminal p.
    circadian p.
    conduction p.
    contractile p.
    early repolarization p.
    intraventricular conduction p.
    juvenile T wave p.
    left ventricular strain p.
    M-shaped mitral valve p.
    Poincaré plot p.
    QR p.
    QS p.
    right ventricular strain p.
    sine-wave p.
    vascular p.
    ventricular contraction p.

paulocardia

pause
  compensatory p.
  noncompensatory p.
  postextrasystolic p.
  preautomatic p.
  sinus exit p.
  ventricular p.

pause-dependent arrhythmia

Pavlov reflex

PAVM
  pulmonary arteriovenous
    malformation

Paykel scale

PCA
  patient-controlled analgesia

PCD
  programmable cardiover-
    ter-defibrillator
    Jewel PCD
      PCD Transvene im-
        plantable cardiover-
        ter-defibrillator sys-
        tem

P cell

PDA
  patent ductus arteriosus
  posterior descending ar-
    tery
    PDA umbrella

PDE isoenzyme inhibitor

PDT
  PDT guide wire
  PDT guiding catheter

PDx pacing and diagnostic
  pacemaker

PE
  pericardial effusion
  pulmonary embolus
  percutaneous endoscopic
  PE Plus II balloon dilatation
    catheter

PE (continued)
  PE Plus II peripheral bal-
    loon catheter

PEA
  pulseless electrical activity

peak
  p. A velocity
  p. circumferential wall
    stress
  p. diastolic filling rate
  p. emptying rate
  p. E velocity
  p. exercise
  p. filling rate
  p. flow velocity
  h p.
  p. incidence
  p. instantaneous gradient
  p. jet flow rate
  p. magnitude
  p.-to-p. pressure gradient
  p. regurgitant flow velocity
  p. systolic gradient
  p. systolic gradient pres-
    sure
  p. systolic pressure
  p. transaortic valve gradi-
    ent
  p.-and-trough levels
  p. velocity of blood flow
  p. work load

peaked P wave

Péan
  P. arterial forceps
  P. clamp
  P. hemostatic forceps
  P. vessel clamp

pearl
  Laënnec p's

pear-shaped heart

Pearson
  P. correlation coefficient
  P.-Clopper value

peau d'orange

pectoral
    p. fremitus
    p. heart
    p. tea

pectoralgia

pectoralis
    p. fascia
    p. major
    p. minor

pectoris
    angina p.
    angor p.
    variant angina p.

pectorophony

pectus
    p. carinatum
    p. deformity
    p. excavatum
    p. gallinatum
    p. recurvatum

pedal
    p. edema
    p. pulses

pedal-mode ergometer

pediatric
    p. cardiomyopathy
    p. hypertension
    p. pigtail catheter
    p. vascular clamp

Pedoff continuous wave transducer

pedunculated thrombus

peel
    pericardial p.

peel-away
    p.-a. banana catheter
    p.-a. catheter
    p.-a. introducer set
    p.-a. sheath

peeling-back mechanism on electrophysiology study

PEEP
    positive end-expiratory pressure

peliosis

Pemco
    P. cannula
    P. prosthetic valve

PE-MT balloon dilatation catheter

Penaz volume-clamp method

pencil percussion

Penderluft syndrome

pendulous heart

pendulum
    cor p.
    p. rhythm

Penfield
    P. dissector
    P. elevator

penicillin prophylaxis

penile-brachial pressure index to assess cardiac disease

Penn State
    P. S. total artificial heart
    P. S. ventricular assist device

PentaCath catheter

pentalogy
    Cantrell p.
    p. of Fallot

PentaPace QRS catheter

peptide
    adrenomedullin p.
    atrial natriuretic p.
    calcitonin gene-related p.
    C-type natriuretic p.
    human atrial natriuretic p.
    procollagen type III amino-terminal p.
    vasoconstrictor p.

Per-C-Cath

perceived exertion

percent of maximum predicted
heart rate

Percor
    P. DL-II intra-aortic balloon
    catheter
    P. intra-aortic balloon cath-
    eter

Percor-Stat-DL catheter

percussion
    p. and auscultation (P&A)
    chest p.
    p. dullness
    fist p.
    p. hammer
    p. note
    p. sound
    p. wave of carotid arterial
    pulse

percutaneous
    p. access kit (PAK)
    p. aortic valvuloplasty
    p. approach
    p. arteriography
    p. balloon angioplasty
    p. balloon aortic valvulo-
    plasty
    p. balloon dilation
    p. balloon mitral valvulo-
    plasty
    p. balloon pericardiotomy
    p. balloon pulmonic valvu-
    loplasty
    p. cardiopulmonary bypass
    p. cardiopulmonary bypass
    support
    p. carotid arteriography
    (PCA)
    p. catheter insertion
    p. catheter introducer kit
    p. coronary rotational ath-
    erectomy
    p. cutting needle
    p. femoral arteriogram
    p. femoral-femoral cardio-
    pulmonary bypass

percutaneous *(continued)*
    p. groin puncture
    p. intra-aortic balloon
    counterpulsation
    p. intra-aortic balloon
    counterpulsation catheter
    p. intrapericardial drug de-
    livery
    p. Judkins technique
    p. laser angioplasty
    p. left heart bypass
    p. mitral balloon commis-
    surotomy
    p. mitral balloon valvotomy
    p. mitral balloon valvulo-
    plasty
    p. mitral commissurotomy
    p. mitral valvuloplasty
    p. patent ductus arteriosus
    closure
    p. puncture technique
    p. radiofrequency catheter
    ablation
    p. retrograde atherectomy
    p. rotational thrombec-
    tomy
    p. rotational thrombec-
    tomy catheter
    p. route
    p. splenoportal venography
    p. stent
    p. subclavian-subclavian
    bypass
    p. subxyphoid pericardial
    access technique
    p. technique
    p. transatrial mitral com-
    missurotomy
    p. transhepatic cardiac
    catheterization
    p. transfemoral arteriogra-
    phy
    p. translumbar aortog-
    raphy
    p. transluminal angioplasty
    p. transluminal angioscopy
    p. transluminal atherec-
    tomy

percutaneous *(continued)*
    p. transluminal balloon dilatation
    p. transluminal balloon valvuloplasty
    p. transluminal coronary angioplasty (PTCA)
    p. transluminal coronary revascularization
    p. transluminal renal angioplasty
    p. transvenous mitral commissurotomy
    p. tunnel

percutaneously
    p. cannulated
    p. inserted
    p. introduced

PerDUCER device

Perez sign

perforating arteries

perforation
    cardiac p.
    guide wire p.
    myocardial p.
    septal p.
    ventricular p.

perforator
    gaiter p's
    ligation of p's
    septal p.
    stripping of p's

performance
    left ventricular systolic p.
    ventricular p.

perfuse

perfusion
    p. abnormality
    p. balloon catheter
    p. bed
    blood p.
    cardiac p.
    coronary artery p.
    p. defect
    extremity p.

perfusion *(continued)*
    mosaic p.
    myocardial p.
    peripheral p.
    p. pressure
    pulsatile p.
    retrograde cardiac p.
    root p.
    tissue p.

periangiitis

periangioma

periaortic
    p. abscess
    p. chain
    p. nodes

periaortitis

periapical

periarterial

periarteritis
    p. gummosa
    p. nodosa
    syphilitic p.

periatrial

periauricular

pericapillary

pericardectomy

pericardiac tumor

pericardial
    p. baffle
    p. basket
    p. biopsy
    p. calcification
    p. cavity
    p. cyst
    p. disease
    p. echo
    p. effusion
    p. fat pad
    p. flap
    p. fluid
    p. fremitus
    p. friction rub
    p. knock

pericardial *(continued)*
    p. lavage
    p. murmur
    p. patch
    p. peel
    p. pleura
    p. puncture
    p. poudrage
    p. pressure
    p. reflex
    p. rub
    p. rupture
    p. sac
    p. sinus
    p. sling
    p. space
    p. tamponade
    p. tap
    p. teratoma
    p. well
    p. window
    p. xenograft

pericardiectomy
    parietal p.
    visceral p.

pericardii
    accretio p.
    concretio p.
    hydrops p.
    paracentesis p.
    synechia p.

pericardiocentesis
    p. needle

pericardiolysis

pericardiomediastinitis

pericardiophrenic

pericardioplasty in pectus exca-
    vatum repair

pericardiopleural

pericardiorrhaphy

pericardioscopy

pericardiosternal ligament

pericardiostomy

pericardiosymphysis

pericardiotomy
    percutaneous balloon p.
    p. scissors
    subxiphoid limited p.
    p. syndrome

pericarditic

pericarditis
    acute benign p.
    acute fibrinous p.
    acute idiopathic p.
    acute nonspecific p.
    adhesive p.
    amebic p.
    bacterial p.
    bread-and-butter p.
    calcific p.
    p. calculosa
    p. callosa
    carcinomatous p.
    cholesterol p.
    chronic constrictive p.
    constrictive p.
    drug-associated p.
    drug-induced p.
    dry p.
    effusive-constrictive p.
    p. with effusion
    p. epistenocardiaca
    p. externa et interna
    external p.
    fibrinous p.
    fibrous p.
    fungal p.
    gram-negative p.
    hemorrhagic p.
    histoplasmic p.
    idiopathic p.
    infective p.
    inflammatory p.
    internal adhesive p.
    ischemic p.
    localized p.
    mediastinal p.
    meningococcal p.
    mycobacterial p.
    neoplastic p.

pericarditis *(continued)*
  p. obliterans
  obliterating p.
  occult p.
  postcardiotomy p.
  postinfarction p.
  post-irradiation p.
  postoperative p.
  purulent p.
  radiation-induced p.
  rheumatic p.
  serofibrinous p.
  serous p.
  p. sicca
  Sternberg p.
  subacute p.
  suppurative p.
  transient p.
  traumatic p.
  tuberculous p.
  uremic p.
  p. villosa
  viral p.
pericarditis-myocarditis syndrome
pericardium *pl.* pericardia
  absent p.
  adherent p.
  bread-and-butter p.
  calcified p.
  congenitally absent p.
  diaphragmatic p.
  dropsy of p.
  empyema of p.
  p. externum
  p. fibrosum
  fibrous p.
  inflamed p.
  p. internum
  parietal p.
  p. serosum
  shaggy p.
  thickened p.
  visceral p.
pericardosis
pericardotomy
pericentriolar

pericyte

perielectrode fibrosis

Periflow peripheral balloon angioplasty-infusion catheter

Periflux PF 1 D blood flow meter

perigraft

Peri-Guard
  P. vascular graft
  P. vascular graft guard

peri-infarction
  p. block
  p. conduction defect
  p. ischemia

perimembranous ventricular septal defect

Perimount RSR pericardial bioprosthesis

perimuscular plexus

perimyocarditis

perimyoendocarditis

perimysial plexus

perimysium

perineal artery

perinodal tissue

perinuclear

period
  absolute refractory p.
  accessory pathway effective refractory p.
  antegrade refractory p.
  atrial effective refractory p.
  atrial refractory p.
  atrioventricular refractory p.
  diastolic filling p.
  effective refractory p.
  ejection p.
  functional refractory p.

period *(continued)*
  G_1 p.
  G_2 p.
  intersystolic p.
  isoelectric p.
  isometric p.
  isometric p. of cardiac cycle
  isometric contraction p.
  isometric relaxation p.
  isovolumetric p.
  isovolumic p.
  p. of isovolumic contraction
  isovolumic relaxation p.
  p. of isovolumic relaxation
  M p.
  pacemaker amplifier refractory p.
  pacemaker refractory p.
  postinfarction p.
  postsphygmic p.
  postventricular atrial refractory p.
  preejection p.
  presphygmic p.
  pulse p.
  rapid filling p.
  p. of rapid ventricular filling
  p. of reduced ventricular filling
  refractory p.
  relative refractory p.
  retrograde refractory p.
  S p.
  sphygmic p.
  systolic ejection p.
  ventricular effective refractory p.
  ventriculoatrial effective refractory p.
  p. of ventricular filling
  vulnerable p.
  Wenckebach p.
periodicity
  AV node Wenckebach p.
periorbital edema

periosteotome
  Alexander-Farabeuf p.

periosteum

peripartum
  p. cardiomyopathy
  p. myocarditis

peripelvic collateral vessel

peripheral
  p. access system
  p. airspaces
  P. AngioJet system
  p. artery bypass
  p. artery disease
  p. arteriosclerosis
  p. atherectomy catheter
  p. atherectomy system
  p. atherosclerotic disease
  p. blood eosinophilia
  p. blood lymphocytes
  p. blood vessel forceps
  p. circulation
  p. cyanosis
  p. edema
  p. laser angioplasty (PLA)
  p. laser recannulation
  p. long-line catheter
  p. neuropathy
  p. perfusion
  p. pulmonic stenosis
  p. pulse
  p. pulse deficit
  p. resistance
  p. stigmata
  p. vascular clamp
  p. vascular disease (PVD)
  p. vascular resistance
  p. vascular retractor

peripherally-inserted central catheter (PICC)

periphlebitic

periphlebitis
  sclerosing p.

periportal

periprosthetic leak

peripylephlebitis

perisystole

perisystolic

perithelium
Eberth's p.

perivalvular leak

perivascular
p. canal
p. edema
p. eosinophilic infiltrates
p. fibrosis
p. spaces

perivasculitis

perivenous

Perma-Flow coronary graft

Perma-Hand
P.-H. braided silk sutures
P.-H. silk sutures

PermaMesh material

permanent
p. cardiac pacing lead
p. demand ventricular pacing system
p. junctional reciprocating
tachycardia
p. pacemaker placement
p. pacing
p. rate-responsive pace-
maker
p. transvenous pacemaker
p. ventricular pacemaker

Permathane Pacesetter lead
pacemaker

PermCath catheter

permeability

permease

Perneczky aneurysm clip

peroneal
p. artery

peroneal (continued)
p.-tibial trunk
p. veins
p. vessels

perpetual arrhythmia

perpetuus
pulsus irregularis p.

Per-Q-Cath percutaneously in-
serted central venous catheter

persistent
p. common atrioventricular
canal
p. ductus arteriosus
p. fetal circulation
p. ostium primum
p. pulmonary hypertension
of newborn
p. truncus arteriosus

Personal Best peak flow meter

Perspex button

Perthes test

pertubation

perturbed
p. autonomic nervous sys-
tem function
p. carotid baroreceptor

peruana
verruga p.

pervenous
p. catheter
p. pacemaker

PES
programmed electrical
stimulation

PET
positron emission tomography
PET balloon
PET balloon atherec-
tomy device
PET scan

Petit sinuses

Peyer patch

Peyrot thorax

PFO
    patent foramen ovale

PFR
    peak filling rate

Pfuhl-Jaffé sign

PFWT
    pain-free walking time

P-H
    P-H conduction time
    P-H interval

pH
    hydrogen ion concentra-
        tion
            pH probe

phacoma

phagocyte

phagocytic function

phagocytosis

Phalen stress test

phaneroplasm

phanerosis
    fat p.

Phaneuf artery forceps

Phantom
    P. cardiac guide wire
    P. 5 Plus ST balloon dilata-
        tion catheter
    P. V Plus catheter

phantom
    p. aneurysm
    p. clamp
    p. limb pain
    p. pacemaker
    p. pain
    p. sponge

phantom *(continued)*
    p. tumor

pharmacoangiography

pharmacodynamics

pharmacokinetics

pharmacologic
    p. cardioversion
    p. stress
    p. stress echocardiography
    p. stress perfusion imaging

pharmacotherapy

phase
    p. angle
    ejection p.
    G_1 p.
    G_2 p.
    p. image
    p. image analysis
    p. imaging
    isovolumetric contrac-
        tion p.
    isovolumic contraction p.
    isovolumetric relaxation p.
    isovolumic relaxation p.
    Korotkoff p.
    M p.
    m p.
    meiotic p.
    plateau p.
    postmeiotic p.
    premeiotic p.
    prereduction p.
    reduction p.
    resting p.
    S p.
    s p.
    supernormal recovery p.
    synaptic p.
    venous p.
    ventricular filling p.
    vulnerable p.
    washout p.

phased
    p. array sector scanner
    p. array sector transducer

phased *(continued)*
    p. array study
    p. array system
    p. array technology
    p. array ultrasonographic
        device

phase-encoded velocity image

phasic sinus arrhythmia

Phemister elevator

phenomenon *pl.* phenomena
    AFORMED p.
    Anrep p.
    Aschner p.
    Ashley p.
    Ashman p.
    Austin Flint p.
    blush p.
    Bowditch staircase p.
    cascade p.
    coronary steal p.
    diaphragm p.
    diaphragmatic p.
    dip p.
    Duckworth p.
    Ehret p.
    embolic p.
    Gallavardin p.
    gap conduction p.
    Gärtner's p.
    Gallavardin p.
    gap conduction p.
    Goldblatt p.
    Gregg p.
    Hering p.
    Hill p.
    Katz-Wachtle p.
    Kienback p.
    Koch p.
    Litten p.
    no-reflow p.
    Raynaud p.
    reentry p.
    R on T p.
    Schellong-Strisower p.
    Splendore-Hoeppli p.
    staircase p.
    steal p.

phenomenon *(continued)*
    treppe p.
    vasovagal p.
    warm-up p.
    washout p.
    Wenckebach p.
    Williams p.
    Woodworth p.

phlebalgia

phlebangioma

phlebarteriectasia

phlebectasia

phlebectasis

phlebectomy

phlebectopia

phlebectopy

phlebemphraxis

phlebexairesis

phlebismus

phlebitic
    p. induration

phlebitis
    adhesive p.
    blue p.
    chlorotic p.
    gouty p.
    p. migrans
    migrating p.
    p. nodularis necrotisans
    p. obliterans
    obliterating p.
    obstructive p.
    plastic p.
    productive p.
    proliferative p.
    puerperal p.
    sclerosing p.
    septic p.
    superficial p.
    suppurative p.

phlebodynamics

phlebofibrosis

phlebogenous

phlebogram

phlebograph

phlebitis
    descending p.

phleboid

phlebolith

phlebolithiasis

phlebology

phlebomanometer

phlebomyomatosis

phlebophlebostomy

phlebopiezometry

phleboplasty

phleborheography

phleborrhaphy

phleborrhexis

phlebosclerosis

phlebosis

phlebostasia

phlebostasis

phlebostenosis

phlebostrepsis

phlebothrombosis

phlebotome

phlebotomist

phlebotomize

phlebotomy
    bloodless p.

phlegmasia
    p. alba dolens
    cellulitic p.
    p. cerulea dolens
    thrombotic p.

phlegmonosa
    angina p.

Phoenix
    P. ancillary valve
    P. cruciform valve
    P. fifth ventricle system
    P. 2 pacemaker
    P. single-chamber pace-
        maker
    P. total artificial heart

phonangiography
    carotid p.

phonarteriogram

phonarteriography

phonangiography

phonocardiogram

phonocardiograph
    linear p.
    logarithmic p.
    spectral p.
    stethoscopic p.

phonocardiographic transducer

phonocardiography
    intracardiac p.

phonocatheter

phonocatheterization
    intracardiac p.

phosphatase
    acid p.
    alkaline p.

phosphinic acid

phosphocreatine

phosphodiesterase
    p. enzyme
    p. inhibitor
    p. isoenzyme inhibitors

phosphofructokinase

phosphokinase
    creatine p. (CPK)

phospholamban

phospholipase
p. A
p. C

phospholipid

phosphomonoesterase

phosphorus
organic p.

phosphorylase
glycogen p.
p. kinase

phosphorylation
oxidative p.

photoablation

photocoagulation

photocoagulator
American Optical p.
argon laser p.
Coherent argon laser p.
infrared ray p.
Mira p.
Novus Omni 2000 p.
Olivella-Garrigosa p.
Ultima 2000 p.
xenon p.
xenon arc p.
Zeiss p.

PhotoDerm VL device

photodisruption

photodynamic therapy

PhotoFix alpha pericardial bioprosthesis

photohemotachometer

photolysis

photometer
HemoCue hemoglobin p.
Kowa laser flare-cell p.
reflectance p.
TUR-Cue p.

photomicrography

photomultiplier

photon
annihilation p.

photopeak

photoplethysmograph

photoplethysmography

photoprotection

photoreactivation

photoresection

photostethoscope

photoreversal

phragmoplast

phrenic
p. artery
p. nerve
p. nerve paralysis
p. veins

phrenocardia

phrenopericardial angle

phrenopericarditis

phthinoid chest

phthisis
aneurysmal p.
bacillary p.
black p.
collier's p.
diabetic p.
fibroid p.
grinders' p.
miner's p.
potter's p.
pulmonary p.
stone-cutter's p.

phycomycosis

phylaxis

Phymos 3D pacemaker

physical
p. inactivity

physical *(continued)*
  p. stimulus

Physical Work Capacity exercise stress test

physiologic
  p. congestion
  p. dead space
  p. dead space ventilation per minute
  p. measurement
  p. monitoring
  p. murmur
  p. overreactivity
  p. pattern release
  p. splitting of S_2
  p. stress
  p. third heart sound

physiology
  constrictive p.
  Damus-Kaye-Stansel procedure for single ventricle p.

phytanic acid accumulation

phytohemagglutinin

phytonadione

PI
  pulmonary insufficiency

piano percussion

piaulement
  bruit de p.

PICA
  posterior inferior communicating artery

PICC
  peripherally-inserted central catheter

pi cell

Pick
  P. and Go monitor
  P. disease
  P. syndrome

Picker
  P. Dyna Mo collimator

Picker *(continued)*
  P. Vista Magnascanner

pickwickian syndrome

Picollion
  P. balloon
  P. Monorail catheter

Pierce-Donachy Thoratec ventricular assist device

Pierre Robin syndrome

piesimeter
  Hales p.

piesis

piezoelectric

pigeon breast deformity

pigtail catheter

Pilling
  P. microanastomosis clamp
  P.-Wolvek sternal approximator

pillow-shaped balloon

Pilotip
  P. catheter
  P. catheter guide

pincushion distortion

pinhole VSD

pink
  pink tetralogy of Fallot

pinked up

Pinkerton balloon catheter

Pinnacle
  P. contact Nd:YAG fiber
  P. introducer sheath
  P. pacemaker

Pins
  P. sign
  P. syndrome

pinocyte

pinocytic

pinocytosis

pinocytotic

pinosome

piriform sinus

Pirogoff angle

pistol-shot femoral sound

piston pulse

pit
    coated p.

pitting edema

P-J interval

PLA
    peripheral laser angio-
        plasty

PLA-1 platelet antigen

placement
    lead p.
    permanent pacemaker p.
    temporary pacemaker p.
    Thoracoport p.

planar
    p. myocardial imaging
    p. thallium scintigraphy
    p. thallium test
    p. xanthoma

plane
    Addison p.
    axial p.
    circular p.
    coronal p.
    cove p.
    frontal p.
    midsagittal p.
    orthogonal p.
    parasagittal p.
    sagittal p.
    short-axis p.
    sternal p.
    sternoxiphoid p.
    transaxial p.
    valve p.

planimeter

planimetry

plantar ischemia test

planocyte

plaque
    arterial p.
    arteriosclerotic p.
    atheromatous p.
    atherosclerotic p.
    calcified p.
    carcinoid p.
    carotid p.
    p. disruption
    eccentric atherosclerotic p.
    echogenic p.
    echolucent p.
    fatty p.
    fibrofatty p.
    fibrotic p.
    fibrous p.
    fissured atheromatous p.
    p. fracture
    Hollenhorst p.
    intraluminal p.
    lipid-rich p.
    MacCallum p's
    myointimal p.
    obstructive p.
    pleural p.
    p. rupture
    sessile p.
    shelf of p.
    stenotic p.
    p. strutting
    submucosal p.
    ulcerated p.
    unstable p.

plaque-cracker
    LeVeen p.-c.

plaquing

plasma
    p. alpha 1-antitrypsin
        (pAAT)
    p. beta-thromboglobulin
    p. catecholamine

plate   391

plasma *(continued)*
    p. coagulation system
    p. colloid osmotic pressure
    p. endothelin
    p. endothelin concentra-
       tion
    p. erythropoietin
    p. exchange column
    p. fibrinogen
    fresh frozen p. (FFP)
    p. glycocalicin
    platelet-poor p.
    platelet-rich p.
    p. renin
    p. renin activity (PRA)
    p. skimming
    p. thromboplastin anteced-
       ent
    p. thromboplastin compo-
       nent
    p. volume
    p. volume expander
    zoster immune p.

plasmagel

plasmahaut

plasmalemma

Plasmalyte A cardioplegic solution

Plasmanate

plasmapheresis

Plasma-Plex bottle

plasmarrhexis

plasma-resistant fiber oxygenator

plasma TFE vascular graft

plasmatic vascular destruction

plasmatogamy

plasmatorrhexis

plasma viscosity

plasma volume expander

plasmic

plasmin

α_2-plasmin inhibitor

plasminogen
    p. activator
    p. activator inhibitor (PAI)
    p. activator inhibitor-1
      (PAI-1)

plasminogen-streptokinase
   complex

plasmogamy

plasmogen

plasmolysis

plasmolytic

plasmolyzability

plasmolyzable

plasmolyze

plasmorrhexis

plasmoschisis

plasmosin

plasmotomy

plasson

plastin

plastic
    p. endocarditis
    p. phlebitis
    p. polymer
    p. sewing ring

plastochondria

plastogamy

plastosome

plasty
    sliding p.

plate
    cell p.
    cuticular p.
    equatorial p.
    metaphase p.

plate *(continued)*
    polar p's
    pole p's
    Strasburger cell p.
    thrombosis p.
    thrombus p.

plateau
    h p.
    p. phase
    p. pulse
    p. response
    ventricular p.

platelet
    p. adhesiveness
    p. aggregation
    p. antibody
    p. count
    p. factor 4
    p. imaging
    p. lysis
    p. receptor glycoprotein
    p. thrombosis
    p. thrombus

platelet-aggregating factor
  (PAF)

platelet-derived growth factor

plateletpheresis

platelet-poor plasma (PPP)

platelet-rich plasma (PRP)

platelike atelectasis

platform
    TomTec echo p.

platinum
    P. PLUS guide wire
    salt of p.

platypnea

platysma

pledget
    cotton p.
    Dacron p.
    Gelfoam p.
    Meadox Teflon felt p.

pledget *(continued)*
    polypropylene p.
    p. sponge
    Teflon p.

pledgeted
    p. Ethibond suture
    p. mattress suture
    p. suture

PlegiaGuard

Plegisol cardioplegic solution

pleomorphic
    p. premature ventricular
      complex
    p. tachycardia

pleomorphism

Plesch
    P. percussion
    P. test

plethora

plethoric

plethysmography
    air p.
    air-cuff p.
    cuff p.
    dynamic venous p.
    face-out, whole-body p.
    impedance p.
    mercury-in-rubber strain
      gauge p.
    segmental p.
    strain-gauge p.
    thermistor p.
    venous occlusion p.

pleura
    mediastinal p.
    parietal p.
    pericardiac p.
    visceral p.

pleural
    p. adhesion
    p. space

pleurodesis

pleuropericardial
    p. incision
    p. murmur
    p. rub
    p. window

pleuropericarditis

PlexiPulse
    P. compression device

plexogenic pulmonary arteriopathy

plexus
    p. arteriae ovaricae
    Batson p.
    brachial p.
    cavernous p. of concha
    Heller p.
    hemorrhoidal p.
    Hovius p.
    intercavernous p.
    Leber p.
    papillary p.
    perimuscular p.
    perimysial p.
    pharyngeal p.
    p. pharyngealis
    presacral p.
    primary p.
    prostatic p.
    prostaticovesical p.
    pudendal p.
    p. pudendalis
    sacral p.
    sacral p., anterior
    Santorini p.
    spermatic p.
    Stensen p.
    subendocardial terminal p.
    subpapillary p.
    Trolard p.
    uterine p.
    p. uterovaginalis
    vaginal p.
    vascular p.
    vascular p., deep
    vascular p., superficial

plexus *(continued)*
    p. venosus mammillae
    p. venosus pterygoideus
    venous p.
    venous p., areolar
    venous p., hemorrhoidal
    venous p., internal carotid
    venous p., prostatic
    venous p., rectal
    venous p., sacral
    venous p., suboccipital
    venous p., uterine
    venous p., vaginal
    venous p., vesical
    venous p. of foot, dorsal
    venous p. of foramen ovale
    venous p. of hand, dorsal
    venous p. of hypoglossal
     canal
    vertebral p.
    vertebral p's, internal
    vesical p.
    p. vesicalis
    vesicoprostatic p.
    vertebral p's, external

plica
    p. venae cavae sinistrae

plication
    annular p.
    p. repair of flail leaflet

plombage

plop
    cardiac tumor p.
    tumor p.

plot
    bull's-eye p.
    Poincaré p.
    polar p.

plug
    Alcock catheter p.
    collagen p.
    decannulation p.
    Dittrich p's
    Ivalon p.
    mucus p.

plug *(continued)*
    Shiley decannulation p.
    Teflon Bardic p.

plumb-line sign

plurinuclear

PMI
    point of maximum impulse

P-mitrale

PML
    posterior mitral leaflet

PND
    paroxysmal nocturnal
        dyspnea

pneocardiac reflex

pneumatic
    p. antishock garment
    p. compression stockings
    p. cuff
    p. tourniquet
    p. trousers

pneumatocardia

pneumocardial

pneumohemia

pneumohemopericardium

pneumohemothorax

pneumohydropericardium

pneumohydrothorax

pneumomediastinography

pneumomediastinum

pneumopericardium

pneumoprecordium

pneumopyopericardium

pocket
    endocardial p.
    pacemaker p.
    regurgitant p.
    retropectoral p.
    subcutaneous pacemak-
        er p.

pocket *(continued)*
    p's of Zahn

Pocket-Dop II

poikilocytosis

Poincaré plot pattern

point
    A p.
    p. of Arrhigi
    Boyd p.
    C p.
    Castellani p.
    cold rigor p.
    p. of critical stenosis
    D p.
    de Mussy p.
    E p.
    Erb p.
    exit p.
    F p.
    Guéneau de Mussy p.
    isoelectric p.
    J p.
    p. of maximal impulse
        (PMI)
    null p.
    O p.
    pressure p.
    Z p.

Poiseuille
    P. law
    P. resistance formula

poisoning
    arsenic p.
    arsine gas p.
    fluorocarbon p.
    lead p.
    mercury p.

polarcardiography

Polaris
    P. electrode
    P. Mansfield/Webster de-
        flectable tip
    P. steerable diagnostic
        catheter

polarity

polarization
    electrochemical p.
    fluorescence p.

polarographic method

Polhemus-Schafer-Ivemark syndrome

polyacrylamide gel electrophoresis

polyacrylonitrile membrane

polyamine

polyangiitis
    microscopic p.

polyarteritis
    disseminated p.
    p. nodosa

polyarthritis

polycardia

polychondritis
    relapsing p.

polyclonal gammopathy

polycrotic

polycrotism

polycythemia
    p. hypertonica
    p. vera

Polydek suture

polyethylene
    p. seat heart valve
    p. terephthalate
    p. terephthalate balloon

PolyFlex
    P. implantable pacing lead
        pacemaker
    P. lead pacemaker

polygelin colloid contrast medium

polygenic
    p. hypercholesterolemia

polygenic *(continued)*
    p. hyperlipidemia

polygonal

polyhedral surface reconstruction

PolyHeme

polykaryocyte

polymer
    plastic p.

polymerase
    p. chain reaction (PCR)
    Taq DNA p.

polymeric endoluminal paving stent

polymorphic
    p. premature ventricular complex
    p. slow wave

polymorphism
    restriction fragment length p.

polymorphonuclear

polymorphous ventricular tachycardia

polymyalgia rheumatica syndrome

polymyositis

polynuclear

polynucleate

polynucleated

polynucleolar

polyolefin copolymer balloon

polyostotic fibrous dysplasia

polyp
    cardiac p.

polypeptide
    atrial natriuretic p. (ANP)
    pancreatic p. (PP)

polyphosphoinositide

polyploidy

Poly-Plus Dacron vascular graft

polypoidal lesion

polypous endocarditis

polypropylene
  p. intracardiac patch
  p. pledget

polysaccharide-iron complex

polysaccharide storage disease

polysomatic

polysomaty

polysome

polysplenia

Polystan
  P. cardiotomy reservoir
  P. perfusion cannula
  P. venous return catheter

polystyrene latex microspheres

polytef

polytetrafluoroethylene

polyurethane
  p. foam embolus
  p. graft
  p. implant material
  p. prosthesis

polyvinyl
  p. chloride (PVC)
  p. chloride balloon
  p. chloride tube
  p. prosthesis

Pompe disease

ponderance
  ventricular p.

Ponstel

Pontiac fever

pool
  blood p.

pooling of blood in extremities

poor R wave progression

popliteal
  p. aneurysm
  p. artery
  p. pulse

Poppen aortic clamp

Poppen-Blalock carotid artery
  clamp

poppet
  ball p.
  disk p.
  prosthetic p.

porcelain aorta

porcine
  p. bioprosthesis
  p. heart valve
  p. heterograft
  p. prosthetic valve
  p. xenograft

pore
  Kohn p's
  nuclear p's

porin

porphyrin

Porstmann technique

port
  chest p.
  Infuse-A-P. p.
  infusion p.
  injection p.
  Luer-Lok p.
  mediastinal p.
  Quinton vascular access p.
  side-arm pressure p.
  supraclavicular p.

porta *pl.* portae

Port-A-Cath
  P. device
  P. implantable catheter
    system

portacaval
  p. anastomosis
  p. H graft
  p. shunt
  p. transposition

port-access
  p.-a. coronary artery by-
    pass grafting
  St. Jude Medical p.-a.

portal
  p. circulation
  p. hypertension
  p. vein
  p. vein thrombosis

Porter sign

Portmanteau test

Portnoy
  P. ventricular cannula
  P. ventricular catheter
  P. ventricular-end shunt

portogram

portography
  computed tomography an-
    giographic p.

portosystemic
  p. anastomosis

Posadas-Wernicke disease

position
  anterior oblique p.
  body p.
  electrical heart p.
  Fowler p.
  left anterior oblique
    (LAO) p.
  left lateral decubitus p.
  levo-transposed p.
  pulmonary capillary wed-
    ge p.
  right anterior oblique
    (RAO) p.
  shock p.
  steep Trendelenburg p.
  Trendelenburg p.

position (continued)
  tricuspid p.
  wedge p.

positive
  p. afterpotential
  p. chronotropism
  p. deflection on ECG
  p. treppe

Positrol
  P. II Bernstein catheter
  P. cardiac device
  P. II catheter

positron emission tomography
  (PET)
  p.e.t. balloon
  p.e.t. balloon atherectomy
    device
  p.e.t. scan

postangioplasty
  p. stenosis

post-balloon angioplasty restenosis

postcapillary

postcardiotomy
  p. intra-aortic balloon
    pumping
  p. syndrome

postcardioversion pulmonary
  edema

postcatheterization

postcava

postcaval

postcommissurotomy syn-
  drome

postdiastolic

postdicrotic

postdiphtheritic stenosis

postdrive depression

postductal

posterior
  p. approach

posterior *(continued)*
  p. auricular branch of external carotid artery
  p. auricular vein
  p. cerebral artery
  p. circumflex artery
  p. circumflex humeral artery
  p. communicating artery
  p. descending artery (PDA)
  p. inferior cerebellar artery
  p. inferior communicating artery (PICA)
  p. intercostal arteries
  p. intercostal veins
  p. leaflet
  p. meningeal artery
  p. myocardial infarction
  p. papillary muscle
  p. scrotal veins
  p. spinal artery
  p. superior alveolar artery
  p. temporal diploic vein
  p. tibial artery
  p. tibial recurrent artery
  p. tibial vein
  p. tympanic artery
  p. vein of left ventricle
  p. vena ventriculi sinistri cordis

posteroinferior dyskinesis

posteroseptal wall

postextrasystolic
  p. aberrancy
  p. beat
  p. pause
  p. potentiation
  p. T wave

postinfarction
  p. angina
  p. course
  p. pericarditis
  p. period
  p. syndrome
  p. ventriculoseptal defect

postinfectious bradycardia

postinflammatory

postintervention

postischemic
  p. heart
  p. myocardium

postmeiotic

postmiotic

postmitotic

postmortem
  p. clot
  p. thrombus

postmyocardial
  p. infarction
  p. infarction syndrome

postoperative pericarditis

postpartum
  p. cardiomyopathy
  p. hypertension

postperfusion
  p. arrhythmia
  p. lung
  p. psychosis
  p. syndrome

postpericardiotomy syndrome

postphlebitic syndrome

postprandial
  p. angina
  p. blood sugar

postpump syndrome

postrenal azotemia

postsphygmic
  p. interval
  p. period

poststenotic dilation

poststreptococcal inflammatory process

posttransfusion syndrome

postural
  p. hypotension

posture
  Stern p.

posturing
  decerebrate p.

Potain sign

potassium (K)
  canrenoate p.
  p. chloride (KCl)
  p. gluconate
  glucose, insulin, and p.
  p. hydroxide (KOH)
  p. inhibition
  p. iodide
  p. ion
  p. wasting

potassium chloride cardioplegia

potassium-sparing effect

potassium-wasting diuretic

potential
  action p.
  after-p.
  bioelectric p.
  cardiac action p.
  electrical p.
  fibrillation p.
  Kent p.
  maximum negative p.
  membrane p.
  monophasic action p.
  pacemaker p.
  putative slow pathway p.
  resting p.
  resting membrane p.
  transmembrane p.
  ventricular late p.

potentiation
  postextrasystolic p.

Pottenger sign

Potts
  P. aneurysm
  P. aortic clamp
  P. anastomosis

Potts *(continued)*
  P. aortic clamp
  P. bulldog forceps
  P. coarctation clamp
  P. coarctation forceps
  P. expansile valvulotome
  P. needle
  P. operation
  P. patent ductus clamp
  P. periosteotome
  P. procedure
  P. pulmonic clamp
  P. rib shears
  P. scissors
  P. shunt
  P. thumb forceps
  P. vascular forceps
  P. vascular scissors
  P.-Cournand angiography
    needle
  P.-Niedner aortic clamp
  P.-Satinsky clamp
  P.-Smith anastomosis
  P.-Smith aortic occlusion
    clamp
  P.-Smith arterial scissors
  P.-Smith bipolar forceps
  P.-Smith dissecting scissors
  P.-Smith monopolar for-
    ceps
  P.-Smith reverse scissors
  P.-Smith scissors
  P.-Smith side-to-side anas-
    tomosis
  P.-Smith tissue forceps
  P.-Smith-Gibson operation

pouch
  Cardio-Cool myocardial
    protection p.
  pacemaker p.
  Parsonnet pulse genera-
    tor p.

poudrage
  Beck epicardial p.
  pericardial p.
  pleural p.
  talc p.

Pourcelot index

powder
  lyophilized p.

powdered tantalum

PPD
  purified protein derivative
  PPD skin test

P-P interval

P pulmonale

P–Q
  P–Q interval
  P–Q segment

P:QRS ratio

P–R
  P–R interval
  prolongation of P–R interval
  shortening of P–R interval
  P–R segment
  depressed P–R segment

PRA
  plasma renin activity

PR-AC measurement

preaortic

prearterioles

preautomatic pause

pre-beta lipoprotein

precapillary
  p. arterioles
  p. sphincter

precardiac
  p. mesoderm

precava

precaval

Preceder interventional guide
  wire

Precept
  P. pacemaker
  P. lead

preclotting
  p. the graft

Preclude pericardial membrane

preconditioning
  ischemic p.

precordial
  p. A wave
  p. bulge
  p. catch syndrome
  p. electrocardiography
  p. heave
  p. honk
  p. leads
  p. motion
  p. movement
  p. palpation
  p. pulse
  p. thrill
  p. thump

precordialgia

precordium
  active p.
  anterior p.
  bulbing of p.
  quiet p.

Predator balloon catheter

prediastole

prediastolic
  p. murmur

predicrotic

predictive value

predose level

preductal coarctation of aorta

preejection
  p. period

preexcitation
  p. syndrome
  ventricular p.

pre-existing condition

pregnancy-induced hypertension

preinfarction
p. angina
p. syndrome

prekallikrein

preload
cardiac p.
p. reduction
p. reserve
ventricular p.

premature
p. atherosclerosis
p. atrial beat
p. atrial complex
p. atrial contraction (PAC)
p. atrioventricular junctional complex
p. excitation
p. junctional beat
p. mid-diastolic closure of mitral valve
p. systole
p. valve closure
p. ventricular beat (PVB)
p. ventricular complex
p. ventricular complex-trigger hypothesis
p. ventricular contraction (PVC)

premedication

premeiotic

premitotic

Premo guide wire

premonitory
p. palpitation
p. syndrome

preparation
Langendorff heart p.

preprandial

prerenal azotemia

preponderance
ventricular p.

prepotential

presacral edema

presbycardia

prescription
exercise p.

preservation
tissue p.

preshaped catheter

presphygmic
p. interval
p. period

pressor drug

pressoreceptive

pressoreceptor

pressosensitive

pressure
"a" wave p.
aortic blood p.
aortic dicrotic notch p.
aortic pullback p.
arterial blood p.
arterial carbon dioxide p.
arterial oxygen partial p.
ascending aortic p.
atmospheres of p.
atrial filling p.
average mean p.
back p.
blood p.
brachial artery end-diastolic p.
brachial artery end-systolic p.
capillary wedge p.
cardiovascular p.
central aortic p.
central venous p.
cerebral perfusion p.
coronary perfusion p.
coronary venous p.
coronary wedge p.
critical closing p.
diastolic blood p.
diastolic filling p.

pressure *(continued)*
  differential blood p.
  distal coronary perfusion p.
  downstream venous p.
  dynamic p.
  elastic recoil p.
  end-diastolic p.
  end-diastolic left ventricular p.
  endocardial p.
  end-systolic left ventricular p.
  femoral artery p.
  filling p.
  p. gradient
  P. guide guidewire
  p. half-time
  p. half-time technique
  high blood p.
  intracardiac p.
  intramyocardial p.
  intrapericardial p.
  intrathoracic p.
  intravascular p.
  intraventricular p.
  jugular venous p. (JVP)
  juxtacardiac pleural p.
  labile blood p.
  left atrial p.
  left subclavian central venous p.
  left ventricular diastolic p.
  left ventricular end-diastolic p.
  left ventricular filling p.
  left ventricular systolic p.
  lower body negative p.
  mean aortic p.
  mean arterial p.
  mean arterial blood p.
  mean blood p.
  mean brachial artery p.
  mean circulatory filling p.
  mean diastolic left ventricular p.
  mean left atrial p.
  mean pulmonary artery p.

pressure *(continued)*
  mean pulmonary artery wedge p.
  mean right atrial p.
  mean systolic left ventricular p.
  p. measurement
  narrowed pulse p.
  p.-natriuresis curve
  negative p.
  normal intravascular p.
  opening p.
  osmotic p.
  p. overload
  PA filling p.
  peak systolic aortic p.
  peak systolic gradient p.
  perfusion p.
  pericardial p.
  plasma colloid osmotic p.
  pullback artery p.
  pulmonary artery systolic p.
  pulmonary artery diastolic p.
  pulmonary artery mean p.
  pulmonary artery peak systolic p.
  pulmonary artery occlusion p.
  pulmonary artery occlusive wedge p.
  pulmonary artery wedge p.
  pulmonary capillary wedge p.
  pulmonary hypertension p.
  pulmonary vascular p.
  pulmonary wedge p.
  pulse p.
  p. recovery
  resting p.
  right atrial p.
  right heart p.
  right subclavian central venous p.
  right ventricular diastolic p.
  right ventricular end-diastolic p.

pressure *(continued)*
>   right ventricular peak sys-
>   tolic p.
>   systemic mean arterial p.
>   systolic blood p.
>   systolic left ventricular p.
>   p. tracing
>   p. transducer
>   transmural p.
>   transmyocardial perfu-
>   sion p.
>   venous p.
>   ventricular diastolic p.
>   ventricular filling p.
>   p. wave
>   p. waveform
>   wedge p.
>   z point p.

pressurelike sensation in chest

Pressurometer blood pressure
>   monitor

Presto
>   P. cardiac device

presystole

presystolic
>   p. gallop
>   p. murmur
>   p. pressure and volume
>   p. pulsation
>   p. thrill

pretibial
>   p. edema
>   p. myxedema

Prevel sign

preventricular stenosis

preventriculosis

Prevue system

Prima
>   P. pacemaker
>   P. Total Occlusion Device

Primacor

primary
>   p. cardiomyopathy

primary *(continued)*
>   p. closure
>   p. pulmonary hypertension
>   murmur
>   p. systemic amyloidosis
>   p. thrombus
>   p. ventricular tachycardia

prime
>   crystalloid p.
>   R-R p.
>   RSR p.

Prime balloon

priming dose

primitive aorta

primordial catheter tube

primum
>   p. atrial septal defect
>   ostium p.
>   persistent ostium p.
>   septum p.

principle
>   Doppler p.
>   Fick p.
>   Frank-Starling p.
>   Frank-Straub-Wiggers-Star-
>   ling p.
>   hemodynamic p.

Prinzmetal
>   P. effect
>   P. variant angina

Prism-CL pacemaker

proANF
>   proatrial natriuretic factor

proarrhythmia

proarrhythmic effect

proatrial natriuretic factor
>   (proANF)

probe
>   AngeLase combined map-
>   ping-laser p.
>   p. balloon catheter
>   blood flow p.

probe *(continued)*
  cardiac p.
  Chandler V-pacing p.
  coronary artery p.
  digoxigenin-labeled DNA p.
  DNA p.
  Doppler flow p.
  Doppler velocity p.
  Dymer excimer delivery p.
  echocardiographic p.
  four-beam laser Doppler p.
  Gallagher bipolar mapping
    p.
  hot-tip laser p.
  Mui scientific 6-channel
    esophageal pressure p.
  nuclear p.
  over-the-wire p.
  Parsonnet coronary p.
  p. patency
  Radiometer p.
  Robicsek vascular p.
  scintillation p.
  Siemens-Elema AB pulse
    transducer p.
  Silverstein stimulator p.
  transesophageal echo p.
  Vasoscope 3 Doppler p.

Probe balloon-on-a-wire dilatation system (USCI)

probing catheter

procaryon

procaryosis

procaryote

procaryotic

Procath electrophysiology catheter

procedure
  Alliston p.
  Anderson p.
  arterial switch p.
  Batiste p.
  Bentall p.
  Bing-Taussig heart p.
  Björk method of Fontan p.

procedure *(continued)*
  Blalock-Taussig p.
  Brock p.
  Charles p.
  cherry-picking p.
  Cockett p.
  compartment p.
  corridor p.
  Damian graft p.
  Damus-Kaye-Stansel p.
  de-airing p.
  debubbling p.
  debulking p.
  domino p.
  Effler-Groves mode of Alli-
    son p.
  endocardial resection p.
  esophageal sling p.
  extended endocardial re-
    section p.
  Fick p.
  Fontan modification of Nor-
    wood p.
  Fontan-Baudet p.
  Fontan-Kreutzer p.
  Gill-Jonas modification of
    Norwood p.
  Glenn p.
  hemi-Fontan p.
  His-Hass p.
  Jacobaeus p.
  Jatene arterial switch p.
  Jonas modification of Nor-
    wood p.
  Junod p.
  Karhunen-Loeve p.
  Ko-Airan bleeding con-
    trol p.
  Kolmogorov-Smirnov p.
  Kono p.
  Lam p.
  Langevin updating p.
  latissimus dorsi p.
  left atrial isolation p.
  Lewis-Tanner p.
  Luke p.
  Lyon-Horgan p.
  maze p.
  Moore p.

procedure *(continued)*
Mustard p.
Nicks p.
Norwood univentricular heart p.
Overholt p.
Potts p.
Quaegebeur p.
Rashkind p.
Rastan-Konno p.
Rastelli p.
Ross p.
Sade modification of Norwood p.
salting-out p.
Schenk-Eichelter vena cava plastic filter p.
Schonander p.
Senning transposition p.
septation p.
Simplate p.
Sondergaard p.
Stansel p.
Sugiura p.
switch p.
Thal p.
Vineberg p.
Waterston-Cooley p.
Womack p.

process
consolidative p.
xiphisternal p.
xiphoid p.

procollagen
type III p.
p. type II aminoterminal peptide

proconvertin
p. blood coagulation factor
p. prothrombin conversion accelerator

prodromal symptom

prodrome

product
Autoplex Factor VIII inhibitor bypass p.

product *(continued)*
calcium p.
fibrinogen degradation p.
fibrinogen-fibrin degradation p.
fibrin split p.
lipid peroxidation p.
rate pressure p.

profile
aortic valve velocity p.
Astra p.
deflated p.
serum lipid p.
ultra-low p.

Profile Plus balloon dilatation catheter

profilin

Profilnine Heat-Treated

Proflex 5 dilatation catheter

Pro-Flo XT catheter

profunda
p. Dacron patchplasty
p. femoris artery
p. femoris vein

profundaplasty

progenitor

progeria

progesterone

progestin

Prograf

Programalith
P. III pacemaker
P. III pulse generator

programmable
p. cardioverter-defibrillator (PCD)
p. implantable medication system
p. pacemaker

programmed electrical stimulation

Programmer
    P. III pacemaker
    Omnicor P.

progression
    poor R wave p.
    R wave p.

progressive
    p. systemic sclerosis
    p. thrombus

pro-inflammatory substance

projection
    anterior p.
    anterior oblique p.
    anteroposterior p.
    left anterior oblique p.
    left lateral p.
    right anterior oblique p.
    spider p.
    steep left anterior obli-
        que p.

projector
    Tagarno 3SD cineangiogra-
        phy p.

prokaryon

prokaryosis

prokaryote

prokaryotic

prolapse
    mitral valve p. (MVP)
    tricuspid valve p.
    valvular p.

prolapsed
    p. mitral valve leaflets
    p. mitral valve syndrome

prolate ellipse

Prolene suture

proliferans
    endocarditis p.

proliferating cell nuclear anti-
    gen

proliferation
    intimal p.
    myxomatous p.
    neointimal p.

Prolith pacemaker

Prolog pacemaker

prolongation
    p. of QRS interval
    p. of QT wave

prolonged Q-T interval syn-
    drome

prometaphase

propagating thrombosis

propagation
    impulse p.
    p. of R wave

Propel
    P. coating
    P. coating cardiac device
    Hi-Torque floppy with P.

propeptide
    aminoterminal p.

property
    p's of lipophilicity
    vagolytic p.

prophylactic
    p. antibiotic therapy
    p. implantation of pace-
        maker

prophylaxis
    endocarditis p.
    subacute bacterial endo-
        carditis (SBE) p.

prophase

prostaglandin

prosthesis *pl.* prostheses
    Alvarez valve p.
    aortic p.
    arterial p.
    ball-and-cage p.

prosthesis *(continued)*
 ball-cage p.
 ball-valve p.
 Barnard mitral valve p.
 Baxter mechanical valve p.
 Beall disk valve p.
 Beall mitral valve p.
 Bentall cardiovascular p.
 bifurcated aortofemoral p.
 bifurcation p.
 bileaflet p.
 Bionit II vascular p.
 Bionit vascular p.
 Björk-Shiley aortic valve p.
 Björk-Shiley convexocon-
   cave 60-degree valve p.
 Björk-Shiley floating disk p.
 bovine pericardial p.
 Braunwald-Cutter ball val-
   ve p.
 bypass p.
 caged-ball valve p.
 Capetown aortic valve p.
 cardiac valve p.
 CarboMedics cardiac valve
   p.
 Carpentier annuloplasty
   ring p.
 Carpentier-Edwards aortic
   valve p.
 Carpentier-Edwards glutar-
   aldehyde-preserved por-
   cine xenograft p.
 Carpentier-Rhone-Poulenc
   mitral ring p.
 Cartwright heart p.
 Cartwright valve p.
 Cartwright vascular p.
 convexoconcave valve p.
 Cooley-Bloodwell mitral
   valve p.
 Cooley-Bloodwell-Cutter p.
 Cooley Dacron p.
 Creech insertion of vascu-
   lar p.
 Cross-Jones disk valve p.
 Cutter aortic valve p.
 Cutter-Smeloff aortic val-
   ve p.

prosthesis *(continued)*
 Cutter-Smeloff cardiac val-
   ve p.
 Dacron arterial p.
 Dacron bifurcation p.
 Dacron vascular p.
 DeBakey ball-valve p.
 DeBakey Vasculour-II vas-
   cular p.
 Delrin frame of valve p.
 Duromedics valve p.
 Edwards seamless p.
 Edwards Teflon intracar-
   diac patch p.
 femorofemoral crossover p.
 Golaski-UMI vascular p.
 Gore-Tex vascular p.
 Gott mitral valve p.
 Gott-Daggett heart valve p.
 Hall-Kaster tilting-disk val-
   ve p.
 Hammersmith mitral p.
 Hancock aortic valve p.
 Hancock mitral valve p.
 Hancock porcine valve p.
 heart valve p.
 hinged-leaflet vascular p.
 hingeless heart valve p.
 Hufnagel disk heart valve p.
 Hufnagel valve p.
 intracardiac patch p.
 Ionescu-Shiley valve p.
 Kaster mitral valve p.
 Kay-Shiley disk valve p.
 Kay-Shiley valve p.
 Kay-Suzuki valve p.
 knitted vascular p.
 Lillehei-Cruz-Kaster p.
 Lillehei-Kaster aortic val-
   ve p.
 Lillehei-Kaster mitral val-
   ve p.
 Lo-Por arterial p.
 low-profile valve p.
 Magnuson valve p.
 Magnuson-Cromie valve p.
 Magovern ball-valve p.
 Magovern-Cromie valve p.
 Meadox woven velour p.

prosthesis *(continued)*
Meadox-Cooley woven low-
porosity p.
Medi-graft vascular p.
Medtronic INTACT porcine
bioprosthesis
Medtronic-Hall tilting-disk
valve p.
Microknit arterial graft p.
Milliknit Dacron p.
Milliknit arterial p.
Milliknit vascular graft p.
mitral valve p.
Monostrut cardiac valve p.
New Weavenit Dacron p.
Omnicarbon heart valve p.
Omniscience single leaflet
cardiac valve p.
Omniscience tilting-disk
valve p.
Orlon vascular p.
Pemco valve p.
polyvinyl p.
porcine heterograft p.
Rashkind double-disk oc-
cluder p.
St. Jude Medical aortic val-
ve p.
St. Jude Medical heart val-
ve p.
St. Jude Medical mitral val-
ve p.
Sauvage filamentous p.
Smeloff-Cutter aortic val-
ve p.
Smeloff-Cutter ball-valve p.
Sorin mitral valve p.
Starr ball heart p.
Starr-Edwards aortic val-
ve p.
Starr-Edwards ball valve p.
Starr-Edwards cardiac val-
ve p.
Starr-Edwards disk valve p.
Starr-Edwards heart val-
ve p.
stentless porcine aortic
valve p.

prosthesis *(continued)*
Sutter-Smeloff heart val-
ve p.
supra-annular p.
sutureless valve p.
Teflon intracardiac
patch p.
Teflon trileaflet p.
tilting-disk aortic valve p.
trileaflet aortic p.
USCI Sauvage Bionit bifurcated vascular p.
vascular graft p.
Vascutek vascular p.
vessel p.
Wada hingeless heart val-
ve p.
Wada valve p.
Weavenit p.
Wesolowski p.
Wesolowski Weavenit vas-
cular p.
woven Teflon p.
woven-tube vascular p.
prosthetic
p. aortic valve
p. ball valve
p. cardiac valve
p. device
p. graft
p. heart valve
p. patch graft
p. poppet
p. ring annuloplasty
p. sizer
p. valve endocarditis
p. valve sewing ring
p. valve suture ring
p. valve thrombosis
p. valve vegetation
protease inhibitor
protease-antiprotease imbalance
protection
myocardial p.
protein
binding p.

protein *(continued)*
 cardiac gap junction p.
 carrier p.
 coagulation p.
 contractile p.
 cytosolic p.
 p. electrophoresis
 G p.
 GTPase-activating p.
 GTP-binding p.
 guanyl-nucleotide-bin-
  ding p.
 insoluble p.
 p. kinase
 membrane transport p.
 thrombus precursor p.
 transport p.

proteinase

α_2-proteinase inhibitor

protein-calorie

proteinosis

proteinuria

proteolytic enzyme

Protex swivel adapter

prothrombin
 p. time (PT)
 p. time/partial thrombo-
  plastin time (PT/PTT)

prothrombinase complex

protocaryon

protocol
 Balke treadmill p.
 Balke-Ware treadmill p.
 Bruce treadmill p.
 cardiac rehabilitation p.
 continuous ramp p.
 Cornell exercise p.
 Ellestad p.
 GUSTO p.
 James exercise p.
 Kattus treadmill p.
 Mayo exercise treadmill p.
 McHenry treadmill exerci-
  se p.

protocol *(continued)*
 modified Bruce p.
 modified Ellestad p.
 Naughton-Balke treadmill p.
 Naughton treadmill p.
 RAMP antitachycardia pa-
  cing p.
 Reeves treadmill p.
 rest metabolism/stress perfusion p.
 SCAN antitachycardia pa-
  cing p.
 Sheffield modification of
  Bruce treadmill p.
 Sheffield treadmill exercise p.
 slow USAFSAM treadmill
  exercise p.
 standard Bruce p.
 TIMI II (thrombolysis in
  myocardial infarction) p.
 USAFSAM treadmill p.
 Weber-Janicki cardiopul-
  monary exercise p.

protodiastolic
 p. gallop
 p. murmur
 p. reversal of blood flow
 p. rumble

protoplasm
 granular p.
 superior p.

protoplast

protozoal myocarditis

protozoan

prourokinase
 p. in myocardial infarction
 p. and t-PA enhancement in
  thrombolysis

Pro-Vent
 P.-V. arterial blood gas kit
 P.-V. arterial blood sam-
  pling kit

proximal
 p. circumflex artery

proximal *(continued)*
p. coronary sinus
p. and distal portion of vessel
p. segment

Pruitt
P. vascular shunt
P.-Inahara balloon-tipped perfusion catheter
P.-Inahara carotid shunt

pruning
branch vessel p.

pseudoaneurysm

pseudoangina

pseudo-AV block

pseudobacterium

pseudoclaudication

pseudocoarctation

pseudodextrocardia

pseudohypotension

pseudoinfarction

pseudointima

pseudomalfunction

pseudomembranous
p. angina

pseudonormalization of T wave

pseudopericarditis

pseudopodium *pl.* pseudopodia

pseudoreduction

pseudotruncus arteriosus

pseudotumoral mediastinal amyloidosis

pseudoxanthoma elasticum

psychocardiac reflex

psychogenic
p. overlay

psychogenic *(continued)*
p. pain

psychosis
postcardiotomy p.
postperfusion p.

PT
prothrombin time

PTAS
percutaneous transluminal angioscopy

PTCA
percutaneous transluminal coronary angioplasty

PTCR
percutaneous transluminal coronary revascularization

PTMC
percutaneous transvenous mitral commissurotomy

PT/PTT
prothrombin time/partial thromboplastin time

PTT
partial thromboplastin time

puerperal
p. phlebitis
p. thrombosis

Puig Massana
P. M. annuloplasty ring
P. M.–Shiley annuloplasty ring
P. M.–Shiley annuloplasty valve

pullback
p. across the aortic valve
left heart p.
p. pressure
p. from ventricle

pulmoaortic canal

pulmonale
atrium p.
cor p.

pulmonale *(continued)*
    P p.
    pseudo–P p.

pulmonary
    p. arterial markings
    p. arterial vent
    p. arterial web
    p. arteriolar resistance
    p. arteriovenous fistula
    p. arteriovenous malforma-
        tion
    p. artery
    p. artery band
    p. artery banding
    p. artery catheterization
    p. artery end-diastolic pres-
        sure
    p. artery pressure
    p. artery sling
    p. artery steal
    p. artery stenosis
    p. artery wedge pressure
    p. autograft valve
    p. AV O_2 difference
    p. blood flow
    p. capillary wedge pressure
    p. circulation
    p. congestion
    p. embolectomy
    p. embolism
    p. embolization
    p. embolus
    p. heart
    p. hypertension
    p. hypertension pressure
    p. murmur
    p. outflow tract
    p. pulse
    p. thromboembolism
    p. valve anomaly
    p. valve area
    p. valve echocardiography
    p. valve gradient
    p. valve restenosis
    p. valve stenosis
    p. valve vegetation
    p. valvular regurgitation
    p. valvular stenosis
    p. valvuloplasty

pulmonary *(continued)*
    p. vascular markings
    p. vascular obstruction
    p. vascular obstructive dis-
        ease
    p. vascular pressure
    p. vascular resistance
    p. vascular resistance in-
        dex
    p. vasculature
    p. vasculitis
    p. vasoconstriction
    p. vein
    p. veno-occlusive disease
    p. venous connection
        anomaly
    p. venous congestion
    p. venous return anomaly
    p. wedge angiography
    p. wedge pressure (PWP)

pulmonic
    p. area
    p. atresia
    p. closure sound
    p. endocarditis
    p. incompetence
    p. insufficiency
    p. murmur
    p. regurgitation
    p. second sound
    p. stenosis
    p. valve
    p. valve closure sound
    p. valve stenosis

pulmonocoronary reflex

Pulmopak pump

Pulsar NI implantable pace-
    maker

pulsatile
    p. abdominal mass
    p. assist device
    p. perfusion

pulsation
    capillary p.
    carotid arterial p.
    expansile p.

pulsation *(continued)*
    jugular venous p.
    precordial p.
    presystolic p.
    suprasternal p.
Pulsator
    P. dry heparin arterial
      blood gas kit
    P. syringe
pulse
    abdominal p.
    abrupt p.
    allorhythmic p.
    alternating p.
    anacrotic p.
    anadicrotic p.
    anatricrotic p.
    arterial pressure p.
    atrial liver p.
    atrial venous p.
    atriovenous p.
    auriculovenous p.
    Bamberger bulbar p.
    biferious p.
    bigeminal p.
    bigeminal bisferious p.
    bisferious p.
    bounding p.
    brachial p.
    bulbar p.
    cannonball p.
    capillary p.
    carotid p.
    catacrotic p.
    catadicrotic p.
    catatricrotic p.
    centripetal venous p.
    collapsing p.
    cordy p.
    Corrigan p.
    coupled p.
    CV wave of jugular ven-
      ous p.
    decurtate p.
    p. deficit
    dicrotic p.
    digitalate p.
    dorsalis pedis p.

pulse *(continued)*
    dropped-beat p.
    elastic p.
    entoptic p.
    epigastric p.
    febrile p.
    femoral p.
    filiform p.
    formicant p.
    F point of cardiac apex p.
    funic p.
    frequent p.
    full p.
    f wave of jugular venous p.
    gaseous p.
    guttural p.
    hard p.
    high-tension p.
    hyperdicrotic p.
    hyperkinetic p.
    hypokinetic p.
    incisura p.
    infrequent p.
    intermittent p.
    irregular p.
    irregularly irregular p.
    jerky p.
    jugular venous p.
    Kussmaul p.
    labile p.
    long p.
    low-tension p.
    Monneret p.
    monocrotic p.
    mouse tail p.
    movable p.
    nail p.
    O point of cardiac apex p.
    p. oximeter
    p. oximetry monitoring
    paradoxic p.
    paradoxical p., reversed
    parvus et tardus p.
    pedal p.
    p. period
    pistol-shot p.
    piston p.
    plateau p.
    polycrotic p.

pulse *(continued)*
    popliteal p.
    precordial p.
    posterior tibial p.
    pressure p.
    pulmonary p.
    quadrigeminal p.
    quick p.
    Quincke p.
    radial p.
    p. rate
    respiratory p.
    retrosternal p.
    reversed paradoxical p.
    Riegel p.
    running p.
    SF wave of cardiac apex p.
    sharp p.
    short p.
    slow p.
    soft p.
    spike-and-dome p.
    strong p.
    tense p.
    thready p.
    tibial p.
    tidal wave p.
    tricrotic p.
    trigeminal p.
    trip-hammer p.
    triple-humped pressure p.
    undulating p.
    unequal p.
    vagus p.
    venous p.
    vermicular p.
    vibrating p.
    water-hammer p.
    p. wave velocity
    p. width
    wiry p.
    y depression of jugular
        venous p.
    y descent of jugular ven-
        ous p.

pulsed
    p. Doppler echocardiogra-
        phy
    p. Doppler flowmetry

pulsed *(continued)*
    p. dye laser
    p. laser ablation

pulsed-wave Doppler mapping

pulseless
    p. bradycardia
    p. disease
    p. electrical activity
    p. idioventricular rhythm

pulsus
    p. abdominalis
    p. alternans
    p. bigeminus
    p. bisferiens
    p. caprisans
    p. catacrotus
    p. catadicrotus
    p. celer
    p. celerrimus
    p. contractus
    p. cordis
    p. debilis
    p. deficiens
    p. deletus
    p. differens
    p. duplex
    p. durus
    p. filiformis
    p. fluens
    p. formicans
    p. fortis
    p. frequens
    p. heterochronicus
    p. inaequalis
    p. incongruens
    p. infrequens
    p. intercidens
    p. intercurrens
    p. irregularis perpetuus
    p. magnus
    p. magnus et celer
    p. mollis
    p. monocrotus
    p. myurus
    p. oppressus
    p. paradoxus
    p. parvus
    p. parvus et tardus

pulsus *(continued)*
- p. plenus
- p. pseudo-intermittens
- p. quadrigeminus
- p. rarus
- p. respiratione intermittens
- p. tardus
- p. tremulus
- p. trigeminus
- p. vacuus
- p. venosus
- p. vibrans

pump
- Abbott infusion p.
- abdominothoracic p.
- Aortic balloon p.
- Asahi blood plasma p.
- AVCO balloon p.
- A-V Impulse foot p.
- balloon p.
- Bard cardiopulmonary support p.
- Bard mini-infuser syringe p.
- Bard Trans-Act intra-aortic balloon p.
- blood p.
- calcium p.
- cardiac balloon p.
- centrifugal p.
- Cobe double blood p.
- Datascope intra-aortic balloon p.
- Datascope system 90 intra-aortic balloon p.
- DeBakey heart p. oxygenator
- disk oxygenator p.
- electrogenic p.
- Emerson p.
- extracorporeal p.
- Flowtron DVT p.
- Gomco thoracic drainage p.
- heart p.
- HeartMate p.
- Hemopump
- hepatic artery infusion p.
- IABP intra-aortic balloon p.
- intra-aortic balloon p. (- IABP)
- ion p.
- IVAC volumetric infusion p.
- Jarvik-7 mechanical p.
- Jobst athrombotic p.
- Jobst extremity p.
- KAAT II Plus intra-aortic balloon p.
- Kontron intra-aortic balloon p.
- left ventricular bypass p.
- muscular venous p.
- p. oxygenator
- p. primed
- pulmonary artery balloon p. (PABP)
- Pulmopak p. for arterial perfusion
- roller p.
- Sarns Siok II blood p.
- sodium p.
- sodium-potassium p.
- venous p.

Pumpette
- Master Flow P.
- Stat 2 P.

punch
- aortic p.
- Brock p.
- circular p.
- Goosen vascular p.
- Hancock aortic p.
- Karp aortic p.
- Medtronic aortic p.
- Mendez-Schubert aortic p.
- Merz aortic p.
- Sparks atrioseptal p.
- Sweet sternal p.

punctate hemorrhage

puncture
- apical left ventricular p.
- arterial p.
- direct cardiac p.
- groin p.
- Kronecker p.
- left ventricular p.
- percutaneous p.

puncture *(continued)*
    transseptal p.
    venous p.
    ventricular p.

pure
    p. flutter
    p. parasystole

purified protein derivative
    (PPD)

Purkinje
    P. cells
    P. conduction
    P. fibers
    P. image tracker
    P. network
    P. system
    P. tumor

Purmann method

purpura
    allergic p.
    anaphylactoid p.
    p. annularis telangiectodes
    fibrinolytic p.
    p. fibrinolytica
    p. fulminans
    p. hemorrhagica
    Henoch p.
    Henoch-Schönlein p.
    idiopathic thrombocyto-
      penic p.
    itching p.
    Majocchi p.
    p. nervosa
    nonthrombocytopenic p.
    p. rheumatica
    Schönlein p.
    Schönlein-Henoch p.
    p. senilis
    p. simplex
    steroid p.
    thrombocytopenic p.
    thrombocytopenic p., idio-
      pathic
    thrombocytopenic p., sec-
      ondary
    thrombotic thrombocyto-
      penic p.

purpura *(continued)*
    thrombopenic p.
    thrombocytopenic p., pri-
      mary

purpuric

purring thrill

pursestring
    p. of black silk
    p. suture

purulent pericarditis

putative slow pathway potential

PV
    pulmonic valve

PVB
    premature ventricular beat

PVC
    premature ventricular con-
      traction
        bigeminal PVC
        early-cycle PVC
        multifocal PVC
        multiform PVC
        paired PVC
        unifocal PVC

PVD
    peripheral vascular disease

PVR
    pulmonary vascular resis-
      tance

P wave
    P w. amplitude
    P w. axis
    bifid P w.
    biphasic P w.
    depressed P w.
    peaked P w.
    retrograde P w.
    P w. triggered ventricular
      pacemaker
    upright P w.

pyelophlebitis

pyemia
    arterial p.
    portal p.

pyemic embolism

pyknoplasson

pyknosis

pyknotic

pylephlebectasis

pylephlebitis
    adhesive p.
    suppurative p.

pylethrombophlebitis

pylethrombosis

pylic

pyopericarditis

pyopericardium

pyopneumopericardium

pyopneumothorax

pyothorax

pyrenolysis

pyriform thorax

pyrogen

Pyrolyte

pyroglycolic acid suture

pyrolytic carbon

pyrophosphate

pyruvic acid

QCA
  quantitative coronary angiography

Q-cath
  Q-c. catheter
  Q-c. catheterization recording system

Q–H interval of jugular venous pulse

Q–M interval

Q–RB interval

Q–R interval

QR pattern

QRS
  QRS alternans
  QRS axis
  QRS changes
  QRS complex
  QRS complex duration
  fusion QRS
  QRS interval
  QRS loop
  QRS morphology
  normal voltage QRS
  preexcited QRS
  slurring of QRS
  QRS synchronous atrial defibrillation shocks
  QRS vector
  QRS wave
  wide QRS

QRS–ST junction

QRS–T
  QRS–T angle
  QRS–T changes
  QRS–T complex
  QRS–T interval
  QRS–T value

QS
  QS complex
  QS deflection
  QS pattern

QS *(continued)*
  QS wave

Q–S$_1$ interval

Q–S$_2$ interval

Q-Stress
  Q-S. treadmill
  Q-S. treadmill stress test

Q-switched
  Q-s. Alexandrite laser
  Q-s. Nd:YAG laser
  Q-s. ruby laser

Q–T
  Q–T interval
  Q–T$_c$ interval (corrected QT interval)
  Q–T interval sensing pacemaker
  Q–T syndrome

QT
  QT corrected for heart rate
  QT dispersion

Q–TU interval syndrome

QU interval

quadrangulation of Frouin

quadricuspid

quadrigeminal
  q. pulse
  q. rhythm

quadrigeminus
  pulsus q.

quadrigeminy

quadripolar
  q. electrode catheter

quadruple rhythm

Quain
  Q. degeneration
  Q. fatty heart

Quanticor catheter

quantitation of ischemic muscle

quantitative
  q. arteriography
  q. computed tomography
  q. coronary angiographic
    analysis
  q. coronary angiography
  q. Doppler
  q. left ventriculography
  q. two-dimensional echo-
    cardiography

Quantum
  Q. pacemaker
  Q. TTC balloon dilator

quartz transducer

quasi-sinusoidal biphasic waveform

Queckenstedt sign

Quénu-Muret sign

Quervain rib spreader

QuickFlash arterial catheter

QuickFurl
  Q. double-lumen balloon
  Q. single-lumen balloon

quiet
  q. chest
  q. heart sounds
  q. precordium

Quik-Chek external pacer tester

Quincke
  Q. disease
  Q. edema
  Q. pulse
  Q. sign

Q–U interval

Quinton
  Q. biopsy catheter
  Q. central venous catheter
  Q. dual-lumen catheter
  Q. PermCath catheter
  Q. Quik-Prep electrode
  Q. tube
  Q. vascular access port
  Q.-Scribner shunt

Q wave
  nondiagnostic Q w.
  Q w. myocardial infarction
  pathologic Q w.
  Q w. regression
  septal Q w.

R
    R on T phenomenon
    R on T ventricular prema-
        ture contraction
    R unit
    R wave
    R wave amplitude
    R wave gating
    R wave progression
    R wave upstroke

RA
    right atrium

RAA
    right atrial appendage

Raaf
    R. Cath vascular catheter
    R. double-lumen catheter
    R. dual-lumen catheter

RAAS
    renin-angiotensin-aldoster-
        one system

rabbit antithymocyte globulin

rabbit-ear sign

racemic epinephrine

racemose aneurysm

Rackley method

racquet incision

RAD
    right axis deviation

rad
    radiation absorbed dose

radarkymography

radial
    r. artery
    r. artery catheter
    r. collateral artery
    r. pulse
    r. recurrent artery

radiation
    r. equivalent in man

radiation *(continued)*
    ionizing r.
    mitogenetic r.
    mitogenic r.
    secondary r.

radiation-induced pericarditis

RadiMedical fiberoptic pres-
    sure-monitoring wire

radiocardiogram

radiocardiography

radiocontrast dye

radiodense

radioelectrocardiogram

radioelectrocardiograph

radioelectrocardiography

Radiofocus Glidewire

radiofrequency (RF)
    r. ablater
    r. ablation (RFA)
    r. catheter ablation
    r. coil
    r. current
    r. hot balloon
    r. pacemaker

radiographic technique

radiography

radioimmunoassay (RIA)

radioisotope
    r. camera
    r. capsule
    CEAker r.
    specific immunoglobulin
        G r.

radioisotopic study

radiolabeled
    r. fibrinogen
    r. microsphere

radiolabeled iodine

radioligand
    r. binding assay

radiologic scimitar syndrome

Radiometer probe

radiomutation

radionuclide
    r. angiocardiography
    r. angiography
    r. angiogram
    r. cineangiocardiography
    r. imaging
    r. scanning
    r. ventriculography

radiopacity

radiopaque
    r. calibrated catheter
    r. ERCP catheter
    r. tantalum stent

radiopharmaceutical

radiotracer

radius
    thrombocytopenia-absent r.

radix
    r. basalis anterior venae basalis communis

RAE
    right atrial enlargement

Raeder-Arbitz syndrome

Raff-Glantz derivative method

railroad track sign

rain of collaterals

rakenangioma

rake retractor

Ramirez shunt

Ramond sign

ramp pacing

ramus *pl.* rami
    r. acetabuli arteriae circumflexae femoris medialis
    r. acromialis arteriae transversae scapulae
    rami anastomotici
    r. anterior arteriae thyroideae superioris
    rami articulares arteriae genus descendentis
    r. atrialis anastomoticus
    rami circumflexi arteriae coronariae sinistrae
    rami atriales arteriae coronariae dextrae
    rami atriales rami circumflexi arteriae coronariae sinistrae
    r. atrialis intermedius arteriae coronariae dextrae
    r. atrialis intermedius rami circumflexi arteriae coronariae sinistri
    rami atrioventriculares
    rami circumflexi arteriae coronariae sinistrae
    r. basalis anterior arteriae pulmonalis dextrae
    r. basalis anterior arteriae pulmonalis sinistrae
    r. basalis lateralis arteriae pulmonalis dextrae
    r. basalis lateralis arteriae pulmonalis sinistrae
    r. basalis medialis arteriae pulmonalis dextrae
    r. basalis medialis arteriae pulmonalis sinistrae
    r. basalis posterior arteriae pulmonalis dextrae
    r. basalis posterior arteriae pulmonalis sinistrae
    rami bronchiales aortae thoracicae
    rami caroticotympanici arteriae carotidis internae

ramus *(continued)*
  r. carpeus dorsalis arteriae
    radialis
  r. carpeus dorsalis arteriae
    ulnaris
  r. carpeus palmaris arteriae
    radialis
  r. carpeus palmaris arteriae
    ulnaris
  r. caudae nuclei caudati ar-
    teriae communicantis
    posterioris
  rami caudati partis trans-
    versae
  rami centrales anteromedi-
    ales arteriae cerebri ante-
    rioris
  r. circumflexus arteriae co-
    ronariae sinistrae
  rami communicantes
  r. coni arteriosi arteriae co-
    ronariae dextrae
  r. coni arteriosi arteriae co-
    ronariae sinistrae
  r. dorsalis venae intercos-
    talis
  rami epiploici arteriae gas-
    troepiploicae dextrae
  rami epiploici arteriae gas-
    troepiploicae sinistrae
  rami esophageales aortae
    thoracicae
  rami esophageales arteriae
    gastricae sinistrae
  rami esophageales arteriae
    thyroideae inferioris
  rami esophageales partis
    thoracicae aortae
  rami gastrici arteriae gas-
    troepiploicae dextrae
  rami gastrici arteriae gas-
    troepiploicae sinistrae
  rami glandulares arteriae
    thyroideae inferioris
  rami glandulares arteriae
    thyroideae superioris
  r. interventricularis ante-
    rior arteriae coronariae
    sinistrae

ramus *(continued)*
  r. interventricularis poste-
    rior arteriae coronariae
    dextrae
  rami interventriculares sep-
    tales arteriae coronariae
    sinistrae
  rami interventriculares sep-
    tales arteriae coronariae
    dextrae
  rami laterales arteriarum
    centralium anterolateral-
    ium
  r. lateralis arteriae pulmon-
    alis dextrae
  r. lateralis interventricu-
    laris anterioris arteriae
    coronariae sinistrae
  r. lingularis arteriae pul-
    monalis sinistrae
  r. lingularis inferior arteriae
    pulmonalis sinistrae
  r. lingularis superior arte-
    riae pulmonalis sinistrae
  rami lobi inferioris arteriae
    pulmonalis dextrae
  rami lobi inferioris arteriae
    pulmonalis sinistrae
  rami lobi medii arteriae
    pulmonalis dextrae
  rami lobi superioris arte-
    riae pulmonalis dextrae
  rami lobi superioris arte-
    riae pulmonalis sinistrae
  r. marginalis dexter arte-
    riae coronariae dextrae
  r. marginalis sinister rami
    circumflexi arteriae co-
    ronariae sinistrae
  r. meatus acustici interni
    arteriae basilaris
  r. medialis arteriae pulmon-
    alis dextrae
  rami mediastinales aortae
    thoracicae
  r. meningeus accessorius
    arteriae meningeae me-
    diae

ramus *(continued)*
- r. meningeus anterior arteriae vertebralis
- r. meningeus posterior arteriae vertebralis
- r. muscularis
- r. nodi atrioventricularis arteriae coronariae dextrae
- r. nodi atrioventricularis rami circumflexi arteriae coronariae sinistrae
- r. nodi sinuatrialis arteriae coronariae dextrae
- r. nodi sinuatrialis rami circumflexi arteriae coronariae sinistrae
- rami esophageales aortae thoracicae
- rami parietales partis abdominalis aortae
- rami parietales partis thoracicae aortae
- rami pericardiaci aortae thoracicae
- rami pharyngei arteriae pharyngeae ascendentis
- rami pharyngei arteriae thyroideae inferioris
- r. plantaris profundus arteriae dorsalis pedis
- rami ad pontem arteriae basilaris
- r. posterior arteriae thyroideae superioris
- r. posterior ventriculi sinistri rami circumflexi arteriae coronariae sinistrae
- r. posterolateralis dexter arteriae coronariae dextrae
- rami subendocardiales
- r. superior lobi inferioris arteriae pulmonalis dextrae
- r. superior lobi inferioris arteriae pulmonalis sinistrae

ramus *(continued)*
- r. tentorii basalis arteriae carotidis internae
- r. tentorii marginalis arteriae carotidis internae
- rami thalamici arteriae cerebri posterioris
- r. thalamicus arteriae communicantis posterioris
- r. transversus arteriae circumflexae femoris medialis
- rami trigeminales et trochleares
- rami tubales arteriae ovaricae
- r. tubalis arteriae uterinae
- r. ventriculi sinistri posterior
- rami viscerales partis abdominalis aortae
- rami viscerales partis thoracicae aortae

Rand microballoon

Randall stone forceps for thromboendarterectomy

randomized
- r. clinical trials

random-zero sphygmomanometer

Ranfac needle

range-alternating current

Ranger
- NC R. over-the-wire balloon catheter
- NC Big R. over-the-wire balloon catheter
- R. over-the-wire balloon catheter
- Quantum R. balloon catheter

Ranke complex

Ransohoff operation

Ranvier
    node of R.

RAO
    right anterior oblique
        RAO angulation
        RAO position
        RAO view

RAP
    right atrial pressure

rape
    bruit de scie ou de r.

rapeseed oil

raphe

rapid
    r. acquisition computed ax-
        ial tomography
    r. atrial pacing
    r. depolarization
    r. filling wave
    r. nonsustained ventricular
        tachycardia
    r. sequence induction
    r. y descent

rapid-burst pacing

rappel
    bruit de r.

rarus
    pulsus r.

Rashkind
    R. balloon
    R. balloon atrial septos-
        tomy
    R. balloon catheter
    R. cardiac device
    R. double-disk occluder
        prosthesis
    R. double umbrella device
    R. procedure
    R. septostomy balloon
        catheter
    R. septostomy needle
    R.-Miller atrial septostomy

Rasmussen aneurysm

Rasor Blood Pumping system

rasp
    Alexander-Faraheuf rib r.
    Beck r.
    Doyen rib r.

raspatory
    Alexander rib r.
    Coryllos rib r.
    rib r.

rasping murmur

rasping pain

Rastan-Kono procedure

Rastan operation

Rastelli
    R. conduit
    R. operation
    R. procedure

rate
    r.-adaptive device
    atrial r.
    auricular r.
    baseline variability of fetal
        heart r.
    basic r.
    beat-to-beat variability of
        fetal heart r.
    complication r.
    circulation r.
    r.-dependent angina
    erythrocyte sedimenta-
        tion r. (ESR)
    expiratory flow r.
    fetal heart r.
    flow r.
    heart r.
    r. hysteresis
    inspiratory flow r.
    left ventricular filling r.
    magnet r.
    maximum predicted
        heart r. (MPHR)
    mean normalized systolic
        ejection r.
    mortality r.

rate *(continued)*
  pacemaker adaptive r.
  peak diastolic filling r.
  peak emptying r.
  peak exercise heart r.
  peak filling r.
  peak jet flow r.
  pulse r.
  QT corrected for heart r.
  repetition r.
  respiratory r.
  r.-responsive pacemaker
  resting heart r.
  sedimentation r.
  slew r.
  stroke ejection r.
  systolic ejection r.
  target heart r.
  time-to-peak filling r.
  ventricular r.
  Westergren erythrocyte se-
    dimentation r.
  Wintrobe sedimentation r.

ratings of perceived exertion

ratio
  albumin-globulin (A-G) r.
  AH-HA r.
  ankle-brachial blood pres-
    sure r.
  AO:AC (aortic valve open-
    ing/aortic valve closing) r.
  aorta-left atrium r.
  aortic root r.
  body-weight r.
  cardiothoracic r.
  conduction r.
  E:A wave r.
  flow r.
  international normalized r.
    (INR)
  karyoplasmic r.
  nucleocytoplasmic r.
  nucleoplasmic r.
  P:QRS r.
  pulmonary to systemic
    blood flow r.
  renal vein renin r.
  resistance r.

ratio *(continued)*
  septal to free wall r.
  shunt r.
  signal-to-noise r.
  systolic velocity r.
  therapeutic r.
  transmitral Doppler E:A r.
  transmitral E:A r.

Ratliff criteria for myocarditis

Rauchfuss triangle

Rautharju ECG criteria

ray
  astral r.
  beta r.
  gamma r.
  necrobiotic r's
  polar r.
  x-r.

Raynaud
  R. disease
  R. phenomenon
  R. syndrome

RayTec x-ray detectable sponge

Razi cannula introducer

RBBB
  right bundle branch block

RBC
  red blood cell

RBC indices
  MCH (mean corpuscular
    hemoglobin)
  MCHC (mean corpuscular
    hemoglobin concentra-
    tion)
  MCV (mean corpuscular
    volume)

RCA
  right coronary artery

RDS
  respiratory distress syn-
    drome

reabsorbable suture

reaction
    accelerated r.
    acute situational r.
    anaphylactic r.
    fibrinolytic r.
    focal r.
    Haber-Weiss r.
    hemoclastic r.
    hexokinase r.
    hunting r.
    inflammatory r.
    Kveim r.
    local r.
    polymerase chain r. (PCR)
    r. recovery time
    reverse transcriptase
      polymerase chain r. (RT-PCR)
    vasovagal r.

reagent
    general r.

Real coronary artery scissors

real-time
    r.-t. three-dimensional echocardiography
    r.-t. ultrasonography

ream out

reanastomosis

rebound
    r. angina
    heparin r.

recalcitrant hypertension

recanalization
    argon laser r.
    r. of artery
    balloon occlusive intravascular lysis enhanced r.
    excimer vascular r.
    peripheral laser r.

recanalized artery

recanalizing thrombosis

recannulization

receptor
    adrenergic r.
    A-II r.
    alpha r.
    beta r.
    beta-adrenergic r.
    cell-surface r.
    cholinergic r.
    chylomicron remnant r.
    endothelin A, B r's
    epithelial 5'-nucleotide r.
    Fc r's
    glycoprotein IIb/IIIa r.
    H1 r.
    juxtacapillary r.
    membrane r.
    nuclear r.

receptor-operated calcium channel

recessed balloon septostomy catheter

reciprocal
    r. beat
    r. bigeminy
    r. changes
    r. rhythm
    r. ST depression

reciprocating
    r. macroreentry orthodromic tachycardia
    r. rhythm

reciprocity

reclosure

recoarctation of aorta

recognition protein

recoil
    catheter r.
    elastic r.
    r. wave

recombinant
    r. alpha$_1$ antitrypsin
    r. alteplase
    r. desulfatohirudin

recombinant *(continued)*
r. hirudin
r. lys-plasminogen
r. tissue plasminogen activator (rt-PA)
r. tissue-type plasminogen activator

reconstitution
r. via collaterals
r. via profunda

reconstruction
aortic r.
arterial r.
bifurcated vein graft for vascular r.
Cabral coronary r.
patch graft r.
transannular patch r.
venous r.

recorder
Avionics two-channel Holter r.
Del Mar Avionics three-channel r.
Eigon CardioLoop r.
event r.
24-hour ambulatory electrocardiographic r.
King of Hearts event r.
Marquette Holter r.
MEDILOG ambulatory ECG r.
Oxford Medilog frequency-modulated r.
pulse volume r.
Vas r.

recovery
r. period of myocardium
pressure r.
sinus node r. time

recrudescence

recruitable collateral vessel

rectocardiac reflex

recurrent
r. artery

recurrent *(continued)*
r. interosseous artery
r. intractable ventricular tachycardia
r. mesenteric ischemia
r. mesenteric vascular occlusion
r. myocardial infarction

recurring ectopic beats

recursion
Levinson-Durgin r.

recurvatum
pectus r.

red
r. atrophy
r. cell aplasia
r. hypertension
r. infarct
r. laser
r. man syndrome
r. rubber catheter
r. thrombus

Redifocus guide wire

RediFurl
R. catheter
R. double-lumen balloon
R. single-lumen balloon
R. TaperSeal IAB catheter

redilatation

redirection of inferior vena cava

redistribution
r. imaging
r. myocardial image
pulmonary vascular r.
vascular r.

reduction
afterload r.
gradient r.
preload r.
stapled lung r.

redundant cusp syndrome

reduplication murmur

Reed ventriculorrhaphy

reedswitch of pacemaker

reendothelialization

reentrant
  r. arrhythmia
  r. atrial tachycardia
  r. circuit
  r. loop
  r. mechanism
  r. pathway
  r. supraventricular tachy-
    cardia

reentry
  anatomical r.
  anisotropic r.
  atrial r.
  atrioventricular nodal r.
  AV nodal r.
  Bachmann bundle r.
  bundle branch r.
  functional r.
  intra-atrial r.
  reflected r.
  SA nodal r.
  sinus nodal r.
  ventricular r.

Reeves treadmill protocol

reference
  r. electrode
  r. value

refill
  transcapillary r.

reflectance oximetry

reflecting level

reflection
  epicardial r.
  guide wire r.
  pericardial r.

reflex
  abdominocardiac r.
  Abrams heart r.
  r. angina
  aortic r.

reflex (continued)
  Aschner r.
  Aschner-Dagnini r.
  atriopressor r.
  auriculopressor r.
  autonomic r.
  Bainbridge r.
  baroreceptor r.
  Bezold r.
  Bezold-Jarisch r.
  bregmocardiac r.
  cardiac depressor r.
  carotid sinus r.
  chemoreceptor r.
  Churchill-Cope r.
  cold pressor r.
  coronary r.
  craniocardiac r.
  Cushing r.
  deep tendon r. (DTR)
  diving r.
  Erben r.
  eyeball compression r.
  eyeball-heart r.
  heart r.
  hepatojugular r.
  Hoffman r.
  hyperactive carotid sinus r.
  hypochondrial r.
  ischemic r.
  Livierato r.
  Loven r.
  McDowall r.
  oculocardiac r.
  oculovagal r.
  orthocardiac r.
  pericardial r.
  pneocardiac r.
  pressoreceptor r.
  pressor r.
  psychocardiac r.
  pulmonocoronary r.
  rectocardiac r.
  sinus r.
  r. sympathoexcitation
  r. tachycardia
  vagal r.
  vascular r.
  vasopressor r.

reflex *(continued)*
  venorespiratory r.
  viscerocardiac r.

Reflex
  R. pacemaker

reflexogenic pressosensitivity

reflux
  abdominojugular r.
  cardioesophageal r.
  erosive r.
  esophageal r.
  r. esophagitis
  extraesophageal r.
  gastroesophageal r.
  hepatojugular r.
  valvular r.
  venous r.

refractory
  r. congestive heart failure
  r. to medical therapy
  r. period, effective
  r. period, functional
  r. period, relative
  r. period of electronic
    pacemaker
  r. tachycardia

Refsum disease

regimen
  dosage r.
  exercise r.
  split-course r.
  stepped-care antihyperten-
    sive r.

region
  AN r.
  N r.
  NH r.
  watershed r.

regional
  r. block anesthesia
  r. cerebral blood flow
  r. ejection fraction image
  r. left ventricular function
  r. myocardial blood flow

regional *(continued)*
  r. myocardial uptake of
    thallium
  r. perfusion
  r. vasodilation
  r. wall motion
  r. wall motion abnormality

regression
  r. analysis
  arteriographic r.
  r. equation
  least-squares r.
  linear r.
  multiple r.
  Q wave r.

regular
  r. rate and rhythm (RRR)
  r. sinus rhythm (RSR)

regularly irregular rhythm

regurgitant
  r. flow
  r. fraction
  r. jet
  r. jet area
  r. mitral valve murmur
  r. murmur
  r. pockets
  r. velocity
  r. wave

regurgitation
  aortic r. (AR)
  aortic valve r.
  congenital mitral r.
  ischemic mitral r.
  mitral r. (MR)
  mitral valve r.
  paravalvular r.
  pulmonary valvular r.
  pulmonic r. (PR)
  semilunar valve r.
  tricuspid r. (TR)
  trivial mitral r.
  valvular r.

rehabilitation
  cardiac r.

rehabilitation *(continued)*
    r. exercises
    work r.

Rehbein rib spreader

Reich-Nechtow clamp

reinfarction

Reinhoff
    R. clamp
    R. rib spreader
    R. swan neck clamp
    R. thoracic scissors

Reinhoff-Finochietto rib
    spreader

Reiter
    R. disease
    R. syndrome

rejection
    acute allograft r.
    r. cardiomyopathy
    cardiac transplant r.
    graft r.
    homograft r.
    no infection-no r. (NI-NR)
    organ r.

relapsing
    r. fever
    r. polychondritis

relation
    concentration-effect r.
    diastolic pressure-volu-
        me r.
    end-systolic pressure-volu-
        me r.
    end-systolic stress-dimen-
        sion r.
    force-frequency r.
    force-length r.
    force-velocity r.
    force-velocity-length r.
    force-velocity-volume r.
    Frank-Starling r.
    interval-strength r.
    length-resting tension r.
    length-tension r.

relation *(continued)*
    pressure-volume r.
    resting length-tension r.
    tension-length r.
    ventilation/perfusion r.
    ventricular end-systolic
        pressure-volume r.

relationship
    Laplace r.
    pressure-flow r.
    stress-shortening r.

relative
    r. cardiac dullness
    r. cardiac volume
    r. incompetence
    r. refractory period
    r. risk
    r. wall thickness

relaxation
    diastolic r.
    dynamic r.
    endothelium-mediated r.
    isovolumetric r.
    isovolumic r.
    left ventricular diastolic r.
    r. loading
    smooth muscle r.
    stress r.
    r. time
    r. time index
    ventricular r.

Relay cardiac pacemaker

Reliavac drain

remission
    Legroux r.

remnant
    chylomicron r.

remodeling
    arterial r.
    concentric r.
    ventricular r.

renal
    r. angiography
    r. arteriography

renal *(continued)*
    r. artery
    r. artery bypass graft
    r. artery clamp
    r. artery disease
    r. artery forceps
    r. artery–reverse saphe-
      nous vein bypass
    r. blood vessel
    r. hypertension
    r. vein
    r. vein renin ratio
    r. venography

renal-splanchnic steal

Rendu
    R.-Osler-Weber disease
    R.-Osler-Weber syndrome

renin
    r.-angiotensin
    r.-angiotensin-aldosterone
    r.-angiotensin-aldosterone
      cascade
    r.-angiotensin-aldosterone
      system (RAAS)
    r.-angiotensin blocker
    r.-angiotensin system
    r. inhibitor
    plasma r.

Renografin contrast medium

renogram study

renography

renomedullary lipid

renoprival hypertension

renovascular
    r. angiography
    r. hypertension

Renovist contrast medium

Rentrop
    R. catheter
    R. classification
    R. infusion catheter

reocclusion

repair
    Brom r.
    DeBakey-Creech aneu-
      rysm r.
    Fontan r.
    pericardioplasty in pectus
      excavatum r.

reparative cardiac surgery

reperfusion
    r. arrhythmia
    r. catheter
    emergency r.
    r. injury
    late r.

reperfusion-induced hemorrhage

repetition
    pulse r.
    r. rate
    r. time (TR)

repetitive
    r. monomorphic ventricu-
      lar tachycardia
    r. paroxysmal ventricular
      tachycardia

replacement
    aortic valve r. (AVR)
    Cosgrove mitral valve r.
    mitral valve r. (MVR)
    supra-annular mitral val-
      ve r.
    valve r.

repletion

replication

repolarization
    atrial r.
    benign early r.
    delayed r.
    early r.
    early rapid r.
    early r.
    final rapid r.
    ventricular r.

repression

reptilase

rescue
  r. angioplasty
  citrovorum r.

ResCue Key

rescuing pacemaker

Research Medical straight multiple-holed aortic cannula

resection
  activation map-guided surgical r.
  atrial septal r.
  r. clamp
  endocardial r.
  endocardial-to-endocardial r.
  infundibular wedge r.
  lesser r.
  myotomy-myectomy-septal r.
  selective subendocardial r.
  septal r.
  transmural r.
  wedge-shaped sleeve aneurysm r.

reserve
  cardiac r.
  cardiopulmonary r.
  contractile r.
  coronary arterial r.
  coronary flow r.
  coronary vascular r.
  coronary vasodilator r.
  diastolic r.
  extraction r.
  Frank-Starling r.
  heart rate r.
  left ventricular systolic function r.
  myocardial r.
  preload r.
  regional contractile r.
  respiratory r.

reserve *(continued)*
  systolic r.
  vasodilator r.
  ventricular r.

reservoir
  Cardiometrics cardiotomy r.
  cardiotomy r.
  Cobe cardiotomy r.
  double bubble flushing r.
  drug delivery r.
  r. face mask
  Intersept cardiotomy r.
  Jostra cardiotomy r.
  Polystan cardiotomy r.
  Sci-Med extracorporeal silicone rubber r.
  Shiley cardiotomy r.
  William Harvey cardiotomy r.

reset nodus sinuatrialis

residual
  r. gradient
  r. jet
  r. stenosis
  r. volume

resistance
  afterload r.
  aortic valve r.
  arteriolar r.
  calculated r.
  cerebrovascular r.
  coronary vascular r.
  elastic r.
  hydraulic r.
  peripheral vascular r.
  pulmonary arteriolar r.
  pulmonary vascular r.
  r. ratio
  systemic vascular r.
  total peripheral r.
  total pulmonary r.
  vascular r.
  vascular peripheral r.
  venous r.

resistant hypertension

resonant to percussion

respiration
aerobic r.
anaerobic r.
cell r.
Cheyne-Stokes r.
Corrigan r.
forced r.
labored r.
unlabored r.

respiratory
r. acidosis
r. alkalosis
r. arrest
r. arrhythmia
r. burst
r. capacity
r. center
r. collapse
r. distress
r. embarrassment
r. excursion
r. failure
r. murmur
r. pulse
r. rate
r. reserve
r. stridor

respiratory-dependent pacemaker

response
antibody immune r.
cardiac r.
cellular-mediated immu-
ne r.
controlled ventricular r.
delayed r.
heart rate r.
vascular r.
rapid ventricular r.
slow ventricular r.

Res-Q
R. ACD
R. ACD implantable cardio-
verter-defibrillator

Res-Q *(continued)*
R. AICD

rest
r. angina
r. ejection fraction
r. and exercise gated nu-
clear angiography
r.-exercise equilibrium radionuclide ventriculogra-
phy
r.-exercise gated nuclear
angiogram
r. hypoxemia
r. metabolism/stress perfusion protocol
r. pain
r. radionuclide angiography

rested state contraction

restenosis
aortic valve r.
false r.
intrastent r.
r. lesion
mitral r.
post-balloon angioplasty r.
pulmonary valve r.
tricuspid r.
true r.

restenotic

resting
r. cardiac output
r. electrocardiogram
r. end-systolic wall stress
r. heart rate
r. length-tension relation
r. membrane potential
r. MUGA scan
r. pulse rate
r. pressure
r. tachycardia
r. value

rest-redistribution thallium 201
imaging

restrictive
r. cardiomyopathy

restrictive *(continued)*
 r. functional impairment
 r. heart disease

resuscitation
 cardiac r.
 cardiopulmonary r. (CPR)
 r. cart
 closed-chest cardiopulmonary r.
 heart-lung r.
 mechanical cardiopulmon-
  ary r.
 mouth-to-mouth r.
 open chest cardiac r.

resuscitator
 Ambu r.
 BagEasy disposable man-
  ual r.
 cardiopulmonary r.
 First Response manual r.
 heart-lung r.
 Hope r.
 Hudson Lifesaver r.
 Kreiselman r.
 Ohio Hope r.
 Robertshaw bag r.
 Safe Response manual r.
 SureGrip manual r.

rete
 r. arteriosum dermidis
 r. arteriosum subpapillare
 articular r.
 articular cubital r.
 articular r. of elbow
 articular r. of knee
 r. canalis hypoglossi
 carpal r., dorsal
 r. cutaneum
 dorsal venous r. of foot
 dorsal venous r. of hand
 r. foraminis ovalis
 malleolar r., lateral
 malleolar r., medial
 r. mirabile
 r. olecrani
 r. of patella
 r. patellae

rete *(continued)*
 plantar r.
 plantar venous r.
 r. subpapillare
 subpapillary r.
 r. vasculosum
 r. venosum

reticularis
 livedo r.

reticular pattern

reticulocyte count

reticuloendothelial system

reticulonodular

reticulum *pl.* reticula
 agranular r.
 Chiari's r.
 endoplasmic r.
 granular r.
 sarcoplasmic r.

retina
 cyanosis retinae

retinal
 r. artery
 r. degeneration
 r. disease
 r. edema
 r. embolism
 r. exudate
 r. infarction
 occlusion of r. arterioles
 r. vasculitis
 r. vessel

retinopathy
 arteriosclerotic r.
 diabetic r.
 exudative r.
 hypertensive r.
 Purtscher angiopathic r.

retisolution

retispersion

retour
 rale de r.

retraction
  intercostal r's
  postrheumatic cusp r.
  sternal intercostal r's
  subcostal r's
  substernal r's
  suprasternal r's
  r. of vena cava

retractor
  abdominal vascular r.
  Ablaza aortic wall r.
  Ablaza-Blanco cardiac
    valve r.
  Adson r.
  Allison r.
  Ankeney sternal r.
  aortic valve r.
  Army-Navy r.
  atrial r.
  atrial septal r.
  Bahnson sternal r.
  Beckman r.
  Burford rib r.
  cardiovascular r.
  Carter mitral valve r.
  Collin sternal self-retain-
    ing r.
  Cooley r.
  Cooley atrial valve r.
  Cooley carotid r.
  Cooley femoral r.
  Cooley-Marz sternal r.
  Cooley mitral valve r.
  Cooley MPC cardiovascu-
    lar r.
  Cooley sternotomy r.
  Coryllos r.
  Cosgrove mitral valve r.
  Crawford aortic r.
  Cushing vein r.
  Darling popliteal r.
  Davidson r.
  Davidson scapular r.
  Deaver r.
  DeBakey-Balfour r.
  DeBakey chest r.
  DeBakey-Cooley r.

retractor (continued)
  DeBakey-Cooley Deaver-
    type r.
  Denver-Wells atrial r.
  Denver-Wells sternal r.
  Desmarres cardiovascu-
    lar r.
  Desmarres vein r.
  epicardial r.
  Favaloro self-retaining ster-
    nal r.
  Finochietto-Geissendorfer
    rib r.
  Frater intracardiac r.
  Garrett peripheral vascu-
    lar r.
  Geissendorfer rib r.
  Gelpi r.
  Gerbode sternal r.
  Ghazi rib r.
  Goligher sternal-lifting r.
  Gross patent ductus r.
  Gross-Pomeranz-Watkins r.
  Haight-Finochietto rib r.
  Haight rib r.
  Harken rib r.
  Harrington-Pemberton r.
  Harrington r.
  Hartzler rib r.
  Hedblom rib r.
  Henley carotid r.
  Hibbs r.
  Himmelstein sternal r.
  intracardiac r.
  Karmody vascular spring r.
  Kelly r.
  Kirklin atrial r.
  Koenig vein r.
  Krasky r.
  Langenbeck-Cushing vein r.
  leaflet r.
  Lemmon self-retaining ster-
    nal r.
  Lemmon sternal r.
  Lemole atrial valve self-re-
    taining r.
  Lemole mitral valve r.
  Liddicoat aortic valve r.
  Lukens thymus r.

retractor *(continued)*
    lung r.
    malleable r.
    Meyerding r.
    Miller-Senn r.
    mitral valve r.
    Morse sternal r.
    Morse valve r.
    neonatal sternal r.
    O'Brien rib r.
    Ochsner vascular r.
    Parsonnet epicardial r.
    patent ductus r.
    peripheral vascular r.
    rake r.
    Richardson r.
    Rochester atrial septal r.
    Ross aortic valve r.
    Rultract internal mammary
      artery r.
    Sachs vein r.
    Sauerbruch r.
    Semb r.
    self-retaining r.
    Senn r.
    Shuletz-Paul rib r.
    sternal r.
    sternotomy r.
    Stille heart r.
    Theis vein r.
    thymus r.
    U.S. Army r.
    vascular spring r.
    vein r.
    vein hook r.
    ventriculogram r.
    Volkmann r.
    Walter-Deaver r.
    Weitlaner r.
    Wylie renal vein r.

retrieval
    intravascular foreign
      body r.

retrocardiac
    r. abnormality
    r. space

retroconduction

retroesophageal aorta

retrograde
    r. aortogram
    r. arteriogram
    r. atherectomy
    r. atrial activation mapping
    r. beat
    r. blood flow across valve
    r. cardiac perfusion
    r. catheter insertion
    r. catheterization
    r. conduction
    r. cardiac perfusion
    r. embolism
    r. fashion
    r. fast pathway
    r. femoral approach
    r. filling
    r. flow
    r. injection
    r. percutaneous femoral ar-
      tery approach
    r. P wave
    r. refractory period
    r. valvuloplasty
    r. valvulotome

retropectoral pocket

retroperfusion
    coronary sinus r.
    r. catheter
    synchronized r.

retrosternal
    r. chest pain
    r. thyroid

retrotracheal space

retrovirus

Retter needle

return
    anomalous pulmonary ven-
      ous r.
    r. extrasystole
    r. flow
    pulmonary venous r.
    rattle of r.

return *(continued)*
   systemic venous r.
   venous r.

returning cycle

Retzius veins

Reul
   R. aortic clamp
   R. coronary artery scissors
   R. coronary forceps

reusable vein stripper

revascularization
   coronary r.
   direct myocardial r.
   heart laser r.
   myocardial r.
   percutaneous transluminal
      coronary r. (PTCR)
   repeat r.
   surgical r.
   transmyocardial r. (TMR)
   transmyocardial laser r.

revascularized

Reveal insertable loop recorder

revehent

reverberation
   r. artifact
   echo r.

reversal
   r. lead

reverse
   r. saphenous vein
   r. transcriptase polymerase
      chain reaction (RT-PCR)
   r. transcriptase polymerase
      chain reaction test

reversed
   r. arm leads
   r. bypass
   r. coarctation
   r. ductus arteriosus
   r. paradoxical pulse
   r. reciprocal rhythm

reversed *(continued)*
   r. rhythm
   r. saphenous vein graft
   r. shunt
   r. 3 sign

reversible
   r. ischemic neurologic de-
      fect

reversion

rewarm

Reye syndrome

Reynolds vascular clamp

Reynolds-Jameson vessel scissors

RF
   radiofrequency
   rapid filling
   rheumatic fever

RF-generated thermal balloon
   catheter

Rh
   Rhesus
      Rh antibody
      Rh factor

rhabdomyolysis

rhabdomyoma
   cardiac r.

rhabdomyosarcoma

RHD
   rheumatic heart disease

rheocardiography

rheography
   light reflection r.

rheologic
   r. change
   r. therapy

rheology

rheumatic
   r. aortitis
   r. arteritis

rheumatic *(continued)*
    r. carditis
    r. endocarditis
    r. fever (RF)
    r. heart disease (RHD)
    r. mitral insufficiency
    r. mitral valve stenosis
    r. myocarditis
    r. pericarditis
    r. valvular disease
    r. valvulitis

rheumatica
    angina r.

rheumatism of heart

rheumatoid
    r. arteritis
    r. arthritis (RA)
    r. factor

rhythm
    accelerated atrioventricular (AV) junctional r.
    accelerated idioventricular r.
    accelerated junctional r.
    agonal r.
    atrial r.
    atrial escape r.
    atrioventricular (AV) r.
    atrioventricular (AV) junctional r.
    atrioventricular (AV) junctional escape r.
    atrioventricular (AV) nodal r.
    auriculoventricular r.
    baseline r.
    bigeminal r.
    cantering r.
    cardiac r.
    circus r.
    concealed r.
    coronary nodal r.
    coronary sinus r.
    converted r.
    coupled r.
    r. disturbance
    ectopic r.

rhythm *(continued)*
    embryocardia r.
    escape r.
    fibrillation r.
    gallop r.
    idiojunctional r.
    idionodal r.
    idioventricular r.
    irregular r.
    irregularly irregular r.
    junctional r.
    junctional escape r.
    lower nodal r.
    midnodal r.
    mu r.
    nodal escape r.
    nodal r.
    nonparoxysmal nodal r.
    normal sinus r. (NSR)
    paced r.
    pacemaker r.
    paroxysmal nodal r.
    parasystolic r.
    pendulum r.
    predominant r.
    pulseless idioventricular r.
    quadrigeminal r.
    quadruple r.
    reciprocal r.
    reciprocating r.
    reentrant r.
    regular rate and r. (RRR)
    regular sinus r. (RSR)
    regularly irregular r.
    reversed reciprocal r.
    reversed r.
    sinoatrial r.
    sinoventricular r.
    sinus r.
    slow escape r.
    r. strip
    supraventricular r.
    systolic r.
    systolic gallop r.
    tic-tac r.
    trainwheel r.
    trigeminal r.
    triple r.
    ventricular escape r.

rhythm *(continued)*
    ventricular r.
    wide complex r.

rhythmicity

RhythmScan

RIA
    radioimmunoassay

rib
    r. approximator
    r. cutter
    r. elevator
    r. guillotine
    r. margin
    r. notching
    r. raspatory
    r. rongeur forceps
    r. stripper

rib contractor
    Adams r. c.
    baby r. c.
    Bailey r. c.
    Bailey-Gibbon r. c.
    Cooley r. c.
    Graham r. c.
    Rienhoff-Finochietto r. c.
    Sellor r. c.
    Waterman r. c.

ribosome

rib shears
    Baer r. s.
    Bethune r. s.
    Brunner r. s.
    Cooley first r. s.
    Coryllos r. s.
    Duval-Coryllos r. s.
    Giertz-Shoemaker r. s.
    Gluck r. s.
    Moure-Coryllos r. s.
    Potts r. s.
    Sauerbruch r. s.
    Shoemaker r. s.
    Stille r. s.
    Stille-pattern r. s.
    Thompson r. s.
    Walton r. s.

rib spreader
    Burford r. s.
    Burford-Finochietto r. s.
    Davis r. s.
    DeBakey r. s.
    Finochietto r. s.
    Gerbode r. s.
    Haight r. s.
    Harken r. s.
    Hertzler baby r. s.
    Lemmon r. s.
    Lilienthal-Sauerbruch r. s.
    Matson r. s.
    McGuire r. s.
    Miltex r. s.
    Nelson r. s.
    Nissen r. s.
    Overholt-Finochietto r. s.
    Rehbein r. s.
    Rienhoff r. s.
    Rienhoff-Finochietto r. s.
    Sweet r. s.
    Sweet-Burford r. s.
    Sweet-Finochietto r. s.
    Theis r. s.
    Tuffier r. s.
    Weinberg r. s.
    Wilson r. s.

Richardson retractor

Richet aneurysm

Ricketts-Abrams technique

rickettsial
    r. endocarditis
    r. myocarditis

Rider-Moeller
    R.-M. cardia dilator

riding
    r. embolism
    r. embolus

Riegel pulse

Rienhoff
    R. arterial clamp
    R. arterial forceps
    R. dissector

Rienhoff *(continued)*
    R. rib spreader

Riesman myocardosis

right
    r. ankle indices
    r. anterior oblique (RAO)
    r. anterior oblique equivalent
    r. anterior oblique position
    r. anterior oblique projection
    r. aortic arch
    r. atrial appendage
    r. atrial enlargement (RAE)
    r. atrial myxoma
    r. atrial pressure
    r. atrial thrombus
    r. atrium (RA)
    r. axis deviation
    r. bundle branch block (RBBB)
    r. common carotid artery
    r. coronary artery (RCA)
    r. coronary catheter
    r. heart
    r. heart bypass
    r. heart catheter
    r. heart catheterization
    r. heart failure
    r. internal jugular artery
    r. internal mammary artery (RIMA)
    r. Judkins catheter
    r. parasternal impulse
    r. pulmonary artery
    r. and retrograde left heart catheterization
    r. subclavian artery
    r.-to-left shunt
    r.-to-left shunt with pulmonic stenosis r. upper sternal border
    r. ventricle (RV)
    r. ventricular apex
    r. ventricular assist device
    r. ventricular cardiomyopathy

right *(continued)*
    r. ventricular decompensation
    r. ventricular diastolic collapse
    r. ventricular diastolic pressure
    r. ventricular dimension
    r. ventricular disease
    r. ventricular dysplasia
    r. ventricular ejection fraction
    r. ventricular end-diastolic pressure
    r. ventricular failure
    r. ventricular function
    r. ventricular heave
    r. ventricular hypertrophy (RVH)
    r. ventricular hypoplasia
    r. ventricular infarction
    r. ventricular inflow obstruction
    r. ventricular lift
    r. ventricular mean
    r. ventricular myocardial dysplasia
    r. ventricular myxoma
    r. ventricular outflow obstruction
    r. ventricular outflow tract
    r. ventricular outflow tract tachycardia
    r. ventricular systolic pressure
    r. ventricular systolic time interval
    r. ventricular wall motion

right-angle
    r.-a. chest catheter
    r.-a. chest tube

right-sided
    r.-s. endocarditis
    r.-s. filling pressures
    r.-s. heart failure

rightward axis

Rigiflex TTS balloon catheter

rigor
    calcium r.

Riley-Cournand equation

Riley-Day syndrome

Riley arterial needle

RIMA
    right internal mammary ar-
        tery

Rindfleisch fold

ring
    aortic r.
    atrial r.
    atrioventricular r.
    atrioventricular valve r.
    Bickel r.
    Carpentier r.
    circumaortic venous r.
    coronary r.
    Crawford suture r.
    double-flanged valve se-
        wing r.
    Duran annuloplasty r.
    fibrous r's of heart
    knitted sewing r.
    Lower r.
    metal sewing r.
    mitral r.
    mitral valve r.
    plastic sewing r.
    prosthetic valve sewing r.
    prosthetic valve suture r.
    Puig Massana annuloplas-
        ty r.
    Puig Massana–Shiley annu-
        loplasty r.
    St. Jude annuloplasty r.
    Sculptor annuloplasty r.
    sewing r.
    supra-annular suture r.
    tricuspid r.
    tricuspid valve r.
    Tru-Arc blood vessel r.
    Universal valve prosthesis
        sewing r.
    Valtrac absorbable biofrag-
        mentable anastomosis r.

ring (continued)
    valve r.
    vascular r.
    r. of Vieussens

Ringer
    R. lactate
    R. solution

risk
    r. assessment
    r.-benefit analysis
    r. category
    empiric r.
    r. factors for cardiac dis-
        ease
    r. factors for coronary ar-
        tery disease
    r. potential
    recurrent r.
    sudden death r.
    surgical r.

Riolan
    anastomosis of R.

rising pulse

Ritchie catheter

Riva-Rocci sphygmomanometer

Rivero
    R.-Carvallo effect
    R.-Carvallo maneuver
    R.-Carvallo sign

Roadrunner PC guide wire

Robertson sign

Robicsek vascular probe

Rochester
    R. aortic vent needle
    R. atrial septal retractor
    R. awl
    R. knife
    R. mitral stenosis knife
    R. needle
    R.-Kocher clamp
    R.-Mixter arterial forceps
    R.-Péan clamp
    R.-Rankin arterial forceps

rocker
  hematology r.

Rockey mediastinal cannula

Rocky Mountain spotted fever

Rodrigo equation

Rodriguez
  R. aneurysm
  R. catheter

Roe aortic tourniquet clamp

roentgenogram
  apical lordotic r.
  chest r.

Roesler-Dressler infarction

Roger
  R. bruit
  bruit de R.
  R. disease
  maladie de R.
  R. murmur

Rogers sphygmomanometer

Roho mattress

Rokitansky disease

roller pump

Rolleston rule

Romano-Ward syndrome

ROMI
  rule out myocardial infarction

rongeur
  aortic valve r.
  Bailey aortic valve r.
  Bethune rib r.
  Brock cardiac dilator r.
  Cushing r.
  Dale thoracic r.
  Giertz r.
  Leksell r.
  Sauerbruch r.
  Semb r.

R on T
  R o. T phenomenon
  R o. T premature ventricu-
    lar contraction

Roos
  R. first-rib shears
  R. procedure for thoracic
    outlet syndrome
  R. test

root
  aortic r.
  aortic r. dimension
  r. injection
  r. perfusion

root-mean-square voltage

Rosai-Dorfman disease

Rosalki technique

rose
  r. spot
  R. tamponade

Rosen guide wire

Rosenbach syndrome

Rosenblum rotating adapter

rosette

Ross
  R. aortic retractor
  R. needle
  R. procedure
  R. retractor
  R. River virus

Rossetti modification of Nissen
  fundoplication

rotablation

Rotablator
  R. atherectomy device
  R. catheter
  Heart Technology R.
  R. wire

Rotacamera

Rotacs
  R. guide wire

Rotacs *(continued)*
    R. motorized catheter
    R. rotational atherectomy
        device
    R. system

rotary atherectomy device

rotating disk oxygenation

rotation
    clockwise r.
    counterclockwise r.
    shoulder r.

rotational
    r. ablation
    r. ablation laser
    r. atherectomy device
    r. atherectomy system
    r. coronary atherectomy
    r. dynamic angioplasty
        catheter

Rotch sign

Rotex
    R. needle
    R. II biopsy needle

Rothschild sign

Roth spot

rotoslide

Roubin-Gianturco flexible coil
    stent

Rougnon-Heberden disease

rouleaux formation

round heart

round-robin classification

rove magnetic catheter

Royal Flush angiographic flush
    catheter

Rozanski precordial lead place-
    ment system

R–P interval

R-Port implantable vascular ac-
    cess system

R–R
    R–R cycle
    R–R interval

R–R'
    R–R' interval
    R–R' pattern

RRR
    regular rate and rhythm

RS4 pacemaker

RS complex

rS deflection

RSR
    regular sinus rhythm

RSR' triphasic pattern on EKG

RS–T
    RS–T interval
    RS–T segment

R-synchronous VVT pacemaker

rt-PA
    recombinant tissue plas-
        minogen activator
    catabolism of rt-PA
    double-chain rt-PA

RT-PCR
    reverse transcriptase
        polymerase chain reac-
        tion

RTV total artificial heart

rub
    friction r.
    pericardial r.
    pericardial friction r.
    pleuropericardial r.
    saddle leather friction r.

rubella syndrome

Rubinstein-Taybi syndrome

rubidium-82 imaging

rubor
    dependent r.

ruby laser

Ruel
    R. aorta clamp
    R. forceps

Rugelski arterial forceps

Ruiz-Cohen round expander

rule
    r. of bigeminy
    Liebermeister r.
    r. out myocardial infarction
        (ROMI)
    Rolleston r.
    Simpson r.

rumble
    Austin Flint r.
    booming r.
    diastolic r.
    filling r.
    mid-diastolic r.
    presystolic r.
    protodiastolic r.

rumbling diastolic murmur

Rumel
    R. cardiac tourniquet
    R. cardiovascular tourni-
        quet
    R. catheter
    R. myocardial clamp
    R. myocardial tourniquet
    R. thoracic clamp
    R. thoracic-dissecting for-
        ceps
    R. thoracic forceps

Rummo disease

Rumpel-Leeds test

runoff
    aortic r.
    aortofemoral arterial r.
    aortogram with distal r.
    arterial r.

runoff (continued)
    r. arteriogram
    digital r.
    distal r.
    venous r.

run
    r's of arrhythmia
    r's of PVCs
    r's of tachycardia
    r's of ventricular tachycar-
        dia

rupture
    abdominal aortic aneu-
        rysm r.
    aortic r.
    balloon r.
    cardiac r.
    chamber r.
    chordae tendineae r.
    chordal r.
    interventricular septal r.
    myocardial r.
    nonpenetrating r.
    papillary muscle r.
    penetrating r.
    pericardial r.
    plaque r.
    traumatic r.
    valve r.
    ventricular free wall r.
    ventricular septal r.

ruptured
    r. abdominal aortic aneu-
        rysm
    r. aortic aneurysm
    r. blood vessels
    r. cerebral aneurysm
    r. sinus of Valsalva

Ruskin forceps

Russian tissue forceps

RV
    right ventricle

RVAD
    right ventricular assist de-
        vice

RVAD *(continued)*
> RVAD centrifugal right ventricular assist device

RVE
> right ventricular enlargement

RVH
> right ventricular hypertrophy

Rx
> Rx perfusion catheter
> Rx Streak balloon catheter

Rx5000 cardiac pacing system

RX stent delivery system

Rychener-Weve electrode

S
   septum

S₁
   first heart sound
      S_1Q_3 pattern
      $S_1Q_3T_3$ pattern
      S_1S_2 interval
      $S_1S_2S_3$ pattern

S₂
   second heart sound
      fixed splitting of S_2
      paradoxical splitting of S_2
      physiological split S_2
      S_2OS interval

S₃
   third heart sound
      S_3 gallop

S₄
   fourth heart sound
      S_4 gallop

S₇
   summation gallop
      S_7 gallop

SA, S-A
   sinoatrial
      SA nodal reentrant tachycardia
      SA node

SAB
   sinoatrial block

Sabin-Feldman dye test

sabot
   coeur en s.
   s. heart

sac
   aneurysmal s.
   aortic s. (AS)
   heart s.
   Hilton s.
   Lap S.
   lateral s.

sac *(continued)*
   Lower's s's
   pericardial s.
   truncoaortic s.

saccular
   s. aneurysm

sacculated
   s. empyema

sacculation
   localized s.

Sachs vein retractor

sacral edema

sacrococcygeal aorta

SACT
   sinoatrial conduction time

saddle
   s. embolism
   s. embolus
   s. leather friction rub
   s. thrombus

Sade modification of Norwood procedure

Sadowsky hook wire

SAECG
   signal-averaged electrocardiogram

Safe-T-Coat heparin-coated thermodilution catheter

Safe-T-Tube
   Montgomery S.

safety
   s. guidewire
   radiation s.
   s. ribbon

SafTouch catheter

sag
   ST s.

sagging ST segment

sagittal
    s. cuts
    s. plane
    s. view

St. Jude
    S. J. annuloplasty ring
    S. J. bileaflet prosthetic
        valve
    S. J. cardiac device
    S. J. composite prosthetic
        valve
    S. J. heart valve prosthesis
    S. J. Medical bileaflet valve
    S. J. Medical bileaflet tilt-
        ing-disk aortic valve
    S. J. Medical Port-Access
    S. J. mitral valve
    S. J. prosthetic aortic valve
    S. J. valve prosthesis

St. Thomas Hospital cardiople-
    gia

St. Thomas solution

St. Vitus dance

Sala cells

Salibi carotid artery clamp

salicylate

saline
    cold s.
    half normal s. (0.45% NaCl)
    heparinized s.
    iced s.
    normal s. (0.9% NaCl)
    s. loading
    s. slush
    s. solution
    topical cold s.

Salkowski test

salt
    dietary s.
    ethylenediaminetetraacetic
        acid disodium s.
    gold s.

salt (continued)
    s. of nickel
    persulfate s.
    s. of platinum
    s. restriction (restricted
        diet)
    s. wasting

salt-and-pepper appearance

salt-and-water dependent hy-
    pertension

saltans
    thrombophlebitis s.

salt-depletion syndrome

salt-free diet

salting-out procedure

saluresis

saluretic agent

salute
    allergic s.

saluting

salvage
    s. balloon angioplasty
    limb s.
    myocardial s.

salves
    tachycardia en s.

salvo
    s. of beats
    s. of premature ventricular
        complexes
    s. of ventricular tachycar-
        dia

SAM
    systolic anterior motion
    systolic aortic motion
        SAM system

Sam Levine sign

sampling
    bioptic s.

sampling *(continued)*
  blood s.
  chorionic villus s.

Samuels
  S. forceps
  S. hemoclip

SAN
  sinoatrial node

San
  S. Joaquin Valley disease
  S. Joaquin Valley fever

Sanborn metabolator

Sanchez-Cascos cardioauditory syndrome

sandbag

Sanders bed

Sandhoff disease

Sandifer syndrome

Sandler-Dodge area-length method

Sandman system

Sandrock test

sandwich
  s. enzyme-linked immuno-sorbent assay
  s. patch
  s. patch enclosure

sanguine

sanguineous

sanguinis
  ictus s.

sanguinous

Sansom sign

SaO$_2$
  arterial oxygen saturation

sap
  cell s.
  nuclear s.

saphena

saphenectomy

saphenofemoral
  s. junction
  s. system

saphenography

saphenous
  greater s. vein
  s. vein
  s. vein bypass graft angiography
  s. vein cannula
  s. vein graft
  s. vein varicosity

sarcoidosis
  cardiac s.

sarcolemmal
  s. calcium channel
  s. level
  s. membrane

sarcolemma lipid

sarcoma
  cardiac s.
  Kaposi s. (KS)
  metastatic s.
  pseudo-Kaposi s.
  soft tissue s.

sarcomatous tumor

sarcomere

sarcoplasmic
  s. reticulum
  s. reticulum-associated glycolytic enzymes

sarcosporidiosis

sarcotubular system

Sarnoff aortic clamp

Sarns
  S. aortic arch cannula
  S. electric saw
  S. intracardiac suction tube

Sarns *(continued)*
S. membrane oxygenator (SMO)
S. soft-flow aortic cannula
S. two-stage cannula
S. ventricular assist device
S. wire-reinforced catheter

Sarot
S. artery forceps
S. bronchus clamp

SART
sinoatrial recovery time

SAS
sleep apnea syndrome

satellite
centriolar s.
chromosomal s.
s. lesion

satellitism

Satinsky
S. aortic clamp
S. clamp
S. scissors
S. vascular clamp
S. vena cava clamp

Satterthwaite method

saturation
arterial s.
arterial oxygen s. (SaO_2)
s. index
mixed venous oxygen s. (SvO_2)
oxygen s.
step-up in oxygen s.
s. time
venous s.

saucerize

Sauerbruch
S. retractor
S. rib shears
S. rongeur

sausaging of vein

Sauvage
S. filamentous prosthesis

Sauvage *(continued)*
S. filamentous velour Dacron arterial graft material

saw
Gigli s.
Hall sternal s.
oscillating s.
oscillating sternotomy s.
Sarns electric s.
sternotomy s.
sternum s.
Stryker s.

sawtooth
s. pattern
s. wave

Sawyer operation

SB
sinus bradycardia

SBE
subacute bacterial endocarditis
SBE prophylaxis

SBF
systemic blood flow

SBP
systemic blood pressure

SCAD
spontaneous coronary artery dissection

SCA-EX
SCA-EX 7F graft
SCA-EX ShortCutter catheter
SCA-EX ShortCutter catheter with rotating blades

scalar
s. electrocardiogram
s. leads

scale
activity s.
Borg numerical s.
Borg treadmill exertion s.
cardiac adjustment s.

scale *(continued)*
    dyspnea s.
    French s.
    Glasgow Coma S.
    gray s.
    Grossman s.
    Health Locus of Control S.
    Holmes-Rahe s.
    Karnovsky rating s.
    Paykel s.
    Psychosocial Adjustment
      to Illness S.
    Tennant distress s.
    Toronto Alexithymia S.
    visual analogue s. (VAS)
    voxel gray s.
    Wigle s.

scalenus anticus syndrome

scalloped commissure

scalloping

scalp
    s. electrode
    s. pH

scalpel

scan
    CardioTec s.
    carotid duplex s.
    cine s.
    s. converter
    CT s.
    dipyridamole thallium-
      201 s.
    duplex s.
    gallium s.
    gated cardiac s.
    gated equilibrium blood
      pool s.
    HRCT s.
    isotope-labeled s.
    M-mode s.
    milk s.
    MUGA (multiple gated ac-
      quisition) blood pool ra-
      dionuclide s.
    perfusion lung s.
    PET s.

scan *(continued)*
    PYP s.
    redistributed thallium s.
    resting MUGA (multiple
      gated acquisition) s.
    R to R s.
    scintillation s.
    sector s.
    sestamibi s.
    SPECT thallium s.
    stress thallium s.
    tebo s.
    teboroxime s.
    technetium-99m hexami-
      bi s.
    technetium-99m pyrophos-
      phate myocardial s.
    thin-slice CT s.
    ultrafast CT s.
    ventilation perfusion s.

Scanlan vessel dilator

scanner
    Biosound wide-angle mono-
      plane ultrasound s.
    CardioData MK-3 Holter s.
    computed tomography s.
    Corometrics Doppler s.
    DelMar Avionics s.
    Diasonics Cardiovue
      SectOR s.
    Imatron C-100 tomograph-
      ic s.
    Imatron Ultrafast CT s.
    phased array section s.
    ultrafast computed tomo-
      graphic s.
    Ultrafast CT s.

scanning
    duplex s.
    electronic s.
    s. electron microscope
      (SEM)
    fluorodopamine positron
      emission tomographic s.
    s. format
    gated blood-pool s.
    infarct avid s.
    interlaced s.

scanning *(continued)*
    MUGA s.
    multiple gated acquisi-
      tion s.
    progressive s.
    radionuclide s.
    thallium s.

scanography

scar
    s. formation on myocar-
      dium
    infarct s.
    infarcted s.
    myocardial s.
    nonviable s.
    well demarcated s.
    zipper s.

scarlatinosa
    angina s.

scarlet fever

Scarpa
    S. fascia
    S. method

scarring
    apical s.

Scatchard plot analysis

scatter
    Compton s.

scattered echo

scattergram

scatterplot smoothing tech-
    nique

scavenger
    s. cell pathway
    lysophosphatidylcholine s.
    oxygen radical s.

scavenging tube

SCD
    sudden cardiac death

Schafer method of artificial res-
    piration

Schapiro sign

Schatz
    S.-Palmaz intravascular
      stent
    S.-Palmaz tubular mesh
      stent

Schaumann disease

Schede thoracoplasty

Scheffé test

Scheie syndrome

Schellong test

Schellong-Strisower phenome-
    non

Schenk-Eichelter vena cava
    plastic filter procedure

Schepelmann sign

Schick sign

Schiff test

Schiller method

Schlesinger solution

Schlichter test

Schmidt-Lanterman clefts

Schmitt-Erlanger model of reen-
    try

Schmorl furrow

Schneider
    S. catheter
    S. index
    S. PTCA instruments
    S. stent
    S. Wallstent
    S.-Meier-Magnum system
    S.-Shiley balloon
    S.-Shiley catheter

Schnidt
    S. clamp
    S. passer

Scholten
  S. endomyocardial bioptome
  S. endomyocardial bioptome and biopsy forceps

Schonander
  S. film changer
  S. procedure
  S. technique

Schoonmaker
  S. catheter
  S. femoral catheter
  S. multipurpose catheter

Schoonmaker-King single catheter technique

Schott treatment

Schüller method

Schultz angina

Schultze test

Schumacher aorta clamp

Schwarten
  S. balloon dilation catheter
  S. LP balloon catheter
  S. LP guidewire

Schwartz clamp

scie
  bruit de s.

Sci-Med
  S. angioplasty catheter
  S. Bandit PTCA catheter
  S. Dispatch over-the-wire catheter
  S. extracorporeal silicone rubber reservoir
  S. guiding catheter
  S. Ranger over-the-wire balloon catheter
  S. skinny catheter
  S. SSC skinny balloon catheter
  S. Transport dilatation balloon catheter

Sci-Med *(continued)*
  S. UltraCross profile imaging catheter

scimitar
  s.-shaped flap
  s. syndrome

scintigram
  pyrophosphate s.

scintigraphic perfusion defect

scintigraphy
  acute infarct s.
  AMA-Fab s.
  dipyridamole thallium-201 s.
  dual intracoronary s.
  exercise thallium s.
  exercise thallium-201 s.
  FFA-labeled s.
  gated blood pool s.
  indium-111 s.
  infarct avid s.
  infarct-avid hot-spot s.
  infarct-avid myocardial s.
  iodine-131 MIBG s.
  labeled FFA s.
  microsphere perfusion s.
  myocardial cold-spot perfusion s.
  myocardial perfusion s.
  myocardial viability s.
  NEFA s.
  perfusion s.
  planar thallium s.
  pulmonary s.
  pyrophosphate s.
  single-photon gamma s.
  SPECT s.
  stress thallium s.
  Tc-PYP s.
  Tc-99 sestamibi s.
  technetium Tc 99m pyrophosphate s.
  thallium-201 myocardial s.
  thallium-201 myocardial perfusion s.
  thallium-201 planar s.
  thallium-201 SPECT s.

scintillating speckle pattern

scintillation
  s. camera
  s. cocktail
  s. probe
  s. scan

scintiphotography

scintiscan
  technetium-99m stannous
    pyrophosphate s.

scintiscanner

scintiview

scirrhous carcinoma

scissors
  bandage s.
  Beall s.
  Beall circumflex artery s.
  Blum arterial s.
  Church s.
  coronary artery s.
  Crafoord thoracic s.
  curved s.
  DeBakey endarterectomy s.
  De Martel s.
  De Martel vascular s.
  Duffield cardiovascular s.
  Dumont thoracic s.
  Finochietto thoracic s.
  Haimovici arteriotomy s.
  Harrington-Mayo thora-
    cic s.
  Howell coronary s.
  iris s.
  Jabaley-Stille Super Cut s.
  Kantrowitz vascular s.
  Karmody venous s.
  Lincoln s.
  Lincoln-Metzenbaum s.
  Litwak mitral valve s.
  Mayo s.
  Metzenbaum s.
  microvascular s.
  Mills arteriotomy s.
  Nelson s.
  pericardiotomy s.

scissors (continued)
  Potts 60° angled s.
  Potts vascular s.
  Potts-Smith vascular s.
  Real coronary artery s.
  right angle s.
  Satinsky s.
  Smith s.
  Snowden-Pencer s.
  Stille-Mayo s.
  straight s.
  Strully s.
  valve s.
  Willauer thoracic s.
  Wilmer s.

sclera
  blue s.

SCL
  sinus cycle length

scleredema
  s. adultorum
  s. of Buschke

sclerodactyly

ScleroLaser

Scleromate

sclerosant

sclerosing
  s. agent
  s. cholangitis
  s. hemangioma
  s. phlebitis
  variceal s.

sclerosis pl. scleroses
  aortic s.
  arterial s.
  arteriocapillary s.
  arteriolar s.
  coronary s.
  endocardial s.
  hyperplastic s.
  medial calcific s.
  Mönckeberg's s.
  multiple s.
  nodular s.

sclerosis *(continued)*
progressive systemic s.
(PSS)
subendocardial s.
tuberous s.
valvular s.
vascular s.
venous s.

sclerotherapy
variceal s.

sclerotic

Scole Alta II 3-channel precali-
brated Holter AM recorder

Scoop 1, 2 catheter

scooping

score
Aldrich s.
APACHE II s.
APACHE III s.
Berning and Steensgaard-
Hansen s.
Brush electrocardiograph-
ic s.
calcium s.
Califf s.
Detsky s.
Dripps-American Surgical
Association s.
Duke treadmill prognos-
tic s.
echo s.
Estes s.
Estes EKG s.
Gensini s.
Gensini coronary artery
disease s.
Goldman cardiac risk in-
dex s.
Hollenberg treadmill s.
jeopardy s.
mean wall motion s.
QRS s.
Romhilt-estes s.
Romhill-Estes left ventricu-
lar hypertrophy s.
Selvester QRS s.

score *(continued)*
TAPSE (tricuspid annular
plane sytolic excursion) s.
VAMC prognostic s.
wall motion s.

scotoma *pl.* scotomata

scout
s. film
s. view

scratch
Lerman-Means s.
Means-Lerman s.

scratchy murmur

screen
collagen vascular s.

screw-in
s.-i. epicardial electrode
s.-i. lead
s.-i. lead pacemaker

screw-on lead

Sculptor annuloplasty ring

SCV-CPR
simultaneous compression
ventilation CPR

SDPS
protamine solution

SE
spin-echo
SE image

SEA
side-entry access
SEA port

sea
s. fronds

seagull
s. bruit
s. murmur

seal
watertight s.

Sealy-Laragh technique

searcher
    Allport-Babcock s.

Sebastiani syndrome

SEC
    spontaneous echo contrast

second
    dyne s's
    s. heart sound (S_2)
    s. messenger
    meters per s. (m/sec)
    s. mitral sound
    s. obtuse marginal artery
        (OM-2)
    s. through fifth shock
        count

secondary
    s. aortic area
    s. asphyxia
    s. cardiomyopathy
    s. chemoprophylaxis
    s. dextrocardia
    s. hypertension
    s. infection
    s. prevention
    s. radiation
    s. thrombus

second-degree
    s.-d. A-V block
    s.-d. heart block

second-look operation

secretor
    gene s.

secretory
    s. leukoprotease inhibitor
        protein
    s. leukoproteinase inhibitor

sector
    s. scan
    s. scan echocardiography

secundum
    s. atrial septal defect
    foramen s.

secundum (continued)
    ostium s.
    septum s.
    s. and sinus venosus de-
        fects

sed (sedimentation) rate

sedentary lifestyle

Seecor pacemaker

seeding
    pumpkin-s.

Seeker guidewire

seesaw murmur

segment
    akinetic s.
    amplitude and slope of
        ST s.
    anterior s.
    anterobasal s.
    anterolateral s.
    apex s.
    apical s.
    apicoposterior s.
    arterial s. of glomeriform
        arteriovenous anastomo-
        sis
    coving of ST s's
    depressed PR s.
    depressed ST s.
    diaphragmatic s.
    distal s.
    dyssynergic myocardial s.
    elevated s.
    flail s's
    hypokinetic s.
    inferior s.
    inferoapical s.
    inferoposterior s.
    noninfarcted s.
    posterobasal s.
    posterolateral s.
    proximal s.
    PR s.
    RS–T s.
    septal wall s.
    septum s.

segment *(continued)*
    ST s.
    Ta s.
    TP s.
    T-P-Q s.
    TQ s.
    venous s. of glomeriform arteriovenous anastomosis
    upsloping ST s.

segmental
    s. arterial disorganization
    s. stenosis
    s. wall motion
    s. wall motion abnormality

segmentation
    k-space s.

segmentectomy

segmented
    s. hyalinizing vasculitis
    s. neutrophils
    s. ring tripolar lead

segmentum
    s. arteriale anastomosis arteriovenosae glomeriformis
    s. venosum anastomosis arteriovenosae glomeriformis

segs
    segmented neutrophils

Sehrt
    S. clamp
    S. compressor

SEI
    subendocardial infarction

seismic wave

seismocardiogram

seismocardiography

seizure

Seldinger
    S. needle

Seldinger *(continued)*
    S. percutaneous technique
    modified S. technique

Selecon coronary angiography catheter

selective
    s. angiography
    s. aortography
    s. arteriogram
    s. arteriography
    s. coronary cineangiography
    s. intracoronary thrombolysis (SICT)
    s. past pathway
    s. visualization

selenium
    s. deficiency
    s. sulfide

self-expanding stent

self-guiding catheter

self-positioning balloon catheter

self-powered treadmill

self-retaining retractor

self-terminating tachycardia

Sellick maneuver

Selman
    S. clamp
    S. vessel forceps

Seloken ZOC

Selvester QRS score

Selverstone
    S. cardiotomy hook
    S. carotid clamp

SEM
    scanning electron microscope
    systolic ejection murmur

Semb
    S. apicolysis

Semb *(continued)*
  S. forceps
  S. lung retractor
  S. rongeur

semidirect leads

semihorizontal heart

semilunar
  s. valve
  s. valve regurgitation

semisynthetic penicillin

semivertical heart

Semliki Forest virus

Semon sign

Sendai virus

senescent
  s. aortic stenosis
  s. heart
  s. myocardium

senile
  s. amyloidosis
  s. arrhythmia
  s. arteriosclerosis

senilis
  arcus s.
  circus s.

senility

Senn retractor

Senning
  S. atrial baffle repair
  S. intra-atrial baffle
  S. operation
  S. transposition procedure

sensation
  elephant-on-the-chest s.
  popping s.
  pressure-like s.

sensing
  afterpotential s.
  integrated bipolar s.
  pacemaker s.
  R wave s.

sensing *(continued)*
  s. spike

sensitivity
  s. analysis
  atrial s.
  aureomycin s.
  chlortetracycline s.
  digitalis s.
  pacemaker s.
  ventricular s.

sensitization
  baroreceptor s.

sensitized cell

Sensolog II, III pacemaker

Sensor pacemaker

sensor
  ClipTip reusable s.

sensorium
  clouded s.

sensorivascular

sensorivasomotor

Sensor Kelvin pacemaker

Sensor Medics metabolic cart

sensory nerve

sentinel node

Sentron pigtail angiographic micromanometer catheter

SEP
  systolic ejection period

separation
  aortic cusp s.
  E point to septal s. (EPSS)
  leaflet s.

Sepracoat coating solution

sepsis
  alcoholism, leukopenia,
    pneumococcal s. (ALPS)
  catheter related s. (CRS)

septal
  s. amplitude

septal *(continued)*
- s. arcade
- s. collateral
- s. defect
- s. dip
- s. dropout
- s. hypertrophy
- s. hyperprofusion on thallium scan
- s. myectomy
- s. myotomy
- s. pathway
- s. perforating arteries
- s. perforation
- s. perforator
- s. perforator branch
- s. resection
- s. separation
- s. wall motion

septation
- s. of heart
- s. procedure

septectomy
- atrial s.
- Blalock-Hanlon atrial s.
- Blalock-Hanlon partial atrial s.
- Edwards s.

septic
- s. embolization
- s. endocarditis
- s. fever
- s. shock

septomarginalis
- trabecula s.

septostomy
- atrial s.
- balloon atrial s.
- blade s.
- blade and baloon trial s.
- Mullins transseptal blade and balloon atrial s.
- Park blade and balloon atrial s.
- Rashkind atrial s.
- Rashkind balloon atrial s.
- Rashkind-Miller atrial s.

septum (S) *pl.* septa
- anteroapical trabecular s.
- asymmetric hypertrophy of s.
- atrial s.
- s. atrioventriculare cordis
- atrioventricular s. of heart
- canal s.
- conal s.
- dyskinetic s.
- infundibular s.
- interarterial s.
- interatrial s.
- s. interatriale cordis
- interlobular septa
- interventricular s.
- s. interventriculare cordis
- membranous s.
- muscular s.
- s. primum
- s. secundum
- sigmoid s.
- s. spurium
- Swiss cheese interventricular s.
- thickened s.
- s. of ventricles of heart
- ventricular s.

sequela *pl.* sequelae

Sequel compression system

sequence
- anaplerotic s.
- direct mapping s.
- FLASH s's
- intra-atrial activation s.
- intracardiac atrial activation s.
- spin-echo imaging s.

sequencing
- DNA s.

sequential
- s. dilations
- s. obstruction

Sequential Compression Device

sequestered lobe of lung

sequestration

Sequicor III pacemaker

SER
    systolic ejection rate

sera (pl. of serum)

serial
    s. changes
    s. cut films
    s. dilatation
    s. EKG tracings
    s. electrophysiologic test-
        ing (SET)
    s. lesions

serialographic filming

series elastic element

seriography

seroconversion

seroeffusive

serofibrinous
    s. pericarditis

serological test

seroma
    graft s.

Seroma-Cath catheter

seronegative spondyloarthropa-
    thy

serosanguineous

serosum
    pericardium s.

serotype
    M-protein s.

serotyping

serous
    s. membranes

serpentine aneurysm

serpiginous

serrated catheter

serum pl. sera
    s. bactericidal titer (SBT)
    s. creatine kinase
    s. electrophoresis
    s. enzyme study
    ERIG s.
    s. iron
    s. level
    s. lipid level
    s. lipid profile
    s. Mgb assay
    s. neopterin
    pericardial s.
    s. prothrombin conversion
        accelerator (SPCA)
    s. renin level
    s. shock
    s. sickness
    s. triglycerides

sessile plaque

sestamibi
    s. imaging
    s. scan
    s. stress test
    Tc-99 s.

set
    Acland-Banis arteriotomy s.
    ACS percutaneous intro-
        ducer s.
    Arrow Hi-flow infusion s.
    Borst side-arm introduc-
        er s.
    Diethrich coronary ar-
        tery s.
    Dotter Intravascular
        Retrieval S.
    Neff percutaneous access s.
    Neo-Sert umbilical vessel
        catheter insertion s.
    Peel-Away introducer s.
    Sobel-Kaplitt-Sawyer gas
        endarterectomy s.

seven-pinhole tomography

Sewall technique

sewing
    s. ring
    s. ring loop

sex
    s. ratio
    s. steroid

sexual
    s. angina
    s. syncope

SFHb
    pyridoxilated stroma-free
        hemoglobin

SF wave of cardiac apex pulse

SFA
    superficial femoral artery

SFHb
    stroma-free hemoglobin,
        pyridoxilated

SFR
    stenotic flow reserve

SGOT
    serum glutamic-oxaloacetic
        transaminase

SGPT
    serum glutamic-pyruvic
        transaminase

Shadow
    S. balloon
    S. over-the-wire balloon
        catheter

shadow
    acoustic s.
    bat wing s.
    butterfly s.
    cardiac s.
    mediastinal s.
    ring s.
    snowstorm s.
    summation s.

shaggy
    s. pericardium

shaggy *(continued)*
    s. ulcertranscript

Shaher-Puddu classification

shake test

shape
    echo-signal s.

Shapiro-Wilks test

sharp waves

Shaver disease

shaver
    s. catheter

shear
    atrial s.
    s. force
    s. rate of blood
    s. stress
    s. thinning

shears
    Bethune rib s.
    Gluck rib s.
    Sauerbruch rib s.
    Shoemaker rib s.
    Stille-Giertz rib s.

sheath
    angioplasty s.
    Arrow s.
    ArrowFlex s.
    arterial s.
    catheter s.
    carotid s.
    check-valve s.
    Cook transseptal s.
    Cordis s.
    crural s.
    Desilets-Hoffman s.
    s. and dilator system
    femoral s.
    femoral artery s.
    French s.
    guiding s.
    Hemaflex s.
    Hemaquet s.
    introducer s.

sheath *(continued)*
888 introducer s.
IVT percutaneous catheter introducer s.
Klein transseptal introducer s.
Mapper hemostasis EP mapping s.
Mullins s.
Mullins transseptal s.
Mullins transseptal catheterization s.
peel-away s.
percutaneous brachial s.
Pinnacle introducer s.
Schweigger-Seidel s.
Super ArrowFlex catheterization s.
tearaway s.
Terumo Radiofocus s.
transseptal s.
USCI angioplasty guiding s.
vascular s.
venous s.

sheath and side-arm

sheath with side-arm adaptor

sheath/dilator
Mullins s.

sheathing
halo s.

Sheehan and Dodge technique

sheep antidigoxin Fab antibody

sheepskin boot

sheet
mucous s's
s. sign

Sheffield
S. exercise stress test
S. exercise test protocol
S. treadmill protocol
S. modification of Bruce treadmill protocol
S. treadmill exercise protocol

Shekelton aneurysm

Sheldon catheter

shelf of plaque

shell
ejection s.

Shenstone tourniquet

shepherd
s's crook deformity
s's hook deformity

Shibley sign

shield
chest s.
face s.
probe s.

shift
axis s.
Doppler s.
mediastinal s.
midline s.
ST segment s.
superior frontal axis s.
s. to the left
s. to the right

shifter
frequency s.

shifting pacemaker

Shiley
S. cardiotomy reservoir
S. catheter
S. convexoconcave heart valve
S. guiding catheter
S. Phonate speaking valve
S. Tetraflex vascular graft
S.-Ionescu catheter

Shimadzu cardiac ultrasound

Shimazaki area-length method

SHJR4
side-hole Judkins right, curve 4
SHJR4 catheter

shock
  biphasic s.
  s. blocks
  burst s.
  cardiac s.
  cardiogenic s.
  chronic s.
  compensated s.
  s. count
  DC electric s.
  DC electrical s.
  declamping s.
  decompensated s.
  defibrillation s.
  diastolic s.
  distributive s.
  high-energy transthora-
    cic s.
  hypovolemic s.
  s. index
  insulin s.
  irreversible s.
  obstructive s.
  oligemic s.
  osmotic s.
  s. position
  QRS synchronous atrial de-
    fibrillation s.
  septic s.
  serum s.
  systolic s.
  s. therapy
  toxic s.
  vasogenic s.

shocky

shoddy fever

Shoemaker rib shears

Shone
  S. anomaly
  S. complex

short
  s. axis (SAX)
  s.-axis parasternal view
  s.-axis plane
  s.-axis plane on echocardi-
    ography

ShortCutter catheter

shortening
  circumferential fiber s.
  fiber s.
  s. fraction
  fractional myocardial s.
  mean rate of circumferen-
    tial s.
  myocardial fiber s.
  s. velocity
  velocity of circumferential
    fiber s.
  ventricular wall s.

short-long-short cycle

shortness of breath

Short Speedy balloon

shortwindedness

Shoshin disease

shot
  fast low-angle s. (FLASH)
  sinus s.

shotty nodes

shoulder
  s. of the heart
  s. horizontal flexion
  s. rotation

shoulder-hand syndrome

shoulder-strap resonance

shower
  embolic s.

Shprintzen syndrome

shrinker
  Juzo s.

SHU-454 contrast medium

SHU-508A contrast agent

shudder
  carotid s.
  s. of carotid arterial pulse

shunt
  Allen-Brown s.

shunt *(continued)*
- aorta to pulmonary artery s.
- aorticopulmonary s.
- aortofemoral artery s.
- aortopulmonary s.
- arteriovenous s.
- ascending aorta-to-pulmonary artery s.
- atrial ventricular s.
- atriopulmonary s.
- balloon s.
- bidirectional s.
- Blalock s.
- Blalock-Taussig s.
- Brenner carotid bypass s.
- cardiac s.
- carotid artery s.
- cardiovascular s.
- cavocaval s.
- Cimino arteriovenous s.
- Cordis-Hakim s.
- s. cyanosis
- Denver pleuroperitoneal s.
- s. detection
- descending thoracic aorta to pulmonary artery s.
- dialysis s.
- distal splenorenal s.
- Drapanas mesocaval s.
- extracardiac s.
- Glenn s.
- Gore-Tex s.
- Gott s.
- Holter s.
- interarterial s.
- intracardiac s.
- intrapericardial aorticopulmonary s.
- intrapulmonary s.
- Javid s.
- Javid endarterectomy s.
- left-to-right s.
- LeVeen peritoneovenous s.
- Marion-Clatworthy sent-to-end vena caval s.
- mesocaval s.
- Model 40-400 Pruitt-Inahara s.

shunt *(continued)*
- modified Blalock-Taussig s.
- net s.
- parallel s.
- s. pathway
- peritoneovenous s.
- portasystemic vascular s.
- portopulmonary s.
- Potts s.
- Pruitt vascular s.
- Pruitt-Inahara carotid s.
- s. quantification
- Quinton-Scribner s.
- Ramirez s.
- s. ratio
- reversed s.
- Reynold-Southwick H-graft portacaval s.
- right-to-left s.
- Simeone-Erlik side-to-end portorenal s.
- splenorenal s.
- subclavian artery to pulmonary artery s.
- Sundt carotid endarterectomy s.
- systemic to pulmonary s.
- Thomas s.
- transjugular intrahepatic portosystemic s. (TIPS)
- USCI s.
- Vascu-Flo carotid s.
- vena cava to pulmonary artery s.
- Vitagraft arteriovenous s.
- Waterston s.
- Waterston-Cooley s.

shunted blood

shunting
- venoarterial s.
- s. of blood

Shy-Drager syndrome

SIADH
- syndrome of inappropriate antidiuretic hormone

sialic acid

sibilance

Sibson
S. notch
S. vestibule

Sicar sign

sicca
pericarditis s.
s. syndrome

sickle
s. cell anemia
s. cell crisis
s. cell disease
s. cell-thalassemia
s. cell trait

sicklemia

sickling

sickness
African sleeping s.
cave s.
compressed-air s.
decompression s.
mountain s.
serum s.
sleeping s.

sick sinus syndrome (SSS)

SICOR cardiac catheterization
recording system

SICT
selective intracoronary
thrombolysis

side
s. arm adapter
s. arm pressure port
s. biting clamp
s. branch compromise
s. branch occlusion
s.-entry access (SEA)
s.-hole catheter
s.-hole Judkins right, curve
4 (SHJR4)
s.-hole Judkins right, curve
4 catheter

side *(continued)*
s.-hole Judkins right, curve
4, short (SHJR4s)
s. port
s. stretching

sideport

siderosis

sidewinder
s. catheter
s. percutaneous intra-aortic
balloon catheter

SIDS
sudden infant death syn-
drome

Siemens
S. BICOR cardioscope
S. electrode
S. HICOR cardioscope
S. open heart table
S. Orbiter gamma camera
S. pacemaker
S. PTCA/open heart table
S. Siecure implantable car-
dioverter-defibrillator
S. ventilator
S.-Albis bicycle ergometer
S.-Elema pacemaker
S.-Elema AB pulse trans-
ducer probe
S.-Pacesetter pacemaker

sigh function

Sigma
S. method
unipolar Pisces S.

sigmoid septum

sign
3-s.
Abrahams s.
ace of spades s.
antler s.
applesauce s.
Aschner s.
atrioseptal s.
Auenbrugger s.
Aufrecht s.

sign *(continued)*
  auscultatory s.
  Baccelli s.
  bagpipe s.
  Bamberger s.
  Bard s.
  Béhier-Hardy s.
  Bethea s.
  Biermer s.
  Biot s.
  Bird s.
  Bouillaud s.
  Boyce s.
  Bozzolo s.
  Branham s.
  Braunwald s.
  bread-and-butter text-
    book s.
  Broadbent s.
  Broadbent inverted s.
  Brockenbrough s.
  Brockenbrough-Braun-
    wald s.
  calcium s.
  Carabello s.
  Cardarelli s.
  cardiorespiratory s.
  Carvallo s.
  Castellino s.
  Cegka s.
  Charcot s.
  Cheyne-Stokes s.
  clenched fist s.
  cooing s.
  Corrigan s.
  Cruveilhier s.
  Cruveilhier-Baumgarten s.
  cuff s.
  D'Amato s.
  Davis s.
  de la Camp s.
  Delbet s.
  Delmege s.
  Demarquay s.
  de Musset s. (aortic aneu-
    rysm)
  de Mussy s. (pleurisy)
  d'Espine s.
  Dew s.

sign *(continued)*
  Dieuaide s.
  Dorendorf s.
  doughnut s.
  Drummond s.
  Duchenne s.
  Duroziez s.
  Ebstein s.
  Ellis s.
  Erni s.
  Ewart s.
  Ewing s.
  Faget s.
  Federici s.
  Fischer s.
  flying W s.
  Friedreich s.
  Glasgow s.
  gooseneck s.
  Gowers s.
  Grancher s.
  Greene s.
  Griesinger s.
  Grocco s.
  Grossman s.
  Gunn s.
  Gunn crossing s.
  Hall s.
  Hamman s.
  Heim-Kreysig s.
  Heimlich s.
  Hill s.
  hilum convergence s.
  hilum overlay s.
  Homans' s.
  Hoover s.
  Hope s.
  Huchard s.
  Intravascular fetal air s.
  Jaccoud s.
  Jackson s.
  jugular s.
  Jürgensen s.
  Karplus s.
  Kellock s.
  knuckle s.
  Korányi s.
  Kreysig s.
  Kussmaul s.

sign *(continued)*
- Laënnec s.
- Lancisi s.
- Landolfi s.
- Levine s.
- Livierato s.
- Lombardi s.
- Löwenberg cuff s.
- Macewen s.
- Mahler s.
- Mannkopf s.
- McCort s.
- McGinn-White s.
- Meltzer s.
- Moschcowitz s.
- Mueller s.
- Müller s.
- Murat s.
- Musset s.
- mute toe s.
- Nicoladoni s.
- Nicoladoni-Branham s.
- Oliver s.
- Osler s.
- pad s.
- Perez s.
- Pfuhl-Jaffé s.
- Pins' s.
- plumb-line s.
- Porter s.
- Potain s.
- Pottenger s.
- Prevel s.
- Prussian helmet s.
- Queckenstedt s.
- Quénu-Muret s.
- Quincke s.
- rabbit-ear s.
- railroad track s.
- Ramond s.
- Raynaud s.
- reversed three s.
- ring s.
- Rivero-Carvallo s.
- Riviere s.
- Robertson s.
- Romaña s.
- Rotch s.
- Rothschild s.

sign *(continued)*
- Sam Levine s.
- Sansom s.
- Schepelmann s.
- Schick s.
- Seitz s.
- Semon s.
- S s. of Golden
- Shapiro s.
- sheet s.
- Shibley s.
- Sicar s.
- silhouette s.
- Skoda s.
- Smith s.
- snake-tongue s.
- square root s.
- steeple s.
- Steinberg thumb s.
- Sterles s.
- Sternberg s.
- string s.
- T s.
- tail s.
- tenting s.
- trapezius ridge s.
- Traube s.
- Trimadeau s.
- Troisier s.
- Trunecek s.
- Unschuld s.
- vein s.
- Walker-Murdoch wrist s.
- Weill s.
- Wenckebach s.
- Westermark s.
- Williams s.
- Williamson s.
- windsock s.
- Wintrich s.

signal
- s.-averaged
- s.-averaged echocardiogram
- s.-averaged echocardiography
- s.-averaged electrocardiogram

signal *(continued)*
s.-averaged electrocardiography
s. averaging
Doppler s.
gating s.
magnetic resonance s.
mosaic-jet s's
s. processing
s.-to-noise ratio

signaling
transmembrane s.

Sigvaris
S. compression stockings
S. medical stockings

Silastic
S. bead embolization
S. catheter
S. electrode casing
S. strain gauge
S. H.P. tissue holder
S. loop
S. tape
S. tubing
S. vessel loop

silence
EKG s.

silent
s. angina
s. electrode
s. gap
s. mitral stenosis
s. myocardial infarction (SMI)
s. myocardial ischemia
s. pericardial effusion

silhouette
cardiac s.
cardiomediastinal s.
s. sign
widened cardiac s.

silica

Silicore catheter

silk
s. guidewire

Silon tent

Silver syndrome

silver (Ag)
s. bead electrode
Grocott methenamine s.
s. sulfadiazine

silver-methenamine stain

silver–silver chloride electrode

Silverstein stimulator probe

silver wire effect

silver-wiring of retinal arteries

Silvester method

SIMA (single internal mammary artery) reconstruction

Simeone-Erlik side-to-end porto-renal shunt

Simons II, III catheter

Simmons-type sidewinder catheter

Simon
S. foci
S. nitinol inferior vena cava (IVC) filter

Simplate procedure

simplex
angina s.
carcinoma s.
herpes s.

Simplus
S. catheter
S. PE/t dilatation catheter

Simpson
S. atherectomy
S. atherectomy device
S. atherectomy catheter
S. Coronary AtheroCath catheter

Simpson *(continued)*
S. Coronary AtheroCath system
S. peripheral AtheroCath
S. PET balloon
S. rule
S. rule method for ventricular volume
S. Ultra Lo-Profile II balloon catheter
S. Ultra Lo-Profile II catheter
S.-Robert catheter
S.-Robert vascular dilation system

Simron

simultaneous compression-ventilation CPR

Sindbis virus

sine wave

sine-wave pattern

Singh
S.–Vaughan Williams antiarrhythmic drug classification
S.–Vaughan Williams classification of arrhythmias

single
s. atrium
s.-balloon valvotomy
s.-balloon valvuloplasty
s.-chamber, rate-responsive
s.-crystal gamma camera
s.-gene disorder s. lumen
s. papillary muscle syndrome
s.-pass lead
s.-photon detection
s.-photon emission
s.-photon emission computed tomography (SPECT)
s.-photon emission tomography (SPET)
s.-photon emission tomography (SPET) imaging

single *(continued)*
s.-photon gamma scintigraphy
s.-plane aortographysingle premature extrastimulation
s.-stage exercise stress test
s. ventricle
s. ventricle malposition
s.-vessel
s.-vessel coronary stenosis
s.-vessel disease

Singley forceps

sinistrocardia

sinistrum
atrium s.
cor s.

sinoaortic baroreflex activity

sinoatrial (SA, S-A)
s. arrest
s. block
s. bradycardia
s. conduction time
s. exit block
s. nodal artery
s. node

sinoauricular
s. block

sinospiral

sinotubular junction

sinoventricular
s. conduction

sinuatrial

sinuatrialis
nodus s. (NS)
nonreset nodus s.
reset nodus s.

sinus
s. aortae
aortic s.
aortic valve s.
s. arrest

sinus *(continued)*
  s. arrhythmia
  basilar s.
  s. bradycardia
  carotid s.
  s. catarrh
  s. coronarius
  coronary s. (CS)
  s. cycle length
  distal coronary s. (DCS)
  s. exit block
  s. exit pause
  s. impulse
  s.-initiated QRS complex
  s. irregularity (SI)
  left coronary s.
  s. mechanism
  middle coronary s. (MCS)
  s. of Morgagni
  s. nodal automaticity
  s. nodal reentrant tachy-
    cardia
  s. nodal reentry
  s. node (SN)
  s. node artery
  s. node automaticity
  s. node/AV conduction ab-
    normality
  s. node disease
  s. node dysfunction
  s. node function
  s. node recovery time
  s. node reentry
  noncoronary s.
  oblique s. of pericardium
  s. obliquus pericardii
  s. pause
  pericardial s.
  s. pericardii
  Petit's s.
  piriform s.
  proximal coronary s. (PCS)
  pulmonary s.
  s. of pulmonary trunk
  s. reflex
  s. rhythm
  s. segment
  s. shot
  s. slowing

sinus *(continued)*
  soleal s's
  s. standstill
  s. tachycardia
  s. thrombosis
  transverse s.
  transverse s. of pericar-
    dium
  s. transversus pericardii
  s. trunci pulmonalis
  s. of Valsalva
  s. of Valsalva aneurysm
  s. of Valsalva aortography
  s. of venae cavae
  s. venarum cavarum
  s. venosus
  s. venosus atrial septal de-
    fect
  venous s.
  s. x-ray

sinuspiral

sinuventricular

siphon
  carotid s.
  Duguet s.
  Moniz carotid s.

Sirius red stain

SIRS
  systemic inflammatory re-
    sponse syndrome

site
  arterial entry S.
  entry S.
  extrapulmonary S.
  target S.

situational syncope

situs
  s. ambiguus
  s. inversus
  s. inversus totalis
  s. solitus
  s. transversus
  visceroatrial s.

size
  French s.

sizer
>   Björk-Shiley heart valve s.
>   Meadox graft s.
>   prosthetic valve s.

sizing
>   s. balloon
>   French s. of catheter

SJM-X-Cell cardiac bioprosthesis

Sjögren syndrome

SK
>   streptokinase

skein

skeletal
>   s. alpha-actin mRNA
>   s. muscle
>   s. muscle plasticity

skeleton
>   cardiac s.
>   fibrous s. of heart
>   s. of heart

skeletonization

skewer technique

skimming
>   plasma s.

skin
>   s. button
>   cool and clammy s.
>   diaphoretic s.
>   s. gun
>   s. heart
>   salmon s.
>   tenting of s.
>   s. turgor
>   s. wheel

Skinny
>   S. dilatation catheter
>   S. over-the-wire balloon catheter

skip graft

skipped beat

skipping a heartbeat

Skoda
>   S. sign

skodaic resonance

SKY epidural pain control system

Skylark surface electrode

Slalom balloon

slant-hole tomography

slaved programmed electrical stimulation

SLE
>   systemic lupus erythematosus

Sleek catheter

sleep
>   s. apnea
>   s. apnea/hypopnea syndrome
>   crescendo s.
>   D s.
>   deep s.
>   s. deprivation
>   desynchronized s.
>   dreaming s.
>   fast wave s.
>   s. hypoxia
>   NREM s.
>   orthodox s.
>   paroxysmal s.
>   REM s.
>   s. spindles
>   s. study
>   synchronized s. (S-sleep)

sleeping
>   s. sickness
>   s. tachycardia

sleeve
>   LocalMed catheter infusion s.

Sleuth
>   CO S.

Sleuth (continued)
 ETO S.
 HBT S.

slew rate

slice
 coronal s.
 transaxial s.

Slider
 S. balloon
 S. catheter

Slidewire extension guide

sliding
 s. filament theory
 s. plasty
 s. rail catheter
 s. scale method

slim disease

sling
 cardiac s.
 pericardial s.
 pressure s.
 pulmonary artery s.
 s. ring complex
 vascular s.

Slinky
 S. balloon
 S. balloon catheter
 S. PTCA catheter

Slip/Stream
 Bennett S.

slit ventricle syndrome

SLMD
 symptomatic left main disease

slope
 closing (on echo) s.
 disappearance s.
 D to E s.
 E to F s.
 flat diastolic s.
 flattened E to F s.
 mitral E to F s.

slope (continued)
 opening (on echo) s.
 ST/HR (ST segment/heart rate) s.
 s. of valve opening

slotted needle

slough

sloughing of skin from necrosis

slow
 s. AV node pathway
 s. channel
 s. channel blocker
 s. escape rhythm
 s.-fast tachycardia
 s. FE
 s.-pathway ablation
 s.-reacting substance of anaphylaxis
 s. response
 s. zone

slowing
 diffuse paroxysmal s.

sludged blood

sludging
 s. of blood

slurred speech

slurring
 s. of ST
 s. of QRS

slurry
 gelatin sponge s.
 talc s.

slush
 ice s.
 saline s.
 topical cooling with ice s.

slushed ice

Sly disease

SM
 sonomicrometry

smallpox vaccine reaction

SMAP
    systemic mean arterial
        pressure

Smart
    S. position-sensing catheter
    S. Trigger

SmartNeedle

SmartTracking on the Marathon
    pacemaker

SMC
    smooth muscle cell

smear
    buffy coat s.

Smec balloon catheter

Smeloff
    S.-Cutter ball-cage pros-
        thetic valve
    S.-Cutter prosthetic valve

SMI
    silent myocardial infarction

Smith-Lemli-Opitz syndrome

Smith scissors

Smith sign

smoking
    pack-years of cigarette s.

smooth
    s. muscle cell
    s. muscle relaxation

smoothing
    digital s.

SMVR
    supra-annular mitral valve
        replacement

SMVT
    sustained monomorphic
        ventricular tachycardiac

snake
    s. graft

snake (continued)
    s. venom

snake-tongue sign

snap
    closing s.
    mitral opening s.
    opening s.
    tricuspid opening s.
    valvular s.

Snaplets-EX

SNAP sleep recorder

snare
    s. catheter
    caval s.
    s. device
    s. technique

sneeze
    s. reflex
    s. syncope

Snider match test

snooze-induced excitation of
    sympathetic triggered activ-
    ity (SIESTA)

Snowden
    S.-Pencer forceps
    S.-Pencer scissors

snowman
    s. abnormality
    s. appearance of heart
    s. heart

snowplow effect

snowstorm shadow

SNRT
    sinus node recovery time
        SNRT-CL

snugged down, suture was

Snuggle Warm convective
    warming system

Snyder Surgivac drainage

^{82}So
   strontium-82

soap
   curd s.

SOB
   shortness of breath

Sobel-Kaplitt-Sawyer gas endarterectomy set

sock array

sodium content (of foods)

sodium pertechnetate Tc 99m

Soemmering
   arterial vein of S.

soft
   s. event
   s. pulse
   s. tissue sarcoma

Soft-EZ reusable electrode

SOF-T guidewire

Softip
   S. catheter
   S. diagnostic catheter

Softouch
   S. guiding catheter
   S. UHF cardiac pigtail cath-
      eter

Softrac
   S.-PTA catheter

Soft-Vu Omni flush catheter

software
   Image-Measure morphome-
      try s.

Sokolow
   S. electrocardiographic
      index
   S.-Lyon voltage
   S.-Lyon voltage criteria

Solcotrans autotransfusion unit

soldered bond

soldering
   s. flux
   s. fumes

soldier
   s. heart
   s. patches

Sole Primeur 33Danalyzer

solid angle concept

solitarius
   nucleus tractus s.

solitary
   s. coronary ostium
   s. pulmonary arteriovenous
      fistula
   s. pulmonary nodule

solitus
   situs s.
   ventricular situs s.
   visceroatrial situs s.

Solo
   S. balloon
   S. catheter

Soludrast contrast material

Solu-Medrol injection

Solus pacemaker

solution
   albumin s.
   antiobiotic s.
   Anti-Sept bactericidal
      scrub s.
   Belzer s.
   Betadine Helafoam s.
   Bretschneider-HTK cardi-
      oplegic s.
   Brompton s.
   Burow s.
   cardioplegic s.
   cold cardioplegic s.
   cold topical saline s.
   Collins s.
   crystalloid cardioplegic s.

solution *(continued)*
  Dakin s.
  Denhardt s.
  dextran s.
  ECS cardioplegic s.
  Euro-Collins cooling s.
  extracellular-like, calcium-
    free s. (ECS)
  Gey s.
  Gey fixative s.
  hand agitated s.
  Hank balanced salt s.
  Hartmann s.
  heparinized s.
  hyperosmotic s.
  ice-cold physiologic s.
  ice slush s.
  ICS cardioplegic s.
  intracellular-like, calcium-
    bearing crystalloid s.
    (ICS)
  Krebs s.
  Krebs-Henseleit s.
  Lugol s.
  Lugol fixative s.
  Massier s.
  Melrose s.
  modified Collins s.
  papaverine s.
  Plasmalyte A cardiopleg-
    ic s.
  Plegisol cardioplegic s.
  priming s.
  Ringer s.
  St. Thomas s.
  saline s.
  Schlesinger s.
  Sepracoat coating s.
  stroma-free hemoglobin s.
  Tyrode s.
  uncrystallized cardiopleg-
    ic s.
  University of Wisconsin s.

soma

somaplasm

SomaSensor
  S. device
  S. pad

somatic

somatomedin

somatoplasm

somniloquism

Sondergaard
  S. cleft (interatrial groove)
  S. procedure

Sones
  S. arteriography technique
  S. brachial cutdown tech-
    nique
  S. cardiac catheterization
  S. Cardio-Marker catheter
  S. catheter
  S. cineangiography tech-
    nique
  S. coronary arteriography
  S. coronary catheter
  S. coronary cineangiogra-
    phy
  S. guidewire
  S. hemostatic bag
  S. Hi-Flow catheter
  S. Positrol catheter
  S. selective coronary arteri-
    ography
  S. technique
  S. woven Dacron catheter

sonicated
  s. contrast agent
  s. dextrose albumin
  s. Renografin-76
  s. Renografin-76 contrast
    medium

Sonicath imaging catheter

sonication technique

sonicator

sonogram

sonography

sonolucency

sonomicrometer piezoelectric
  crystals

sonomicrometry

Sonos
S. 500 imaging system
S. 2000 ultrasound imager
S. 5500 ultrasound
imagerCVC

Sopha Medical gamma camera

Sophy high-resolution collimator

Sorenson thermodilution catheter

Sorin
S. mitral valve prosthesis
S. pacemaker
S. prosthetic valve

soroche

sorter
cell s.

SOS guidewire

sotalol
s. hydrochloride

souffle
cardiac s.
fetal s.
funic s.
mammary s.

soufflet
bruit de s.

sound
A_2 (aortic closure) heart s.
adventitious heart s.
aortic closure s.
aortic ejection s.
aortic second s.
atrial s.
auscultatory s.
bandbox s.
Beatty-Bright friction s.
bell s.
bellows s.
booming diastolic rum-
ble s.

sound *(continued)*
bottle s.
cannon s.
cardiac s.
coin s.
cracked-pot s.
crunching s.
distant heart s.
double-shock s.
eddy s.
ejection s.
first s.
first heart s.
fixed splitting of second
heart s.
flapping s.
fourth s.
fourth heart s.
friction s.
gallop s.
heart s.
heart s. S_1
heart s. S_2
heart s. S_3
heart s. S_4
hippocratic s.
Korotkoff s.
M_1 (mitral valve closure)
heart s.
mammary souffle s.
mitral first s. (M_1)
mitral second s. (M_2)
muffled heart s.
nonejection systolic s.
P_2 (pulmonic closure)
heart s.
pacemaker s.
pacemaker heart s.
paradoxical splitting of second heart s.
paradoxically split S_2 s.
percussion s.
pericardial friction s.
physiologic heart s.
physiologic third heart s.
physiologically split S_2 s.
physiologic splitting of second heart s.
physiologic third heart s.

sound *(continued)*
  pistol-shot s.
  pistol-shot femoral s.
  prosthetic valve s.
  puffing s.
  pulmonary component of
    second heart s.
  pulmonic closure s.
  pulmonic ejection s.
  pulmonic second s.
  pulmonic valve closure s.
  quiet heart s's
  reduced s.
  S_3 gallop s.
  S_4 gallop s.
  sail s.
  second s.
  second heart s.
  second mitral s.
  souffle heart s.
  shaking s.
  split heart s.
  splitting of heart s's
  squeaky-leather s.
  succussion s's
  systolic ejection s's
  T_1 (tricuspid valve closure)
    heart s.
  tambour s.
  third s.
  third heart s.
  tic-tac heart s.
  tick-tack s's
  to-and-fro s.
  tricuspid valve closure s.
  tumor plop s.
  valvular ejection s.
  vascular ejection s.
  water-wheel s.
  s. wave cycle
  weak heart s.
  widely split second heart s.
  xiphisternal crunching s.
S/P
  status post
SP1005
  Cardiomyostimulator
    SP1005

space
  antecubital s.
  s. of Burns
  echo-free s.
  epicardial s.
  extrapleural s.
  fifth intercostal s.
  H s.
  His perivascular s.
  Holzknecht s.
  intercostal s.
  intercristal s.
  interstitial s.
  Larrey s's
  left fifth intercostal s.
  left intercostal s. (LICS)
  mediastinal s.
  mitochondrial membrane s.
  pericardial s.
  perivascular s.
  perinuclear s.
  physiological dead s.
  pleural s.
  Poiseuille's s.
  popliteal s.
  posterior septal s.
  prevertebral s.
  retrocardiac s.
  subphrenic s.
  Traube semilunar s.
  Westberg's s.
  Zang s.

SpaceLabs
  S. Event Master
  S. Holter monitor
  S. pulse oximeter

Spacemaker balloon dissector

spacer
  Ellipse compact s.

spacing

spadelike configuration

SPAF
  Stroke Prevention in Atrial
    Fibrillation

Span-FF

sparing
   myocardial s.

spark erosion

sparkling appearance of myocardium

Sparks mandrel technique

spasm
   arterial s.
   carpopedal s.
   catheter induced s.
   catheter induced coronary
     artery s.
   catheter-related peripheral
     vessel s.
   catheter-tip s.
   coronary s.
   coronary artery s.
   diffuse arteriola s.
   ergonovine-induced s.
   post-bypass s.
   vascular s.
   venous s.

spatial
   s. intensity
   s. resolution
   s. tracking
   two-dimensional s.
   s. vector
   s. vectorcardiography

spatula

SPCA
   serum prothrombin con-
     version accelerator

speckled pattern

Spearman
   S. nonparametric univariate
     correlation
   S. rho test

Spears laser balloon

specificity

speckling

SPECT
   single-photon emission
     computed tomography
   adenosine ^{99m}Tc sestamibi
     SPECT
   SPECT scintigraphy
   stress perfusion and rest
     function by sestamibi-
     gated SPECT
   SPECT thallium scan
   SPECT tomography

spectra (*plural of* spectrum)

Spectra-Cath STP catheter

Spectraflex pacemaker

spectral
   s. analysis
   S. Cardiac Status Test
   s. envelope
   s. leakage
   pattern s. analysis
   s. phonocardiograph
   s. power
   s. temporal mapping
   s. turbulence mapping
   s. waveform

Spectranetics
   S. P23 Statham transducer
   S. laser
   S. laser sheath for lead ex-
     traction
   S. Prima FX laser wire
   S. Vitesse C catheter
   S. Vitesse E excimer laser
     catheter

Spectraprobe

Spectrax
   S. SX, SX-HT, SXT, VL, VM,
     VS pacemaker
   S. programmable Med-
     tronic pacemaker

spectrophotometer
   Hitachi U-2000 s.
   liquid scintillation s.

spectroscopy
    electron paramagnetic res-
      onance s.
    flame emission s.
    fluorescence s.
    magnetic resonance s.
    near-infrared s.
    NMR s.
    proton s.
    Raman s.

spectroscopy-directed laser

SpectRx test

specular echo

Speedy balloon catheter

spell
    blackout s.
    grayout s.
    hypercyanotic s.
    hypoxic s.
    presyncopal s.
    syncopal s.
    tet s.
    tetrad s.

Spembly cryoprobe

Spencer plication of vena cava

Spens syndrome

sphere
    attraction s.

sphericity index

spheroplast

sphincter
    cardioesophageal s.
    hepatic s.
    precapillary s.

sphygmic
    s. interval

sphygmocardiograph

sphygmocardioscope

sphygmochronograph

sphygmodynamometer

sphygmogram

sphygmograph

sphygmographic

sphygmography

sphygmoid

sphygmology

sphygmomanometer
    Ayers s.
    cuff s.
    Erlanger s.
    Faught s.
    Hawksley random zero
      mercury s.
    Mosso s.
    Physio-Control Lifestat s.
    random-zero s.
    Riva-Rocci s.
    Rogers s.

sphygmomanometry

sphygmometer

sphygmometroscope

sphygmo-oscillometer

sphygmopalpation

sphygmophone

sphygmoplethysmograph

sphygmoscope
    Bishop's s.

sphygmoscopy

sphygmosystole

sphygmotonograph

sphygmotonometer

sphygmoviscosimetry

spider
    s. angioma
    arterial s.

spider *(continued)*
    s. burst
    s. projection
    vascular s.
    s. venom
    s. x-ray view

spike
    s. activity
    atrial s.
    s.-and-dome configuration
    s.-and-dome pulse
    H s.
    H and H' s.
    pacemaker s.
    sensing s.
    wave s.

spillover
    jugular venous catechol s.

spin
    s. density
    s.-echo
    s.-echo imaging
    s.-echo imaging sequence
    s.-echo MRI
    s.-lattice time

spinal needle

spindle
    aortic s.
    Bütschli's nuclear s.
    central s.
    His' s.
    mitotic s.
    nuclear s.
    sleep s.

spiral
    Curschmann s's
    s. dissection

spireme

spirochetal
    s. disease
    s. infection
    s. myocarditis

spirochete

spirometer
    Tissot s.
    incentive s.

Spitzer theory

splanchnic
    s. bed perfusion
    s. blood flow
    s. vessel

splanchnicotomy

Splendore-Hoeppli phenome-
    non

splenomegaly
    congestive s.
    thrombophlebitic s.

splenoportal hypertension

splenoportography

splenorenal shunt

splice
    breakaway s.

splinter hemorrhages

splinting

split
    paradoxic s. of S_2
    physiological s. of S_2

split-sheath introducer

splitter
    beam s.

splitting
    commissural s.
    fixed s. of S_2
    s. of heart sounds
    reversed s. of S_2
    s. of S_1
    s. of S_2
    wide s. of S_2

spondylitis
    ankylosing s.

spondyloarthropathy
    seronegative s.

sponge
- 4 × 4 s.
- Collostat s.
- Collostat hemostatic s.
- Ivalon s.
- laparotomy s.
- phantom s.
- RayTec s.
- stick s.

spongioplasm

spontaneous
- s. coronary artery dissection
- s. echo contrast
- s. reentrant sustained ventricular tachycardia

spot
- Brushfield s.
- café-au-lait s.
- Campbell de Morgan s.
- cold s.
- cotton-wool s.
- De Morgan s's
- Horder s's
- hot s.
- milk s.
- rose s.
- Roth s.
- soldier's s.
- tendinous s.
- ventricular milk s's
- white s.

spray
- Hurricaine s.
- Nitrolingual Translingual S.

spread
- lymphangitic s.
- venous s.

spreader
- Bailey rib s.
- Burford rib s.
- Burford-Finochietto rib s.
- Davis rib s.
- DeBakey rib s.

spreader (continued)
- Favaloro-Morse rib s.
- Finochietto rib s.
- Haight rib s.
- Harden rib s.
- Harken rib s.
- Lemmon sternal s.
- Lilienthal rib s.
- Medicon s.
- Miltex s.
- Morse sternal s.
- Nelson rib s.
- Rehbein rib s.
- Reinhoff-Finochietto rib s.
- Tuffier rib s.
- Weinberg rib s.
- Wilson rib s.

spring
- s. catheter
- disk s.

spring-loaded stent

Sprint catheter

SPTI
- systolic pressure time index

spur
- calcific s.

spuria
- angina s.

spurious aneurysm

spurium
- septum s.

sputum
- blood-tinged s.
- frothy s.
- pink s.
- rusty s.

S–QRS interval

square
- s. wave response
- s. wave stimulus

squatting
  s. to relieve dyspnea

squeak

squeaky-leather sound

squeeze
  s. effect
  thoracic s.
  tussive s.

SR (slew rate)

Sramek formula

SR calcium ATPase

SRT (segmented ring tripolar)
  lead

ST
  ST alterations
  ST interval
  ST junction
  ST sag
  slurring of ST
  ST vector
  ST wave

stab
  s. incision
  s. wound

stability

stab-in epicardial electrode

stable angina

staccato pain

Stachrom PAI chromogenic assay

Stack
  S. autoperfusion balloon
  S. perfusion catheter
  S. perfusion coronary dila-
    tion catheter

Stadie-Riggs microtome

stage
  knäuel s.
  resting s.
  vegetative s.

Stage I-VII of Bruce protocol

staging
  TMN s.

stain
  calcofluor s.
  Dieterle s.
  Diff-Quik s.
  endocardial s.
  Gomori methenamine sil-
    ver s.
  Gram s.
  H&E s.
  hematoxylin-eosin s.
  immunoperoxidase s.
  Kinyoun s.
  Mallory s.
  Masson trichrome s.
  May-Grünwald-Giemsa s.
  Miller elastic s.
  Movat s.
  mucicarmine s.
  Pizzolatto s.
  silver-methenamine s.
  Sirius red s.
  TTC s.
  van Gieson s.
  Wright s.
  Ziehl-Neelsen s.

staining

stainless
  s. steel guidewire
  s. steel mesh stent
  s. steel staples

staircase phenomenon

Stairmaster mobile stairs

Stamey test

Stansel procedure

stand-alone laser treatment

standard
  Boehringer Mannheim s.
  s. Bruce protocol
  s. deviation
  s. error
  s. Lehman catheter

standard *(continued)*
   s. limb lead
   s. needle
standby
   s. pacemaker
   s. pulse generator
standstill
   atrial s.
   auricular s.
   cardiac s.
   sinus s.
   ventricular s.
Stanford
   S. biopsy method
   S. bioptome
   S. treadmill exercise protocol
   S.-type aortic dissection
   S.-Caves bioptome
Stanicor pacemaker
Stannius ligature
staphcidal drug
staphylococcal
   s. endocarditis
stapler
   Androsov vascular s.
   Auto-Suture surgical s.
   Inokucki vascular s.
star
   daughter s.
   mother s.
   polar s.
   s. of Verheyen
Starling
   S. curve
   S. equation
   S. force
   S. law
   S. mechanism
Starr
   S.-Edwards aortic valve prosthesis
   S.-Edwards ball-and-cage valve

Starr *(continued)*
   S.-Edwards ball valve prosthesis
   S.-Edwards cardiac valve prosthesis
   S.-Edwards disk valve prosthesis
   S.-Edwards heart valve prosthesis
   S.-Edwards mitral prosthesis
   S.-Edwards mitral valve
   S.-Edwards pacemaker
   S.-Edwards prosthetic valve
   S.-Edwards Silastic valve
Star Sync
stasis *pl.* stases
   s. cirrhosis
   s. dermatitis
   s. edema
   s. of blood flow
   pressure s.
   s. ulcer
   venous s.
state
   cardiovascular steady s.
   gradient-recalled acquisition in the steady s.
   hypercoagulable s.
   hyperdynamic s.
   inotropic s.
   postabsorptive s.
   postictal s.
Statham
   S. electromagnetic flowmeter
   S. strain-gauge transducer
static dilation technique
statins
station pull-through
statistic
   Gehan s.
   Lee-Desu s.
   Mantel-Haenszel s.
   Wei-Lachin s.

Stat 2 Pumpette

stathmokinesis

status
    s. angiosus
    cardiac s.
    functional s.
    mental s.
    work s.

staxis

ST depression
    downsloping ST d.
    horizontal ST d.
    reciprocal ST d.

steal
    coronary s.
    endoperoxide s.
    iliac s.
    s. mechanism
    s. phenomenon
    pulmonary artery s.
    renal-splanchnic s.
    subclavian s.
    transmural s.

steam autoclaved

steatorrhea

steatosis
    s. cardiaca
    s. cordis
    macrovesicular s.
    microvesicular s.

Steell murmur

steel-winged butterfly needle

steep Trendelenburg position

steeple sing

steerable
    s. angioplastic guidewire
    s. electrode catheter
    s. guidewire catheter

Steerocath catheter

Stegemann-Stalder method

Steidele complex

Steinberg thumb sign

Steinert disease

Stela electrode lead

stellate
    s. ganglion
    s. ganglion blockade

stellectomy

Stellite
    S. ring material
    S. ring material of pros-
        thetic valve

stellula
    s. of Verheyen
    s. verheyenii

stem
    transposition of arterial s's

stenocardia

stenosal murmur

stenosing ring of left atrium

stenosis
    American Heart Associa-
        tion classification of s.
    aortic s.
    aortic valvular s.
    aortoiliac s.
    s. area
    bottle-neck s.
    branch pulmonary s.
    branch pulmonary artery s.
    buttonhole mitral s.
    calcific aortic s.
    calcific bicuspid valvular s.
    calcific mitral s.
    calcific nodular aortic s.
    caroticovertebral s.
    carotid s.
    carotid aortic s.
    chronic aortic s.
    cicatricial s.
    congenital aortic s.
    congenital aortic valvular s.
    congenital mitral s.
    congenital pulmonary s.
    congenital tricuspid s.

stenosis *(continued)*
 coronary artery s.
 coronary luminal s.
 coronary ostial s.
 critical s.
 critical coronary s.
 critical valvular s.
 s. diameter
 discrete subvalvular aortic s.
 distal s.
 Dittrich s.
 double aortic s.
 dynamic subaortic s.
 eccentric s.
 enucleation of subaortic s.
 fibromuscular subaortic s.
 fibrous subaortic s.
 fish-mouth mitral s.
 fixed-orifice aortic s.
 flow-limiting s.
 focal eccentric s.
 geometry of s.
 granulation s.
 hemodynamically significant s.
 high-grade s.
 hourglass s.
 hypertrophic infundibular subpulmonic s.
 hypertrophic subaortic s.
 idiopathic hypertrophic subaortic s. (IHSS)
 infundibular s.
 infundibular pulmonic s.
 innominate artery s.
 s. length
 linear s.
 luminal s.
 membranous s.
 mitral s.
 mitral valve s.
 muscular subaortic s.
 napkin-ring s.
 noncalcified s.
 noncalcified coronary s.
 noncritical s.
 orificial s.
 nonrheumatic aortic s.

stenosis *(continued)*
 peripheral arterial s.
 peripheral pulmonary artery s.
 peripheral pulmonic s.
 point of critical s.
 postangioplasty s.
 postdiphtheritic s.
 preangioplasty s.
 preventricular s.
 pulmonary s.
 pulmonary artery s.
 pulmonary artery branch s.
 pulmonary branch s.
 pulmonary valve s.
 pulmonary valvular s.
 pulmonic s.
 pulmonic valve s.
 renal artery s.
 residual s.
 rheumatic aortic s.
 rheumatic aortic valvular s.
 rheumatic mitral valve s.
 rheumatic tricuspid s.
 renal artery s.
 segmental s.
 senescent aortic s.
 severe s.
 silent mitral s.
 single-vessel coronary s.
 stenotic s.
 subaortic s.
 subpulmonary s.
 subpulmonic s.
 subpulmonic infundibular s.
 subvalvar aortic s.
 subvalvular s.
 subvalvular aortic s.
 subvalvular mitral s.
 supra-aortic s.
 supravalvar s.
 supravalvular s.
 supravalvular aortic s.
 tight s.
 tricuspid s.
 tricuspid valve s.
 tubular s.
 unicusp aortic s.

stenosis *(continued)*
    valvar aortic s.
    valvular aortic s.
    valvular pulmonic s.
    valvular s.
    vascular s.
    s. with a spastic component

stenotic
    s. coronary artery
    s. lesion

stent
    ACS Multi-Link coronary s.
    activated balloon expandable intravascular s.
    s. apposition
    Atkinson tube s.
    AVE Micro s.
    bailout s.
    balloon-expandable flexible coil s.
    balloon-expandable intravascular s.
    biodegradable s.
    CardioCoil coronary s.
    carotid s.
    Carpentier s.
    coil s.
    coil vascular s.
    Cook intracoronary s.
    Cordis radiopaque tantalum s.
    Dacron s.
    s. deployment
    double-J s.
    Dynamic Y s.
    eluting s.
    emergency bailout s.
    Endocoil s.
    endoluminal s.
    s. expansion
    Flex s.
    Freitag s.
    Gianturco s.
    Gianturco Z s.
    Gianturco-Roubin s.
    heat-activated recoverable temporary s.

stent *(continued)*
    heat-expandable s.
    helical coil s.
    Hood stoma s.
    Hood-Westaby T-Y s.
    s. implantation
    InStent CarotidCoil s.
    interdigitating coil s.
    intravascular s.
    Medivent self-expanding coronary s.
    Medivent vascular s.
    Medtronic interventional vascular s.
    mesh s.
    Micro s.
    6 Micro S. PL
    Multi Link s.
    Neville s.
    nitinol mesh s.
    nitinol thermal memory s.
    Novastent s.
    Orlowski s.
    Palmaz s.
    Palmaz balloon-expandable iliac s.
    Palmaz vascular s.
    Palmaz-Schatz balloon-expandable s.
    Palmaz-Schatz coronary s.
    Palmaz-Schatz Crown balloon expandable s.
    polymeric endoluminal paving s.
    radiopaque tantalum s.
    Reduced Anticoagulation in Vein Graft S. (RAVES)
    Roubin-Gianturco flexible coil s.
    Schatz-Palmaz intravascular s.
    Schatz-Palmaz tubular mesh s.
    Schneider s.
    self-expanding s.
    spring-loaded s.
    spring-loaded vascular s.
    stainless steel mesh s.

stent *(continued)*
 Strecker balloon-expandable s.
 Strecker coronary s.
 Strecker tantalum s.
 s. strut
 tantalum s.
 thermal memory s.
 Tower s.
 T-Y s.
 Ultraflex self-expanding s.
 VascuCoil peripheral vascular s.
 Wallstent flexible, self-expanding wire-mesh s.
 Wallstent spring-loaded s.
 Wiktor coronary s.
 wire mesh self-expandable s.
 Y s.
 Z s.
 zigzag s.

stenting
 bailout s.
 coronary s.
 endoluminal s.

stentless
 s. porcine aortic valve
 s. porcine aortic valve prosthesis
 s. porcine xenograft

stent-mounted
 s.-m. allograft valve
 s.-m. heterograft valve

step-down therapy

step-down unit

stepped-care antihypertensive regimen

step
 Krönig s's

stepwise

stereocilium

stereoplasm

Sterges carditis

Steri-cath catheter

Sterles sign

Sterna-Band self-locking suture

sternad

sternal
 s. angle of Louis
 s. border
 s. dehiscence
 left s. border
 s. notch
 s. plane
 s. splitting
 s. synchondrosis
 s. wire
 s. wiring

sternalgia

sternal-splitting incision

Sternberg
 S. myocardial insufficiency
 S. pericarditis
 S. sign

sternochondral junction

sternoclavicular angle

sternocleidomastoid
 s. artery

sternocostal triangle

sternodynia

sternomastoid

sternotome

sternotomy
 median s.

sternoxiphoid plane

Stern posture

sternum
 burning sensation over s.
 s. saw
 wiring of s.

steroid
 s. aerosol
 anabolic s.

steroid *(continued)*
    high-dose s.
    sex s.

steroid-eluting pacemaker lead

steroid-sparing agent

Stertzer
    S. brachial guiding catheter
    S. guiding catheter

Stertzer-Myler extension wire

stethoscope
    bell of s.
    diaphragm of s.
    nuclear s.

Stevens-Johnson syndrome

Stewart-Hamilton cardiac output technique

sthenic fever

ST/HR slope

STI
    systolic time interval

stick
    arterial s.
    s. tie
    venipuncture s.

stiff
    s. heart
    s. heart syndrome

stiffness
    active dynamic s.
    chamber s.
    diastolic s.
    elastic s.
    s. index
    muscle s.
    myocardial s.
    vascular s.
    volume s.

stigma *pl.* stigmata
    malpighian s.
    peripheral s.

stigmata

Stilith implantable cardiac pulse generator

Still
    S. disease
    S. murmur

Still-Crawford clamp

Stille-Giertz rib shears

Stille-Mayo scissors

stimulant
    adrenergic s.

stimulation
    alpha-adrenergic s.
    atrial single and double extra s.
    β-adrenergic s.
    beta-adrenergic s.
    beta adrenoceptor s.
    noninvasive programmed s. (NIPS)
    paired electrical s.
    programmed electrical s. (PES)
    slaved programmed electrical s.
    subthreshold s.
    supramaximal tetanic s.
    s. threshold
    s. threshold of pacemaker
    transcutaneous electrical s.
    transesophageal atrial s.
    ultrarapid subthreshold s.
    vagal s.
    ventricular-programmed s.
    ventricular single and double extra s.

stimulator
    Arzco model 7 cardiac s.
    Atrostim phrenic nerve s.
    Bloom DTU 201 external s.
    Bloom programmable s.
    Grass S88 muscle s.

stimulus *pl.* stimuli
    afterpotential s.
    chemical s.
    heterotopic s.

stimulus *(continued)*
>   neurohumoral s.
>   nomotopic s.
>   pacing s.
>   paired s.
>   physical s.
>   premature s.
>   psychological s.
>   square wave s.
>   triple s.

stippling
>   s. of lung fields

stitch
>   anchoring s.

stochastic risk

Stockert cardiac pacing electrode

stocking-glove distribution

stockings
>   antiembolism s.
>   A-T antiembolism s.
>   Bellavar medical support s.
>   Camp-Sigvaris s.
>   Carolon life support antiembolism s.
>   compression s.
>   Comtesse medical support s.
>   elastic s.
>   Fast-Fit vascular s.
>   Florex medical compression s.
>   graduated compression s.
>   Jobst s.
>   Jobst VPGS s.
>   Jobst-Stride support s.
>   Jobst-Stridette support s.
>   Juzo s.
>   Kendall compression s.
>   Linton elastic s.
>   Medi vascular s.
>   Medi-Strumpf s.
>   pneumatic compression s.
>   Sigvaris compression s.
>   Sigvaris medical s.
>   Stride support s.

stockings *(continued)*
>   TED antiembolism s.
>   TED (thromboembolic disease) s.
>   thigh-high antiembolic s.
>   True Form support s.
>   Twee alternating cut-off compressor s.
>   Vairox high compression vascular s.
>   VenES II Medical s.
>   Venofit medical compression s.
>   Venoflex medical compression s.
>   venous pressure gradient support s.
>   Zimmer antiembolism support s.

stocking-seam incision

stoichiometric fashion

Stokes
>   collar of S.
>   S.-Adams disease
>   S.-Adams syndrome

Stokvis-Talma syndrome

stoma
>   coronary artery s.

stone
>   s. heart
>   vein s.

stone-cutter's phthisis

stool
>   melenic s's

stopcock
>   three-way s.

store
>   myocyte magnesium s's

storm
>   thyroid s.

Storz needle cannula

straddling
>   s. aorta

straddling *(continued)*
  s. atrioventricular valve
  s. embolism
  s. thrombus
  s. tricuspid valve

straight
  s. AP pelvic injection
  s. back syndrome
  s. flush percutaneous cath-
    eter
  s. hemostat

straight-line EKG

strain
  0157-H7 s.
  cell s.
  s. gauge
  s.-gauge plethysmography
  Lagrangian s.
  left ventricular s.
  mercury-in-Silastic s. gauge
  s. pattern n EKG
  right ventricular s.

strand
  iridium s.

stranding

strandy infiltrate

strangulation

strap muscles

stratification
  risk s.

stratified thrombus

Stratus cardiac troponin I test

Strauss method

streak
  fatty s.

streaky infiltrate

stream
  axial s.

streaming
  cytoplasmic s.
  protoplasmic s.

Strecker
  S. balloon-expandable stent
  S. coronary stent
  S. tantalum stent

strength
  Bayer Low Adult S.

strenuous exercise

strep throat

streptococcal sore throat

streptococcus
  group A s.

Streptococcus pyogenes

stress
  circumferential wall s.
  S. Echo bed
  s. echocardiography
  emotional s.
  s.-induced
  s.-injected sestamibi-gated
    SPECT with echocardiog-
    raphy
  left ventricular end-systol-
    ic s.
  left ventricular wall s.
  s. management
  mental s.
  meridional wall s.
  s. MUGA electrocardiogram
  s. perfusion and rest func-
    tion by sestamibi-gated
    SPECT
  pharmacologic s.
  physiological s.
  s.-redistribution-reinjection
    thallium-201 imaging
  s.-related arrhythmia
  s.-related hypertension
  s. relaxation
  shear s.
  s.-shortening relationship
  tensile s.
  s. test
  s. thallium-201 myocardial
    perfusion imaging
  s. thallium scan
  s. thallium scintigraphy

stress *(continued)*
  s. thallium study
  ventricular wall s.
  wall s.
  s. washout myocardial per-
    fusion image

Stretch
  S. balloon
  S. cardiac device
  S. receptor

stretching
  side s.
  s. syncope

stria *pl.* striae

Striadyne

striation
  tabby cat s.
  tigroid s.

Stride
  S. cardiac pacemaker
  S. support stockings

strident

string sign

strip
  bovine pericardium s.
  cardiac monitor s.
  Cover-S. wound closure
  EKG monitor s.
  felt s.
  Flu-Glow s.
  rhythm s.
  transtelephonic rhythm s.

stripe
  subepicardial fat s.

stripper
  Alexander rib s.
  Babcock vein s.
  Cole polyethylene vein s.
  Doyle vein s.
  Dunlop thrombus s.
  Emerson vein s.
  endarterectomy s.
  external vein s.

stripper *(continued)*
  hydraulic vein s.
  internal vein s.
  Kurten vein s.
  Matson rib s.
  Mayo vein s.
  Meyer vein s.
  Nabatoff vein s.
  New Orleans endarterecto-
    my s.
  olive-tipped s.
  thrombus s.
  Trace vein s.
  vein s.
  Webb vein s.
  s. with bullet end
  Zollinger-Gilmore intralumi-
    nal vein s.

stripping
  s. of multiple communica-
    tors
  varicose vein s.

stroke
  back s.
  cardioembolic s.
  effective s.
  s. ejection rate
  embolic s.
  heart s.
  heat s.
  s. index
  lacunar s.
  s. output
  s. power
  recovery s.
  thromboembolic s.
  s. volume
  s. volume index
  s. work
  s. work index

stroma-free hemoglobin solution

Strong unbridling of celiac artery axis

stromuhr

strontium-82

Stroop color word conflict test

Strouhal number

structure
    echo-dense s.
    tubuloreticular s.
    wall s.

Strully scissors

struma
    Riedel s.

strut
    George Washington s.
    stent s.
    tricuspid valve s.
    valve outflow s.

strutting
    plaque s.

Stryker saw

ST segment
    ST s. abnormality
    ST s. alternans
    ST s. changes
    coved ST s.
    depressed ST s.
    ST s. depression
    ST s. displacement
    elevated ST s.
    ST s. elevation
    isoelectric ST s.
    sagging ST s.
    ST s. shift
    upsloping ST s.
    ST s. vector forces

ST-T
    ST-T deviation
    ST-T wave
    ST-T wave changes

Stuart
    S. coagulation factor
    S.-Prower blood coagulation factor
    S.-Prower factor

Student-Newman-Keuls test

Student *t* test

study
    altitude simulation s.
    amyl nitrite s.
    atrial pacing s.
    cardiac electrophysiologic s.
    cardiac wall motion s.
    case-control s.
    cohort s.
    Doppler s.
    Doppler flow s.
    electrophysiologic s.
    enzyme s.
    equilibrium-gated blood-pool s.
    first-pass s.
    Framingham s.
    gated blood pool s.
    hemodynamic-angiographic s.
    hypertension optimal treatment s.
    hypoxic response s.
    imaging s.
    interventional s.
    intracardiac electrophysiologic s.
    muscle immunocytochemical s.
    myocardial perfusion s.
    nuclear ventricular function s.
    periorbital Doppler s.
    phased array s.
    polysomnographic s.
    radioisotopic s.
    radionuclide s.
    serum enzyme s.
    sleep s.
    stress thallium s.
    VeHF s.
    wall motion s.

stump
    cardiac s.
    s. pressure

stunned
  s. atrium
  s. myocardium

stunning
  myocardial s.

Sturge-Weber syndrome

stuttering
  s. myocardial infarction
  s. of perfusion

stylet
  Bing s.
  cardiovascular s.
  straight s.
  transmyocardial pacing s.
  transseptal s.

Stylus cardiovascular suture

sub
  subendocardial

Sub-4
  S.-4 Platinum Plus wire kit
  S.-4 small vessel balloon
    dilatation catheter

subacute
  s. bacterial endocarditis
  s. infective endocarditis
  s. myocardial infarction
  s. pericarditis
  s. tamponade

subannular
  s. mattress suture
  s. region

subaortic stenosis

subclavian
  s. approach for cardiac
    catheterization
  s. arteriovenous fistula
  s. artery
  s. artery bypass graft
  s. lymphatic
  s. murmur
  s. peel-away sheath

subclavian (continued)
  s. steal
  s. steal syndrome
  s. triangle
  s. vein

subclavian-carotid bypass

subclavian-subclavian bypass

subclavicular murmur

subcostal
  s. approach
  s. view
  s. zone

subcutaneous
  s. pocket
  s. suture
  s. tunnel
  s. tunneling device

subcuticular suture

subendocardial
  s. infarction (SEI)
  s. ischemia
  s. layer
  s. myocardial infarction
  s. resection
  s. zone

subendocardium

subepicardial
  s. fat stripe

suberosis

subfascially

subintimal

subjunctional heart block

sublingual nitroglycerin

submassive pulmonary embolism

submucosa

submucosal
  s. gland hypertrophy
  s. plaque

submucous

suboptimal visualization

suboptimally visualized

subpectoral
s. implantation of cardioverter-defibrillator
s. implantation of pulse
generator

subphrenic space

subplasmalemmal

subpulmonary
s. obstruction
s. stenosis

subpulmonic stenosis

Sub-Q-Set subcutaneous continuous infusion device

Subramanian clamp

subsarcolemmal cisternae

subsartorial tunnel

subsidiary atrial pacemaker

substance
chromidial s.
interfibrillar s. of Flemming
interfilar s.
interspongioplastic s.
myocardial depressant s.
neurotransmitter s.
s. P
paramagnetic s.
pro-inflammatory s.
thiobarbituric acid reac-
tive s.
vasodepressor s.

substantia
s. hyalina
s. opaca

substernal

substitutional cardiac surgery

substrate
arrhythmogenic s.
tachyarrhythmic s.

subthreshold stimulation

subtraction
s. angiography
digital s.
functional s.
intraoperative digital s.
mask-mode s.

subtype
Reston s.
Sudan s.
Zaire s.

subvalvular
s. aortic stenosis
s. mitral stenosis
s. obstruction
s. stenosis

subxiphoid
s. approach
s. area
s. echocardiography view
s. limited pericardiotomy

sucker
Churchill s.
intracardiac s.

sucking wound

Sucquet-Hoyer anastomosis

suction
diastolic s.
Pleur-evac s.

Sudan subtype

sudden
s. cardiac death
s. infant death syndrome

suffocating chest pain

Sugiura
S. procedure
S. vascular surgery procedure for esophageal vari-
ces

suicide ventricle

suit
anti-G s.
Life S.
MAST s.

sulcus *pl.* sulci
atrioventricular s.
bulboventricular s.
s. coronarius cordis
coronary s. of heart
costophrenic sulci
interventricular s., anterior
interventricular s., inferior
interventricular s., posterior
interventricular s. of heart
s. interventricularis anterior
s. interventricularis inferior
s. interventricularis posterior
longitudinal s. of heart, anterior
longitudinal s. of heart,
posterior
pulmonary s.
s. terminalis
s. terminalis atrii dextri
s. terminalis cordis
terminal s. of heart
terminal s. of right atrium

sulfur colloid
technetium bound to s. c.

SULP II balloon catheter

sum
ray s.

Sumida cardioangioscope

Summagraphics digitizing tablet

summation
s. beat
s. gallop (S₇)
impulse s.
s. shadow

summit
ventricular septal s.

sump pump

sundowning

Sundt carotid endarterectomy
shunt

Sundt-Kees clip for aneurysms

Super-9
S.-9 guiding cardiac device
S.-9 guiding catheter

Super ArrowFlex catheterization sheath

superdicrotic

superficial
s. femoral artery
s. femoral artery occlusion
s. phlebitis

Superflow guiding catheter

superimposed echodensity

superimposition

superior
s. carotid artery
s. mesenteric artery bypass
s. mesenteric artery syn-
drome
s. mesenteric vascular occlusion
s. QRS axis
s. thyroid artery
s. vena cava (SVC)
s. vena cava syndrome

supernatant

supernormal recovery phase

superoinferior heart

superoxide
s. anion
s. dismutase

Superselector Y-K guidewire

SuperStat hemostatic agent

supertension

supersystemic pulmonary artery pressure

supine
    s. bicycle stress echocardiography
    s. exercise
    s. rest gated equilibrium image

supply
    energy s.
    myocardial oxygen s.

support
    Abee s.
    advanced cardiac life s. (ACLS)
    advanced life s. (ALS)
    advanced trauma life s. (ATLS)
    basic cardiac life s. (BCLS)
    basic life s. (BLS)
    biventricular s. (BVS)
    cardiopulmonary s. (CPS)
    Dr. Gibaud thermal health s.
    extracorporeal life s. (ECLS)
    IMP-Capello arm s.
    inotropic s.
    percutaneous cardiopulmonary s. (PCPS)
    percutaneous cardiopulmonary bypass s. (PCBS)

suppression
    s. of arrhythmia
    overdrive s.

suppurative
    s. pericarditis

supra-annular
    s. constriction
    s. mitral valve replacement
    s. prosthesis
    s. suture ring

supra-aortic ridge

supraceliac aorta

supraclavicular
    s. fossa

supracristal ventricular septal defect

supra-Hisian block

supramaximal tetanic stimulation

supranormal
    s. conduction
    s. excitability
    s. excitation

suprasellar aneurysm

suprasternal
    s. examination
    s. notch view on echocardiogram
    s. pulsation
    s. view

supravalvar
    s. aortic stenosis-infantile hypercalcemia syndrome
    s. aortic stenosis syndrome
    s. stenosis

supravalvular
    s. aortic stenosis
    s. aortic stenosis–infantile hypercalcemia syndrome
    s. aortic stenosis syndrome
    s. aortogram

supraventricular
    s. arrhythmia
    s. crest
    s. ectopy
    s. ectopic levels
    s. extrasystole
    inducible sustained orthodromic s. tachycardia
    s. premature contraction
    s. tachyarrhythmia
    s. tachycardia (SVT)

supraventricularis
    crista s.

surcingle
    Von Lackum s.

surdocardiac syndrome

surf
    Human S.
    s. test

surface
    anterior s. of heart
    Carmeda BioActive S.
    diaphragmatic s. of heart
    inferior s. of heart
    left s. of heart
    pulmonary s. of heart
    right s. of heart
    sternocostal s. of heart

surfactant
    bovine lavage extract s.
    s. deficiency
    hydrolysis of s.
    pulmonary s.

surgery
    ablative cardiac s.
    bypass s.
    cardiac s.
    cardiothoracic s. (CTS)
    excisional cardiac s.
    keyhole s.
    open heart s.
    palliative s.
    reparative cardiac s.
    substitutional cardiac s.

surgical
    s. intervention

Surgica K6 laser
    surgical revascularization

Surgical Nu-Knit

Surgicel
    S. gauze

Surgiclip
    Auto Suture S.

Surgicraft
    S. pacemaker electrode
    S. suture

Surgilase 150 laser

Surgilene suture

Surgilon suture

Surgitool prosthetic valve

Surgitron unit

surveillance angiography

susceptibility

suspended
    s. heart
    s. heart syndrome

sustained
    s. monomorphic ventricular tachycardia
    s. reciprocating tachycardia
    s. release

susurrus

Sutter-Smeloff heart valve

Sutton law

suture
    absorbable s.
    anchoring s.
    angle s.
    atraumatic s.
    black s.
    braided silk s.
    bridle s.
    buried s.
    Cardioflon s.
    cardiovascular silk s.
    catgut s.
    chromic s.
    chromic catgut s.
    circular s.
    coated s.
    collagen s.
    continuous s.
    Cooley U s's
    cotton s.
    Dacron s.
    Dacron-bolstered s.
    deep s.
    Deklene s.
    Dermalene s.

suture *(continued)*
- Dermalon s.
- Dexon s.
- Dexon Plus s.
- double-armed s.
- doubly ligated s.
- dural tenting s.
- Endoknot s.
- end-to-side s.
- EPTFE vascular s.
- Ethibond s.
- Ethicon s.
- Ethiflex s.
- Ethilon s.
- everting mattress s.
- figure-of-eight s.
- Flexon steel s.
- Frater s.
- Gregory stay s.
- gut s.
- heavy silk s.
- heavy wire s.
- horizontal s.
- horizontal mattress s.
- imbricating s.
- intermittent s.
- interrupted s.
- interrupted pledgeted s.
- intracuticular s.
- inverted s.
- inverting s.
- Lembert s.
- ligature s.
- locked s.
- locking s.
- looped s.
- mattress s.
- Maxon s.
- Mersilene s.
- Mersilene braided nonabsorbable s.
- monofilament absorbable s.
- monofilament polypropylene s.
- nonabsorbable s.
- noneverting s.
- Novofil s.
- Nurolon s.

suture *(continued)*
- nylon s.
- over-and-over whip s.
- patch reinforced mattress s.
- pericostal s.
- Perma-Hand s.
- plain s.
- plastic s.
- pledgeted s.
- pledgeted Ethibond s.
- pledgeted mattress s.
- Polydek s.
- polypropylene s.
- pop-off s.
- Potts tie s.
- preplaced s.
- Prolene s.
- pursestring s.
- pyroglycolic acid s.
- reabsorbable s.
- retention s.
- running s.
- seromuscular-to-edge s.
- silk s.
- simple s.
- single-armed s.
- skin staples s.
- stainless steel wire s.
- staples s.
- Steri-Strips s.
- Sterna-Band self-locking s.
- stitch s.
- Stylus cardiovascular s.
- subannular mattress s.
- subcutaneous s.
- subcuticular s.
- Surgicraft s.
- Surgilene s.
- Surgilon s.
- synthetic s.
- Teflon s.
- Teflon pledgeted s.
- tenting s.
- Tevdek pledgeted s.
- through-and-through continuous s.

suture *(continued)*
    through-the-wall mattress s.
    Ti-Cron s.
    traction s.
    transfixion s.
    Trumbull s.
    Tycron s.
    U double-barrel s.
    umbilical tape s.
    undyed s.
    U s's
    vertical s.
    Vicryl s.
    whipstitch s.
    white s.
    wire s.

suturing
    coupled s.

SV
    stroke volume

SVAS
    supravalvular aortic stenosis

SVC
    slow vital capacity
    superior vena cava

SVG
    saphenous vein graft

SVI
    stroke volume index

SVM
    syncytiovascular membrane

SVPC
    supraventricular premature contraction

SVR
    systemic vascular resistance

SVRI
    systemic vascular resistance index

SVT
    supraventricular tachycardia

swallow
    barium s.
    s. syncope
    wet s.

Swan
    S. aortic clamp
    S.-Ganz balloon flotation catheter
    S.-Ganz bipolar pacing catheter
    S.-Ganz catheter
    S.-Ganz flow-directed catheter
    S.-Ganz Guidewire TD catheter
    S.-Ganz Pacing TD catheter
    S.-Ganz pulmonary artery catheter
    S.-Ganz syndrome
    S.-Ganz technique for cardiac catheterization
    S.-Ganz thermodilution catheter

Swank high-flow arterial blood filter

S wave
    deep S w.
    slurred S w.
    wide S w.

sweat
    s. chloride
    s. chloride test

sweating

sweep

Sweet
    S. sternal punch
    S. Tip lead

SWI
    Stroke work index

swimmer's view

swinging heart

Swiss
    S. cheese defect
    S. cheese interventricular
        septum
    S. Kiss intrastent balloon
        inflation device

switch
    DNA s.
    isoactin s.
    isomyosin s.
    s. operation
    s. procedure

switching
    automatic mode s.
    mode s.

Swyer-James syndrome

Sydenham chorea

Sylvest disease

Sylvius
    valve of S.

Symbion
    S. cardiac device
    S. Jarvik-7 artificial heart
    S. J-7 70-mL ventricle total
        artificial heart
    S. pneumatic assist device

Symbion/CardioWest 100 mL total artificial heart

Symbios 7006 pacemaker

Symcor

symmetrical phased array

sympathectomy
    cervicothoracic s.
    high thoracic left s.
    lumbar s.
    regional cardiac s.

sympathetic
    s. activity
    s. nervous system

sympathoadrenal system

sympathoexcitation
    reflex s.

sympathoexcitatory

sympathoinhibition

sympatholytic

sympathomimetic
    s. amine
    s. drug

sympathovagal
    s. balance
    s. imbalance
    s. transition

Symphony patient monitoring
system

symphysis *pl.* symphyses
    cardiac s.
    s. pubis

symplasmatic

symport

symptom
    Baumès s.
    Buerger's s.
    Burghart s.
    Duroziez s.
    Fischer s.
    Kussmaul s.
    s.-limited exercise test
    Oehler's s.
    prodromal s.
    s. reproduced with exer-
        tion
    Trunecek s.

symptomatic digitalis-induced
bradyarrhythmia

symptom-free interval

symptom-limited treadmill exercise test

synapsis

Synapse electrocardiographic
cream

synaptene

synaptic

Sync
    Star S.

synchondrosis
    sternal s.

SynchroMed programmable
    pump

synchronization

synchronized DC cardioversion

synchronizer
    CardioSync cardiac s.

synchronous mode of pace-
    maker

synchrony
    atrial s.
    atrioventricular (AV) s.
    S. I pacemaker
    S. II pacemaker

synchrotron-based transvenous
    angiography

syncopal
    s. migraine
    s. migraine headache
    s. spell

syncope
    Adams-Stokes s.
    s. angiosa
    cardiac s.
    cardiogenic s.
    cardioinhibitory s.
    carotid sinus s.
    cerebrovascular s.
    cough s.
    defecation s.
    deglutition s.
    diver's s.
    exertional s.
    glossopharyngeal vagal s.
    hypoglycemic s.
    hypoxic s.

syncope *(continued)*
    hysterical s.
    local s.
    micturition s.
    migraine s.
    mixed neurally mediated s.
    near-s.
    neurally-mediated s.
    neurocardiogenic s.
    neuromediated s.
    noncardiac s.
    orthostatic s.
    positional s.
    postmicturition s.
    posttussive s.
    postural s.
    sexual s.
    situational s.
    sneeze s.
    Stokes-Adams s.
    stretching s.
    swallow s.
    toilet-seat s.
    transient s.
    tussive s.
    vasodepressor-cardioinhi-
        bitory s.
    vasovagal s.
    X s.

syncytial virus

syncytiovascular membrane

syndactyly

syndesis

syndrome
    acute retroviral s.
    Adams-Stokes s.
    adrenogenital s.
    Albright s.
    Alport s.
    ALPS s.
    amniotic fluid s.
    Andersen s.
    angina with normal coron-
        aries s.
    anomalous first thoracic
        rib s.

syndrome *(continued)*
   antiphospholipid s.
   aortic arch s.
   aortic arteritis s.
   apallic s.
   Apert s.
   apical systolic click-mur-
     mur s.
   arteriohepatic dysplasia s.
   Asherson s.
   Ask-Upmark s.
   atypical chest pain s.
   Austrian s.
   Ayerza s.
   Babinski's s.
   Babinski-Vaquez s.
   ballooning mitral cusp s.
   ballooning mitral valve s.
   ballooning posterior leaf-
     let s.
   bangungut s.
   Bannayan-Zonana s.
   Bannwarth s.
   Barlow's s.
   Barsony-Polgar s.
   Barth s.
   Bartter s.
   Bauer s.
   beer and cobalt s.
   Behçet s.
   Bernheim's s.
   Beuren s.
   billowing mitral valve s.
   billowing posterior leaf-
     let s.
   Blackfan-Diamond s.
   Bland-Garland-white s.
   Bloom s.
   blue finger s.
   blue toe s.
   blue velvet s.
   Boerhaave s.
   Bouillaud's s.
   Bouveret's s.
   Bradbury-Eggleston s.
   bradycardia-tachycardia s.
   brady-tachy s.
   bradytachycardia s.
   bradytachydysrhythmia s.

syndrome *(continued)*
   Brett s.
   Brugada s.
   Budd-Chiari s.
   Bürger-Grütz s.
   capillary leak s.
   Caplan s.
   carcinoid s.
   cardioauditory s.
   cardiofacial s.
   carotid sinus s.
   carotid steal s.
   Carpenter s.
   CATCH 22 s.
   cauda equina s.
   cervical rib s.
   Charcot's s.
   Charcot-Weiss-Baker s.
   CHARGE s.
   Chiari s.
   Chiari-Budd s.
   Chinese restaurant s.
   chronic hyperventilation s.
   Churg-Strauss s.
   click s.
   click-murmur s.
   Cockayne s.
   Cogan s.
   compartment s.
   compartmental s.
   concealed Wolff-Parkinson-
     White s.
   congenital central hypov-
     entilation s.
   Conn s.
   Conradi-Hünermann s.
   coronary steal s.
   Cornelia de Lange s.
   costochondral s.
   costoclavicular s.
   costoclavicular rib s.
   costosternal s.
   CREST s.
   cri-du-chat s.
   cryptophthalmos s.
   Curracino-Silverman s.
   Cushing's s.
   cutis laxa s.
   Cyriax s.

syndrome *(continued)*
   DaCosta s.
   declamping shock s.
   DeGimard s.
   de Lange s.
   Determann s.
   DiGeorge s.
   Down s.
   Dressler's s.
   drowned newborn s.
   drug-induced lupus s.
   Duncan s.
   Dysshwannian s.
   Eaton-Lambert s.
   effort s.
   Ehlers-Danlos s.
   Eisenmenger's s.
   elfin facies s.
   Ellis-van Creveld s.
   eosinophilia-myalgia s.
   eosinophilic pulmonary s.
   epibronchial right pulmonary artery s.
   euthyroid sick s.
   external carotid steal s.
   familial cholestasis s.
   fat embolism s.
   fetal alcohol s.
   fibrinogen-fibrin conversion s.
   flapping valve s.
   Fleischner s.
   floppy valve s.
   Forney s.
   Forrester s.
   four-day s.
   Gailliard s.
   Gaisböck s.
   Gasser's s.
   gastrocardiac s.
   Gerhardt s.
   Goldenhar s.
   Goodpasture s.
   Gorlin s.
   Gowers s.
   Grönblad-Strandberg s.
   Guillain-Barré s.
   Gulf War s.
   Halbrecht s.

syndrome *(continued)*
   Hamman-Rich s.
   hand-arm vibration s.
   Hare s.
   heart and hand s.
   heart-hand s.
   Hegglin s.
   Heiner s.
   hemangioma-thrombocytopenia s.
   hemolytic uremic s.
   hemopleuropneumonia s.
   Henoch-Schönlein s.
   Hermansky-Pudlak s.
   Herner s.
   heterotaxy s.
   holiday heart s.
   Holt-Oram s.
   homocystinuria s.
   Horner s.
   Horton's s.
   Howel-Evans s.
   Hughes-Stovin s.
   Hunter s.
   Hunter-Hurler s.
   Hurler s.
   hyperabduction s.
   hyperapolipoprotein B s.
   hypereosinophilia s.
   hypereosinophilic s.
   hyperkinetic heart s.
   hypersensitive carotid sinus s.
   hyperventilation s.
   hyperviscosity s.
   hypoplastic left heart s.
   hypoplastic right heart s.
   hypothenar hammer s.
   idiopathic hypereosinophilic s.
   idiopathic long Q-T interval s.
   s. of inappropriate antidiuretic hormone
   incontinentia pigmenti s.
   intermediate coronary s.
   ischemic heart disease s.
   Ivemark s.
   Jackson s.

syndrome *(continued)*
- Janus s.
- Jervell and Lange-Nielsen s.
- Jeune s.
- Job s.
- Kallmann s.
- Kartagener s.
- Kasabach-Merritt s.
- Kawasaki s.
- Kearns s.
- Kearns-Sayre s.
- Kimmelstiel-Wilson s.
- Klein-Waardenburg s.
- Klinefelter s.
- Klippel-Feil s.
- Klippel-Trenaunay-Weber s.
- Kostmann s.
- Kugelberg-Welander s.
- Kussmaul s.
- LAMB s.
- Landouzy-Déjérine s.
- Landry-Guillain-Barré s.
- Laubry-Soulle s.
- Laurence-Moon-Bardet-Biedl s.
- Laurence-Moon-Biedl s.
- Leitner s.
- Lenègre s.
- Lenz s.
- LEOPARD s.
- Leredde s.
- Leriche's s.
- Lev s.
- Libman-Sacks s.
- Löffler s.
- long Q–T s.
- long Q–TU s.
- Lown-Ganong-Levine s.
- low cardiac output s.
- low-salt s., low-sodium s.
- Lutembacher's s.
- Macleod s.
- malignant carcinoid s.
- Mallory-Weiss s.
- Marfan s.
- Marie s.
- Marie-Bamberger s.
- Maroteaux-Lamy s.
- Martorell's s.

syndrome *(continued)*
- mastocytosis s.
- Maugeri s.
- McArdle s.
- Meadows s.
- Meigs s.
- Mendelson s.
- Mèniére s.
- metastatic carcinoid s.
- midsystolic click s.
- midsystolic click-late systolic murmur s.
- mitral valve prolapse s.
- Mondor s.
- Morgagni-Adams-Stokes s.
- Morquio s.
- Mounier-Kuhn s.
- Moynahan s.
- multiple lentigines s.
- MVP s.
- myocardial ischemic s.
- Naffziger's s.
- NAME s.
- nephrotic s.
- Noonan s.
- Opitz s.
- Ortner's s.
- Osler-Weber-Rendu s.
- pacemaker s.
- pacemaker twiddler's s.
- Paget-Schroetter s.
- Paget-von Schroetter s.
- Paget-von Schrötter s.
- Pancoast s.
- papillary muscle s.
- paraneoplastic s.
- Penderluft s.
- pericardiotomy s.
- pericarditis-myocarditis s.
- Pick s.
- pickwickian s.
- PIE s.
- Pierre Robin s.
- Pins s.
- Plummer-Vinson s.
- P mitral s.
- Polhemus-Schafer-Ivemark s.
- polyangiitis overlap s.

syndrome *(continued)*
  polymyalgia rheumatica s.
  post-cardiac injury s.
  postcardiotomy s.
  postcardiotomy psychos-
    is s.
  postcommissurotomy s.
  postinfarction s.
  post-myocardial infarc-
    tion s.
  postperfusion s.
  postpericardiotomy s.
  postphlebitic s.
  postpump s.
  post-thrombotic s.
  posttransfusion s.
  P pulmonale s.
  precordial catch s.
  preexcitation s.
  preinfarction s.
  premonitory s.
  primary mitral valve pro-
    lapse s.
  prolapsed mitral valve s.
  prolonged QT interval s.
  pseudoclaudication s.
  pseudoxanthoma elasti-
    cum s.
  pulmonary infarction s.
  pulmonary sling s.
  Q–T s.
  Q–TU interval s.
  radiologic scimitar s.
  Raeder-Arbitz s.
  Raynaud s.
  redman s.
  redundant cusp s.
  Reiter s.
  Rendu-Osler-Weber s.
  Reye s.
  Riley-Day s.
  Romano-Ward s.
  Rosenbach s.
  Roussy-Lévy s.
  rubella s.
  Rubinstein-Taybi s.
  salt-depletion s.
  Sanchez-Cascos cardioaudi-
    tory s.

syndrome *(continued)*
  Sandifer s.
  scalenus s.
  scalenus anterior s.
  scalenus anticus s.
  Scheie s.
  Schönlein-Henoch s.
  scimitar s.
  Sebastiani s.
  shoulder-hand s.
  Shprintzen s.
  Shy-Drager s.
  sicca s.
  sick sinus s.
  Silver s.
  single papillary muscle s.
  Sjögren s.
  sleep apnea s.
  sleep apnea/hypopnea s.
  slipping rib s.
  slit ventricle s.
  Smith-Lemli-Opitz s.
  Spens' s.
  splenic flexure s.
  stiff heart s.
  Stokes' s.
  Stokes-Adams s.
  Stokvis-Talma s.
  straight back s.
  Sturge-Weber s.
  subclavian steal s.
  sudden infant death s.
  superficial vena cava s.
  superior mesenteric ar-
    tery s.
  superior vena cava s.
  supravalvar aortic stenos-
    is s.
  supravalvar aortic stenosis-
    infantile hypercalcemia s.
  supravalvular aortic sten-
    osis s.
  supravalvular aortic steno-
    sis-infantile hypercalcem-
    ia s.
  surdocardiac s.
  suspended heart s.
  Swan-Ganz s.
  Swyer-James s.

syndrome *(continued)*
    systemic inflammatory response s.
    systolic click-late systolic murmur s.
    systolic click-murmur s.
    tachybradycardia s.
    tachycardia-bradycardia s.
    tachycardia-polyuria s.
    Takayasu's s.
    TAR s.
    Taussig-Bing s.
    Taybi s.
    thoracic endometriosis s.
    thoracic outlet s.
    thoracic outlet compression s.
    thrombocytopenia-absent radius s.
    thromboembolic s.
    Tietze s.
    toxic oil s.
    trash foot s.
    Treacher Collins s.
    trisomy D s.
    Trousseau s.
    Turner s.
    twiddler's s.
    Uhl s.
    Ullmann s.
    VACTERL s.
    vascular s.
    vascular leak s.
    vasculocardiac s. of hyperserotonemia
    vasovagal s.
    VATER association s.
    velocardiofacial s.
    vena cava s.
    venolobar s.
    Vernet s.
    Villaret s.
    Vogt-Koyanagi-Harada s.
    Volkmann's s.
    von Willebrand s.
    Waardenburg s.
    Ward-Romano s.
    wasting s.
    Watson s.

syndrome *(continued)*
    Weber-Osler-Rendu s.
    Werner s.
    West s.
    white clot s.
    Williams s.
    Williams-Campbell s.
    Wilson-Mikity s.
    Wiskott-Aldrich s.
    Wolff-Parkinson-White s.
    WPW s.
    Wright's s.
    s. X
    XO s.
    XXXX s.
    XXX s.
    yellow nail s.
    Yentl s.
    Young s.

synechia *pl.* synechiae
    s. pericardii

synergenesis

synergism

synergistic

Synergyst
    S. DDD pacemaker
    S. II pacemaker

synezesis

syngenesioplastic transplant

synizesis

Synthaderm dressing

synthesis
    thromboxane s.

synthetase
    pantothenate s.

synvinolin

syphilis
    bejel s.
      cardiovascular s.
      tertiary s.

syphilitic
    s. aortic aneurysm

syphilitic *(continued)*
>   s. aortic valvulitis
>   s. aortitis
>   s. arteritis
>   s. endarteritis
>   s. endocarditis
>   s. myocarditis

syringe
>   anaerobic Pulsator s.
>   Concord line draw s.
>   Namic angiographic s.
>   Osciflator balloon inflation s.
>   Pulsator s.
>   Raulerson s.
>   Ultraject prefilled s.

system
>   Abiomed biventricular support s.
>   ABL 625 s.
>   ABL 520 blood gas measurement s.
>   ACS Concorde over-the-wire catheter s.
>   Acuson cardiovascular s.
>   adrenergic nervous s.
>   Advanced Cardiovascular S's (ACS)
>   Advanced Catheter S's (AC)
>   Aladdin infant flow s.
>   Alcon Closure S.
>   ANCOR imaging s.
>   Angio-Jeg rapid thrombectomy s.
>   annular phase array s.
>   Arcomax FMA cardiac angiography s.
>   Atakr s.
>   atrioventricular conduction s.
>   Atrium Blood Recovery s.
>   automated cervical cell screening s.
>   automatic exposure s.
>   autonomic nervous s.
>   Autotrans s.
>   autotransfusion s.

system *(continued)*
>   BACTEC s.
>   Bard cardiopulmonary support s.
>   Bard percutaneous cardiopulmonary support s.
>   Baylor autologous transfusion s.
>   Beta-Cath s.
>   BiliBlanket phototherapy s.
>   Biodex S.
>   Biosound Phase 2 ultrasound s.
>   blood-vascular s.
>   Bonchek-Shiley vein distention s.
>   BosPac cardiopulmonary bypass s.
>   brachiocephalic s.
>   BRAT s.
>   Burette multiple patient delivery s.
>   Cadence tiered therapy defibrillator s.
>   Capintex VEST s.
>   cardiac conduction s.
>   CardiData Prodigy s.
>   Cardiofreezer cryosurgical s.
>   cardioscope U s.
>   cardiovascular s.
>   Cardiovascular Angiography Analysis S.
>   Cardiovit AT-10 ECG/spirometry combination s.
>   CASE computerized exercise EKG s.
>   catheter-snare s.
>   catheter-tip micromanometer s.
>   Cath-Finder catheter tracking s.
>   Cell Saver autologous blood recovery s.
>   Cell Saver Haemonetics Autotransfusion s.
>   Cenflex central monitoring s.

system *(continued)*
    CGR biplane angiograph-
        ic s.
    chemoreceptor s.
    cine-pulse s.
    CineView Plus Freeland s.
    Circulaire aerosol drug de-
        livery s.
    circulatory s.
    circulatory support s.
    CMS AccuProbe 450 s.
    Cobe Spectra apheresis s.
    codominant s.
    COER-24 delivery s.
    CO_2ject s.
    complement s.
    complete pacemaker pa-
        tient testing s.
    conducting s. of heart
    conduction s.
    conduction s. of heart
    coordinate s.
    COROSKOP C cardiac imag-
        ing s.
    CPS s.
    Cragg Endopro s.
    C-VEST radiation detec-
        tor s.
    CVIS/InterTherapy intravas-
        cular ultrasound s.
    cytochrome P450 s.
    Dallas Classification S.
    DCI-S automated coronary
        analysis s.
    Desilets introducer s.
    Diasonics/Sonotron Ving-
        med CFM 800 imaging s.
    dilator-sheath s.
    Dinamap s.
    dominant left coronary ar-
        tery s.
    DUPEL drug delivery s.
    Dymer excimer delivery s.
    echocardiographic auto-
        mated boundary detec-
        tion s.
    echocardiographic scor-
        ing s.
    Echovar Doppler s.

system *(continued)*
    electrode s.
    Elscint tomography s.
    endocrine s.
    Endotak lead s.
    EnGuard double-lead ICD s.
    EnGuard pacing and defib-
        rillation lead s.
    EPT-1000 cardiac abla-
        tion s.
    Erie S.
    Estes point s.
    Estes-Romhilt EKG point-
        score s.
    Fiberlase s.
    fiberoptic catheter deliv-
        ery s.
    fibrinolytic s.
    fixed-wire balloon dilata-
        tion s.
    Flowtron DVT pump s.
    FMA cardiovascular imag-
        ing s.
    Frank lead s.
    Frank EKG lead place-
        ment s.
    Frank XYZ orthogonal
        lead s.
    gastrointestinal therapeu-
        tic s.
    gated s.
    General Electric Advantx s.
    GenESA closed-loop deliv-
        ery s.
    Guidant TRIAD three-elec-
        trode energy defibrilla-
        tion s.
    Gyroscan HP Philips 15S
        whole-body s.
    Haemolite autologous
        blood recovery s.
    Haemonetics Cell Saver s.
    HeartMate implantable
        pneumatic left ventricular
        assist s.
    HEARTrac I Cardiac Moni-
        toring s.
    hematopoietic s.

system *(continued)*
Hewlett-Packard 5 MHz phased-array TEE s.
Hewlett-Packard Sonos 1000, 1500 ultrasound s.
hexaxial reference s.
His-Purkinje s.
Hombach lead placement s.
IDIS s.
Image-View s.
Imatron C-100 s.
implantable left ventricular assist s.
INCA s.
Infiniti catheter introducer s.
infra-Hisian conduction s.
Innovator Holter s.
integrated lead s.
INTEGRIS cardiac imaging s.
Intra-Op autotransfusion s.
Irri-Cath suction s.
Irvine viable organ-tissue transport s.
isocenter s.
Jinotti closed suctioning s.
kallikrein-bradykinin s.
kallikrein-kinin s.
Kiethly-DAS series 500 data-acquisition s.
King double umbrella closure s.
KK s.
lead s.
left ventricular assist s.
Leocor hemoperfusion s.
Leukotrap red cell storage s.
Liposorber LA-15 s.
Luxtec fiberoptic s.
Magnum-Meier s.
Marquette Case-12 electrocardiographic s.
Marquette Case-12 exercise s.
Mason-Likar 12-lead EKG s.
M/D 4 defibrillator s.

system *(continued)*
MEDDARS cardiac catheterization analysis s.
MedGraphics Cardio O2 s.
Medi-Facts s.
Medi-Tech catheter s.
Medtronic Interactive Tachycardia Terminating s.
Medtronic Transvene endocardial lead s.
Meier-Magnum s.
Metrix atrial defibrillation s.
MicroHartzler ACS balloon catheter s.
micromanometer catheter s.
MIDA 1000 monitoring s.
Mobin-Uddin filter s.
Monaldi drainage s.
Mullins sheath s.
Myocardial Infarction Data Acquisition S.
nervous s.
nonthoracotomy defibrillation lead s.
Novacor left ventricular assist s.
Omni tract retractor s.
OptiHaler drug delivery s.
orthogonal lead s.
over-the-wire balloon dilatation s.
Oximetrix 3 S.
Oxycure topical oxygen s.
Oxyfill oxygen refilling s.
Paceart complete pacemaker patient testing s.
pacemaker code s.
pacemaker tester s.
parasympathetic nervous s.
Patil stereotactic s.
PCA s.
PCD Transvene implantable cardioverter-defibrillator s.
PDB preperitoneal distention balloon s.

system *(continued)*
  Pelorus stereotactic s.
  peripheral access s.
  Peripheral AngioJet s.
  peripheral atherectomy s.
  phased array s.
  plasma coagulation s.
  Pleur-evac autotransfu-
    sion s.
  Port-A-Cath implantation
    catheter s.
  portal s.
  Portex Soft-Seal cuff s.
  Prevue s.
  Probe balloon-on-a-wire di-
    lation s.
  programmable implantable
    medication s.
  PulseSpray infusion s.
  Purkinje s.
  Q-cath catheterization re-
    cording s.
  Quinton computerized ex-
    ercise EKG s.
  Rasor Blood Pumping s.
  Remac s.
  renin-angiotensin-aldoster-
    one s.
  reticuloendothelial s.
  Rfb s.
  Romhilt-Estes point scor-
    ing s.
  Rotacs s.
  rotational atherectomy s.
  Rozanski lead placement s.
  R-Port implantable vascular
    access s.
  Rx5000 cardiac pacing s.
  SAM s.
  Sandman s.
  saphenofemoral s.
  sarcotubular s.
  Schneider-Meier-Magnum s.
  Sequel compression s.
  Sequestra 1000 s.
  sheath and dilator s.
  SICOR cardiac catheteriza-
    tion recording s.

system *(continued)*
  Simpson Coronary
    AtheroCath s.
  Simpson-Robert vascular
    dilation s.
  single chamber cardiac
    pacing s.
  SKY epidural pain con-
    trol s.
  Snuggle Warm convective
    warming s.
  Sonos 500 imaging s.
  sympathetic nervous s.
  sympathoadrenal s.
  Symphony patient monitor-
    ing s.
  T s.
  TAM s.
  Transtelephonic ambula-
    tory monitoring s.
  Thora-Klex chest drain-
    age s.
  Thoratec VAD S.
  Thrombolytic Assess-
    ment s.
  Thumper CPR s.
  Total Synchrony S.
  transluminal lysing s.
  transtelephonic ambula-
    tory monitoring s.
  triaxial reference s.
  TRON 3 VACI cardiac imag-
    ing s.
  two-bottle thoracic drain-
    age s.
  Unilink s.
  USCI Probe balloon-on-a-
    wire dilatation s.
  Vario s.
  vascular s.
  VDD pacing s.
  Ventak PRx defibrillation s.
  Ventak PRx III/Endotak s.
  Ventritex TVL s.
  vessel occlusion s.
  Veterans Affairs Medical
    Center scoring s.
  Viagraph EKG s.
  video s.

system *(continued)*
    Vingmed CFM 800 echocar-
      diographic s.
    V_1-like ambulatory lead s.
    V_5-like ambulatory lead s.
    White s.
    Xillix ACCESS s.
    XYZ lead s.
    Yellow IRIS s.

systema
    s. cardiovasculare
    s. conducens cordis

systemic
    s. AV O_2 difference
    s. blood flow (SBF)
    s. circulation
    s. collateral
    s. heart
    s. hemodynamic parame-
      ters
    s. hemodynamics
    s. infection
    s. inflammatory response
      syndrome
    s. lupus erythematosus
      (SLE)
    s. mean arterial pressure
    s. necrotizing vasculitis
    s. pressure
    s. to pulmonary artery
      anastomosis
    s. to pulmonary connection
    s. to pulmonary shunt
    s. resistance
    s. and topical hypothermia
    s. vascular hypertension
    s. vascular resistance
    s. vascular resistance index
    s. venous hypertension
    s. venous return

systole
    aborted s.
    s. alternans
    anticipated s.
    atrial s.
    auricular s.
    cardiac s.
    coupled premature s.

systole *(continued)*
    electrical s.
    electromechanical s.
    extra s.
    frustrate s.
    hemic s.
    isovolumic s.
    late s.
    premature s.
    premature atrial s.
    premature junctional s.
    premature ventricular s.
    total s.
    total electromechanical s.
    ventricular s.
    ventricular ectopic s.

systolic
    s. anterior motion
    s. anterior motion of mitral
      valve
    s. apical impulse
    s. apical murmur
    s. blood pressure
    s. bruit
    s. click
    s. click-murmur syndrome
    s. current
    s. current of injury
    s. doming
    s. ejection murmur
    s. ejection period
    s. ejection rate
    s. fractional shortening
    s. function
    s. gallop
    s. gallop rhythm
    s. gradient
    s. heart failure
    s. honk
    s. hypertension
    S. Hypertension in the El-
      derly
    s. left ventricular pressure
    s. pressure
    s. pressure time index
    s. regurgitant murmur
    s. reserve
    s. shock
    s. thrill

systolic *(continued)*
    s. time interval
    s. trough
    s. upstroke time
    s. velocity ratio

systolic *(continued)*
    s. whipping
    s. whoop

systolometer

T
- T artifact
- T cells
- T loop
- T sign
- T system
- T-tube
- T vector
- T wave
- T wave alternans
- T wave changes
- T wave flattening
- T wave inversion
- upright T waves

T2
- T2 relaxation time
- T2 weighted image

T_4
- thyroxine

t test

T1 weighted image

Ta
- tantalum

tabacosis

tabby
- t. heart
- t. cat striation

tabetic cuirass

table
- anterior t.
- Diamond-Forrester t.
- Kaplan-Meier life t.
- Siemens open heart t.
- tilt t.

tablet
- buccal t.
- enteric-coated t.
- scored t.
- sublingual t.

tabourka
- bruit de t.

TAC atherectomy catheter

tache
- t. blanche
- t's laiteuses

tachogram

tachography study

tachyarrhythmia
- supraventricular t.
- ventricular t.

tachybrady arrhythmia

tachybradycardia syndrome

tachycardia
- accelerated t.
- alternating bidirectional t.
- antidromic atrioventricular (AV) reciprocating t.
- antidromic circus-movement t.
- antidromic t.
- atrial t. (AT)
- atrial chaotic t.
- atrial ectopic t.
- atrial paroxysmal t.
- atrial reentry t.
- atrial ventricular nodal reentry t.
- atrial ventricular reciprocating t.
- atrioventricular junctional reciprocating t.
- atrioventricular (AV) nodal t.
- atrioventricular nodal reentrant t.
- atrioventricular reciprocating t.
- atrioventricular t.
- auricular t.
- automatic atrial t.
- automatic ectopic t.
- AV junctional t.
- AV nodal reentry t.
- AV node reentrant t.
- AV reciprocating t.
- bidirectional ventricular t.
- bundle branch reentrant t.

tachycardia *(continued)*
  chaotic atrial t.
  circus-movement t.
  Coumel t.
  t. cycle length
  double t.
  drug-refractory t.
  ectopic atrial t.
  ectopic t.
  endless loop t.
  t. en salves
  entrainment t.
  essential t.
  exercise-induced t.
  familial t.
  fascicular t.
  fetal t.
  idiopathic ventricular t.
  idioventricular t.
  inducible polymorphic ventricular t.
  intra-atrial reentrant t.
  junctional t.
  junctional ectopic t.
  junctional reciprocating t.
  macroreentrant atrial t.
  Mahaim-type t.
  malignant ventricular t.
  monoform t.
  monomorphic ventricular t.
  multifocal atrial t.
  narrow-complex t.
  nodal paroxysmal t.
  nodal reentrant t.
  nodal t.
  nonparoxysmal atrioventricular junctional t.
  nonparoxysmal ventricular t.
  nonsustained ventricular t.
  orthodromic atrioventricular (AV) reciprocating t.
  orthodromic atrioventricular (AV) reentrant t.
  orthodromic circus-movement t.
  orthostatic t.
  pacemaker-mediated t.
  parasystolic atrial t. (PAT)

tachycardia *(continued)*
  parasystolic ventricular t.
  paroxysmal junctional t.
  paroxysmal nodal t.
  paroxysmal reentrant supraventricular t.
  paroxysmal sinus t.
  paroxysmal supraventricular t.
  paroxysmal t.
  paroxysmal ventricular t.
  t. pathway mapping
  permanent junctional reciprocating t.
  pleomorphic t.
  polymorphous ventricular t.
  primary ventricular t.
  rapid nonsustained ventricular t.
  reciprocating t.
  reciprocating macroreentry t.
  reentrant atrial t.
  reentrant supraventricular t.
  reflex t.
  refractory t.
  repetitive monomorphic ventricular t.
  repetitive paroxysmal ventricular t.
  salvo of ventricular t.
  S-A nodal reentrant t.
  self-terminating t.
  sinus nodal reentrant t.
  sinus reentrant t.
  sinus t.
  sleeping t.
  slow-fast t.
  spontaneous reentrant sustained ventricular t.
  supraventricular t. (SVT)
  sustained monomorphic ventricular t.
  t. traumosa exophthalmica
  ventricular t.
  wide QRS t.
  t. window

tachycardia *(continued)*
    Wolff-Parkinson-White
      reentrant t.

tachycardiac

tachycardia-dependent aberrancy

tachycardia-dependent block

tachycardia-induced cardiomyopathy

tachycardia-polyuria syndrome

tachycardia-terminating pacemaker

tachycardic

tachycrotic

tachydysrhythmia

Tachylog pacemaker

tachypacing

tachyphylactic

tachyphylaxis

tachypnea
    nervous t.

tachyrhythmia

tachysystole
    atrial t.
    auricular t.

tack
    biodegradable surgical t.
    Effler t.

tacrolimus

Tactilaze angioplasty

TAD guide wire

taenia (tenia)
    taenia terminalis

tag
    epicardial fat t.

Tagarno 3SD cineangiography projector

TAH
    total artificial heart
    Berlin TAH
    CardioWest TAH
    Penn State TAH
    University of Akron TAH
    Utah TAH
    Vienna TAH

tail sign

Takayasu
    T. aortitis
    T. arteritis
    T. disease
    T. syndrome
    T.-Ohnishi disease

takeoff of a vessel

tambour
    bruit de t.
    t. sound

tamponade
    t. action
    acute t.
    atypical t.
    balloon t.
    cardiac t.
    chronic t.
    esophageal t.
    heart t.
    low-pressure t.
    nontraumatic t.
    pericardial t.
    regional t.
    Rose t.
    t. sounds
    subacute t.
    traumatic t.

tandem
    T. cardiac device
    t. lesion
    t. stent

Tangier disease

tantalum (Ta)
    t. balloon-expandable stent

tantalum *(continued)*
   radioactive t.
   t. stent

tap
   bloody t.
   mitral t.
   pericardial t.

Tapcath esophageal electrode

tape
   Cath-Secure t.
   Silastic t.

tapered
   t. movable core curved
      wire guide
   T. Torque guide wire

Taper guide wire

Taperseal hemostatic device

tapotage

Tapsul pill electrode

tardus
   pulsus t.
   pulsus parvus et t.

target
   t. heart rate
   T. Tip lead

Tascon prosthetic valve

task
   metabolic equivalents of t.
      (METS)

taurinum
   cor t.

Taussig
   T.-Bing anomaly
   T.-Bing complex
   T.-Bing disease
   T.-Bing malformation
   T.-Bing syndrome
   Blalock-T. operation

Taybi disease

Tay-Sachs disease

Tc
   technetium

Tc-99
   technetium 99

tcu-PA
   2-chain urokinase plasmin-
      ogen activator

tear
   intimal t.
   neointimal t.

teardrop heart

TEC
   transluminal endarterec-
      tomy catheter
   transluminal extraction
      catheter
      TEC atherectomy de-
         vice

technetium (Tc)
   t. 99m furifosmin
   t. hexakis 2-methoxyisobu-
      tyl isonitrile (Tc-99 sesta-
      mibi)
   t. 99m hexamibi scan
   t. 99m imaging
   t. 99m MIBI imaging
   t. 99m pyrophosphate
   t. 99m sestamibi
   t. 99m sestamibi stress test
   t. 99m stannous pyrophos-
      phate scintiscan
   t. 99m teboroxime

technique
   ablative t.
   Amplatz t.
   antegrade double balloon/
      double wire t.
   antegrade/retrograde cardi-
      oplegia t.
   anterior sandwich patch t.
   anterograde transseptal t.
   anti-aliasing t.
   apex cardiography t.
   Araki-Sako t.
   arterial switch t.

technique *(continued)*
- atrial well t.
- background subtraction t.
- Bentall inclusion t.
- biplane ventriculography t.
- bootstrap two-vessel t.
- Brecher and Cronkite t.
- button t.
- catheterization t.
- Copeland t.
- coronary flow reserve t.
- Creech t.
- cutdown t.
- digital subtraction t.
- dilator and sheath t.
- direct insertion t.
- dye dilution t.
- ECG signal-averaging t.
- en bloc vein resection t.
- exchange t.
- Exorcist t.
- Fick t.
- first-pass t.
- flow mapping t.
- flush t.
- Fourier-acquired steady-state t. (FAST)
- gated t.
- George Lewis t.
- Goris background subtraction t.
- Grüntzig t.
- immunofluorescent t.
- immunostaining t.
- indicator dilution t.
- Indocyanine Green t.
- Jantene arterial switch t.
- J loop t.
- Judkins t.
- Judkins Sones t.
- kissing balloon t.
- Lown t.
- minimal leak t.
- modified brachial t.
- modified Seldinger t.
- Mullins blade t.
- Mustard transposition of great vessels t.
- no-leak t.

technique *(continued)*
- Norwood t.
- partial encircling endocardial ventriculotomy t.
- percutaneous t.
- Porstmann t.
- pressure half-time t.
- radionuclide t.
- Rashkind balloon t.
- Schoonmaker-King single catheter t.
- Sheehan Dodge t.
- Seldinger t.
- Sones t.
- Stewart-Hamilton cardiac output t.
- thermal dilution t.
- thermodilution t.
- transfixion t.
- Trusler aortic valve t.
- two-patch t.
- upgated t.
- velocity catheter t.
- Waldhausen subclavian flap t.

TED
thromboembolic disease
TED antiembolism stockings

tedding device

TEE
transesophageal echocardiography
Omniplane TEE
TEE probe

TEEP
transesophageal echocardiography with pacing

Tefcor movable core straight wire guide

Teflon
T. catheter
T. coating
T. graft
T. intracardiac patch

Teflon *(continued)*
> T. intracardiac patch prosthesis
> T. pledget
> T. pledget suture buttress
> T. sheath
> T. trileaflet prosthesis
> T. woven prosthesis

Teflon-coated
> T.-c. Dacron suture
> T.-c. guide wire
> T.-c. needle

Teflon-covered needle

Teflon-pledgeted suture

Teflon-tipped catheter

TEGwire
> T. balloon dilatation catheter
> T. guide

Teichholz
> T. ejection fraction

telangiectasia
> essential t.
> hemorrhagic t.
> hereditary hemorrhagic t.

telangiectasis

telangiectatic

telangiectodes

telangiitis

telangion

telangiosis

telecardiogram

telecardiography

telecardiophone

Telectronics
> T. ATP implantable cardioverter-defibrillator
> T. Guardian ATP 4210 device

Telectronics *(continued)*
> T. Guardian ATP II ICD
> T. leads
> T. lithium pacer
> T. pacemaker

telelectrocardiogram

telelectrocardiograph

telemetry
> cardiac t.
> t. electrocardiogram
> t. monitoring
> multiple-parameter t.
> t. receiver
> t. system

telesystolic

Teletrast gauze

telopeptide

temperature
> basal body t.
> core t.
> t. probe
> reduced blood t.

temperature-sensing pacemaker

temporal
> t. arteritis
> t. arteriole of retina
> t. diploic vein
> t. field defect
> t. vein
> t. venule of retina

temporary
> t. aortic shunt subclavian-subclavian bypass
> t. magnet
> t. pacemaker placement
> t. pacing
> t. pacing catheter
> t. pacing wire
> t. pervenous lead
> t. transvenous pacemaker
> t. unilateral pulmonary artery occlusion
> t. vascular clip

temporary *(continued)*
  t. vessel clip

Ten balloon

tendinea
  macula t.

tendineae
  chordae t.

tendinosum
  xanthoma t.

tendinous
  t. spot
  t. xanthoma
  t. zones of heart

tendo
  t. infundibuli

tendon
  t. of conus
  coronary t's
  t. of infundibulum
  t. of Todaro

Tennis Racquet angiographic
  catheter

tense
  t. abdomen
  t. edema
  t. pulse
  t. time index

tensile strength

tension
  arterial oxygen t.
  left ventricular t.
  myocardial t.
  wall t.

tension-free anastomosis

tensionless anastomosis

teratoma
  pericardial t.

terminal
  t. aorta
  t. edema

terminal *(continued)*
  t. endocarditis
  t. groove
  t. Purkinje fibers
  t. vein
  central t t. of Wilson

termination
  underdrive t.

tertiary contractions

Terumo
  T. AV fistula needle
  T. Doppler fetal heart rate
    monitor
  T. Glidewire
  T. hydrophilic guide wire
  T. Radiofocus sheath
  T. SP coaxial catheter
  T. ST hydrophilic-polymer-
    coated microcatheter
  T. Surflow intravenous
    catheter

tetracrotic

tetrad
  Fallot t.

tetralogy
  Eisenmenger t.
  t. of Fallot
  pink t. of Fallot

TGA
  transposition of the great
    arteries

TGF
  transforming growth factor

thallium
  t. perfusion imaging
  t. scan

thallium-201
  t.-201 exercise stress test
  t.-201 perfusion scintigra-
    phy
  t.-201 scan
  t.-201 SPECT scintigraphy

THC:YAG laser

thebesian
    t. circulation
    t. foramina
    t. valve
    t. vein

theca
    t. cordis

Theden method

Theis rib retractor

theorem
    Ba t.
    Bernoulli t.

theory
    aging t. of atherosclerosis
    Bayliss t.
    Cannon t.
    closed circulation t.
    closed-open circulation t.
    cross-linkage t.
    encrustation t.
    fast circulation t.
    metabolic t. of atheroscle-
        rosis
    myogenic t.
    open circulation t.
    open-closed circulation t.
    reentry t.
    response-to-injury t.
    Spitzer t.

therapeutic
    t. intervention
    t. phlebotomy
    t. thoracentesis

therapy
    ablation t.
    adjunctive t.
    angina-guided t.
    anti-anginal t.
    antiarrhythmic t.
    anticoagulant t.
    antiendotoxin t.
    antihypertensive t.
    antimicrobial t.
    antiplatelet t.
    augmentation t.

therapy (continued)
    beta-blocker t.
    combination t.
    compression t.
    conservative t.
    diet t.
    digitalis t.
    diuretic t.
    embolization t.
    empiric t.
    fibrinolytic t.
    immunosuppression t.
    intrathecal t.
    ischemia-guided medical t.
    maintenance t.
    oral anticoagulant t.
    palliative t.
    prophylactic t.
    radiation t.
    step-down t.
    thrombolytic t.
    transcatheter t.
    vasodilator t.

Thera-SR pacemaker

thermal
    t. angiography
    t. balloon system
    t. dilution catheter
    t. dilution technique
    t. memory stent

thermal/perfusion balloon an-
    gioplasty

Thermedics
    T. HeartMate 1001P left an-
        terior assist device
    T. left ventricular assist de-
        vice

thermistor
    t. plethysmography
    t. thermodilution catheter

Thermo Cardiosystems left ven-
    tricular assist device

thermodilution
    t. balloon catheter
    t. cardiac output computer
    t. catheter

thermodilution *(continued)*
    t. catheter introducer kit
    coronary sinus t.
    Kim-Ray t.
    t. pacing catheter
    t. Swan-Ganz catheter
    t. technique
    t. test

thermoexpandable stent

thermography
    infrared t.
    t. study

Thermos pacemaker

thermostromuhr

thiamine deficiency

thickened
    t. aortic valve
    t. pericardium
    t. valve leaflets

thickening
    cardiac wall t.
    endocardial t.
    intimal t.
    leaflet t.
    wall t.

thickness
    intimal-medial t.
    relative wall t.
    wall t.

thigh-high antiembolic stockings

thinning
    infarct t.
    shear t.
    ventricular wall t.

thin-walled
    t.-w. catheter
    t.-w. needle

third-degree heart block

third heart sound (S₃)

Thoma ampulla

Thomas shunt

Thomsen disease

thoracalgia

thoracalis
    aorta t.

thoracentesis
    Argyle-Turkel t.
    t. needle

thoracic
    t. aneurysm
    t. aorta
    t. aortic aneurysm
    t. aortic dissection
    t. arch aortography
    t. artery forceps
    t. axis
    t. cardiac nerve
    t. cage
    t. duct
    t. ganglia
    t. inferior vena cava
    t. outlet compression
    t. outlet syndrome
    t. rib syndrome
    t. vein

thoracica
    aorta t.
    arteria t. interna
    arteria t. lateralis
    arteria t. suprema
    vena t. lateralis

thoracicus
    ductus t.

thoracoabdominal
    t. aortic aneurysm
    t. dyssynchrony
    t. paradox

thoracocardiography

thoracocentesis

thoracodorsal artery

thoracolumbar

thoracophrenolaparotomy

Thoracoport

thoracoscope
    Boutin t.
    Coryllos t.

thoracosternotomy

thoracostomy

thoracotomy

Thoratec
    T. biventricular assist de-
        vice
    T. cardiac device
    T. pump
    T. right ventricular assist
        device
    T. ventricular assist device

thorax *pl.* thoraces
    barrel-shaped t.
    pyriform t.

Thorek scissors

Thorek-Feldman scissors

Thorel
    T. bundle
    T. pathway

thready pulse

three-block claudication

three-chambered heart

three-channel electrocardio-
    gram

three-dimensional
    t.-d. echocardiography
    t.-d. Fourier transform

three-legged cage heart valve

three-pillow orthopnea

three-turn epicardial lead

three-vein graft

threshold
    aerobic t.
    anaerobic t.
    anginal perceptual t.
    atrial capture t.

threshold *(continued)*
    atrial defibrillation t.
    defibrillation t.
    t. of discomfort
    fibrillation t.
    ischemic t.
    pacemaker t.
    pacing t.
    pain t.
    sensing t.
    ventricular capture t.

thrill
    aneurysmal t.
    aortic t.
    arterial t.
    coarse t.
    dense t.
    diastolic t.
    harsh t.
    palpable t.
    parasternal systolic t.
    precordial t.
    presystolic t.
    prominent t.
    systolic t.

throbbing aorta

thrombasthenia

thrombectomize

thrombectomy
    t. catheter
    percutaneous rotational t.

thrombin
    clot-bound t.
    t. generation

thrombin-antithrombin
    t.-a. III complex

thrombin clotting time

thrombin-soaked Gelfoam

thromboangiitis obliterans

thromboaortopathy
    occlusive t.

thromboarteritis
    t. purulenta

thromboclasis

thromboclastic

thrombocyst

thrombocystis

thrombocytapheresis

thrombocythemia

thrombocytopenia
    drug-induced t.
    essential t.
    idiopathic t.
    malignant t.
    t. with absence of radius

thrombocytosis

thromboelastogram

thromboelastograph

thromboembolectomy

thromboembolia

thromboembolic
    t. disease (TED)
    t. disease stockings
    t. pulmonary hypertension
    t. syndrome

thromboembolism
    pulmonary t.
    venous t.

thromboendarterectomy (TEA)

thromboendarteritis

thromboendocarditis

thrombogenesis

thrombogenic

thrombogenicity

thromboglobulin
    beta t.

thromboid

thrombolic

thrombokinesis

thrombolus

thrombolymphangitis

thrombolysoangioplasty

thrombolysis
    T. and Angioplasty in Myo-
        cardial Infarction (TAMI)
    T. and Angioplasty in Un-
        stable Angina (TAUSA)
    coronary t.
    intracoronary t.
    T. in Myocardial Infarction
        (TIMI)
    selective intracoronary t.

thrombolytic
    t. agent
    t. therapy

thrombomodulin

thrombophilia

thrombophlebitis
    iliofemoral t.
    t. migrans
    migratory t.
    t. purulenta
    t. saltans

thromboplastin
    partial t. time (PTT)
    t. time (TT)

thrombopoiesis

thrombopoietic

thrombopoietin

thromboresistance

thrombosed

thrombosis *pl.* thromboses
    agonal t.
    aortic t.
    aortoiliac t.
    arterial t.
    atrophic t.
    brachial t.
    brachial artery t.
    cardiac t.

thrombosis *(continued)*
    catheter-induced t.
    cavernous sinus t.
    central splanchnic venous t.
    cerebral t.
    cerebrovascular t.
    coagulation t.
    compression t.
    coronary artery t.
    creeping t.
    deep venous t. (DVT)
    dilatation t.
    dilation t.
    effort-induced t.
    embolic t.
    femoral artery t.
    femoral venous t.
    iliac vein t.
    incomplete t.
    infective t.
    intramural t.
    t. of jugular bulb
    jumping t.
    laser-induced t.
    t. of lateral sinus
    marantic t.
    mesenteric arterial t.
    mesenteric venous t.
    mural t.
    Paget-Schroetter venous t.
    plate t.
    platelet t.
    portal vein t.
    propagating t.
    prosthetic valve t.
    puerperal t.
    recanalizing t.
    renal vein t.
    Ribbert t.
    t. of sigmoid sinus
    sinus t.
    traumatic t.
    vascular t.
    venous t.
thrombostasis
thrombotic
    t. endocarditis

thrombotic *(continued)*
    t. microangiopathy
    t. occlusion
    t. thrombocytopenic purpura

thrombus *pl.* thrombi
    agglutinative t.
    agonal t.
    annular t.
    atrial t.
    ball t.
    ball valve t.
    basilar artery t.
    blood plate t.
    blood platelet t.
    calcified t.
    coral t.
    currant jelly t.
    fibrin t.
    globular t.
    hyaline t.
    infective t.
    intracardiac t.
    intramural thrombi
    intravascular t.
    laminated t.
    lateral t.
    Laënnec t.
    marantic t.
    marasmic t.
    mixed t.
    mural t.
    obstructive t.
    occluding t.
    occlusive t.
    organized t.
    pale t.
    parietal t.
    pedunculated t.
    plate t.
    platelet t.
    postmortem t.
    primary t.
    progressive t.
    propagated t.
    red t.
    right atrial t.
    saddle t.
    secondary t.

thrombus *(continued)*
    straddling t.
    stratified t.
    t. stripper
    traumatic t.
    valvular t.
    ventricular t.
    white t.

through-and-through
    t.-a.-t. continuous sutures
    t.-a.-t. myocardial infarction

through-the-wall mattress suture

Thruflex
    T. balloon
    T. PTCA balloon catheter

ThurLumen lumen

thrush
    t. breast
    t. breast heart

thulium-holmium:YAG laser

thulium-holmium-chromium:
    YAG laser (THC:YAG laser)

thump
    chest t.
    precordial t.

thumpversion

thymectomize

thymectomy
    video-assisted thoracoscopic t.

thymoma

thyrocalcitonin

thyrocardiac
    t. disease

thyroid
    aberrant t.
    accessory t.
    t. antibody
    t. artery

thyroid *(continued)*
    t. bruit
    t. cachexia
    t. deficiency
    diffusely enlarged t.
    t. disease
    t. function test
    t. hormone
    intrathoracic t.
    t. isthmus
    t. notch
    overactive t.
    palpable t.
    t. profile
    retrosternal t.
    t. storm
    substernal t.
    t. vein

thyroidectomy

thyroiditis
    chronic lymphocytic t.
    de Quervain t.
    granulomatous t.
    Hashimoto t.
    Riedel t.
    subacute diffuse t.
    woody t.

thyrointoxication

thyromegaly

thyrotoxic
    t. cardiopathy
    t. goiter
    t. heart disease

thyrotoxicosis

TI
    tricuspid incompetence
    tricuspid insufficiency

TIA
    transient ischemic attack

Tibbs arterial cannula

tibial
    t. artery
    t. pulse

tibioperoneal vessel angioplasty

tic-tac
    t.-t. rhythm
    t.-t. sounds

tidal
    t. wave pulse

tiered-therapy
    t.-t. antiarrhythmic device
    t.-t. programmable cardio-
      verter-defibrillator

Tietze syndrome

tiger
    t. heart
    t. lily heart

tight stenosis

tightness
    chest t.

tilting-disk
    t.-d. aortic valve prosthesis
    t.-d. heart valve
    t.-d. occluder
    t.-d. prosthetic valve

tilt-table test

tilt test

timbre
    t. métallique

time
    acceleration t.
    acquisition t.
    activated clotting t.
    activated coagulation t.
    activated partial thrombo-
      plastin t. (aPTT)
    A-H conduction t.
    atrioventricular t.
    bypass t.
    cardiopulmonary bypass t.
    carotid ejection t.
    circulation t.
    clot retraction t.
    coagulation t.

time *(continued)*
    conduction t.
    corrected sinus node re-
      covery t.
    cross-clamp t.
    dead t.
    deceleration t.
    donor organ ischemic t.
    doubling t.
    Duke bleeding t.
    echo t.
    echo delay t.
    ejection t.
    euglobulin clot lysis t.
    flushing t.
    generation t.
    H-R conduction t.
    H-V conduction t.
    interpulse t.
    intra-atrial conduction t.
    inversion t.
    isovolumic relaxation t.
    Ivy bleeding t.
    left ventricular ejection t.
    lysis t.
    P-A conduction t.
    partial thromboplastin t.
      (PTT)
    P-H conduction t.
    prothrombin t. (PT)
    prothrombin t./partial
      thromboplastin t. (PT/
      PTT)
    relaxation t.
    repetition t.
    sinoatrial conduction t.
    sinoatrial recovery t.
    sinus node recovery t.
    thromboplastin t.
    tincture of t.
    transmitral E-wave deceler-
      ation t.
    ventricular activation t.

time-averaged peak velocity

time-gain

time-of-flight echoplanar imaging

TIMI
   thrombolysis in myocardial
      infarction
         TIMI classification

tined
   t. lead pacemaker
   t. ventricular electrode

tinkle
   Bouillaud t.
   metallic t.

tip
   aortographic suction t.
   Bovie coagulation t.
   cannula t.
   catheter t.
   coronary perfusion t.
   irrigating t.
   leaflet t.
   Mayo coronary perfusion t.
   t. occluder
   olive t.
   papillary muscle t.
   valve t.
   venous cannula t.

tip-deflecting
   t.-d. catheter
   t.-d. wire

TIPS
   transjugular intrahepatic
      portosystemic shunt

tirofiban

tissue
   t. ablation
   adhesive t.
   adventitial t.
   aortic t.
   atrioventricular conduc-
      tion t.
   avascular t.
   blood supply to t.
   caseated t.
   connective t.
   t. factor pathway inhibitor
   granulation t.
   junctional t.

tissue *(continued)*
   His-Purkinje t.
   interfascicular fibrous t.
   myocardial t.
   t. necrosis
   nodal t.
   perinodal t.
   t. plasminogen activator (t-
      PA)
   t. preservation
   t. valve
   vascular t.

titanium
   t. cage
   t. ball-cage heart valve
   T. VasPort

titer
   agglutination t.
   antiheart antibody t.
   anti-Rho-D t.
   antistreptolysin t.
   antistreptolysin O t.
   bactericidal t.
   hemagglutination t.
   Lyme t.
   rubella t.

titrate dosage

titrated inital dose

titration

TKO-type IV

Tl
   thallium

T-loop

TMR
   transmyocardial revascu-
      larization

to-and-fro
   t.-a.-f. friction sound
   t.-a.-f. murmur

tobacco heart

Todaro's tendon

Toennis
   T. anastomosis scissors

Toennis *(continued)*
  T. dissecting scissors

toilet-seat
  t.-s. angina
  t.-s. syncope

tolerance
  exercise t.
  exercise t. test
  hemodynamic t.

tomographic study

tomography
  atrial bolus dynamic computer t.
  axial computed t.
  axial transverse t.
  biplanar t.
  cine computed t.
  computerized t. (CT)
  computerized axial t. (CAT)
  focal plane t.
  gated computed t.
  high resolution computed t.
  positron emission t. (PET)
  positron emission transaxial t.
  rapid acquisition computed axial t.
  single-photon emission computed t. (SPECT)
  Ultrafast CT electron beam t.
  xenon-enhanced computed t. (XECT)

TomTec echo platform

tone
  heart t's
  t. and rhythm
  Traube double t.
  vascular t. and elasticity

tonography
  carotid compression t.

tonometer
  Gärtner t.

tonometer *(continued)*
  hemostatic t.
  Recklinghausen t.

tonometry
  applanation t.

tonsillaris
  angina t.

top-hat supra-annular aortic valve

topical
  Bactroban T.
  t. anesthesia
  t. cooling
  t. coronary vasodilator
  Efudex T.
  Gelfoam T.
  t. hypothermia
  t. medication
  t. thrombin

Torcon
  T. angiographic catheter
  T. NB selective angiographic catheter

Torek resection of thoracic esophagus

Torktherm torque control catheter

toroidal valve

Toronto
  T. SPV aortic valve
  T. SPV bioprosthesis

torque-control balloon catheter

Torricelli orifice equation

torsades de pointes

tortuosity

tortuous
  t. aorta
  t. varicosities
  t. veins
  t. vessel

torulosis

torus
    t. aorticus

tortuosity

Toshiba
    T. biplane transesophageal
        transducer
    T. electrocardiography ma-
        chine

total
    t. absence of circulation on
        4-vessel angiography
    t. alternans
    t. anomalous pulmonary
        venous connection
    t. anomalous pulmonary
        venous drainage
    t. anomalous pulmonary
        venous return
    t. artificial heart
    t. blood volume
    t. cardiopulmonary bypass
    t. cavopulmonary connec-
        tion
    t. cholesterol
    t. circulatory arrest
    t. coronary flow
    T. Cross balloon catheter
    t. end-diastolic diameter
    t. end-systolic diameter
    t. peripheral resistance
    t. pulmonary blood flow

Toupet hemifundoplication

Tourguide guiding catheter

tourniquet
    automatic rotating t.
    Esmarch t.
    garrote t.
    t. ischemia
    Medi-Quet t.
    pneumatic t.
    Rumel t.
    Spanish t.
    torcular t.

Tower stent

toxic
    t. cardiopathy
    t. myocarditis

toxicity
    cardiac t.
    digitalis t.
    digoxin t.
    drug t.
    procaine t.

toxicosis
    hemorrhagic capillary t.

TP
    TP interval
    TP segment

t-PA
    tissue plasminogen activa-
        tor

T-P-Q segment

TpT
    thrombus precursor pro-
        tein

TQ segment

TR
    tricuspid regurgitation

trabecula *pl.* trabeculae
    trabeculae carneae cordis
    trabeculae cordis
    fleshy trabeculae of heart
    t. septomarginalis

trabecular
    t. hypertrophy
    t. vein

trabeculation

tracheal tug

trachealis
    angina t.

tracing
    carotid pulse t.
    diamond-shaped t.
    electrocardiogram t.

tracing *(continued)*
    fetal heart monitor t.
    jugular venous pulse t.
    pressure t.
    venous pulse t.

Tracker-18 Soft Stream catheter

Tracker Soft Stream side-hole microinfusion catheter

tract
    atriodextrofascicular t.
    atriofascicular t.
    atrio-Hisian t's
    atrionodal bypass t.
    concealed bypass t.
    flow t. of the heart
    internodal t's
    James accessory t's
    left ventricular outflow t.
    nodo-Hisian bypass t.
    nodoventricular t.
    outflow t.
    right ventricular outflow t.
    Wolff-Parkinson-White bypass t.

traction aneurysm

trailing edge

training effect

trains of ventricular pacing

trainwheel rhythm

Trakstar balloon catheter

trans
    t. fatty acids

transaortic
    t. valve gradient

transatrial
    t. pacing

transaxial
    t. plane
    t. tomography

transbrachial arch aortogram

transcapillary refill

transcatheter
    t. ablation
    t. arterial chemoembolization
    t. brachytherapy
    t. closure of atrial septal defect
    t. embolization
    t. therapy
    t. umbrella

transcranial
    t. contrast Doppler sonography
    t. Doppler probe
    t. Doppler velocities

transcutaneous pacemaker

transducer
    Acuson multiple TEE t.
    t. aperture
    Doppler t.
    echocardiographic t.
    M-mode t.
    Pedoff continuous wave t.
    phased array sector t.
    phonocardiographic t.
    Spectranetic P23 Statham t.
    Toshiba biplane transesophageal t.
    ultrasound t.

transducer-tipped catheter

transduction
    mechanoelectrical t.
    signal t.

transesophageal
    t. atrial pacing
    t. atrial stimulation
    t. contrast echocardiography
    t. dobutamine stress echocardiography
    t. echocardiography (TEE)
    t. echocardiography with pacing

transesophageal *(continued)*
    t. echo probe

transfemoral catheter

transferase

transferrin

transfixion suture

transforming growth factor-β

transhepatic
    t. embolization
    t. portacaval shunt

transient
    t. asystole
    t. cardiac arrest
    t. cerebral vein thrombosis
    t. depolarization
    t. heart block
    t. ischemia
    t. ischemic attack
    t. mesenteric ischemia
    t. pericarditis
    t. syncope

transition
    forced ischemia-reperfusion t.

transjugular intrahepatic portosystemic shunt (TIPS)

translocase

translumbar aortography

transluminal
    t. angioplasty
    t. angioplasty catheter
    t. balloon
    t. balloon angioplasty
    t. coronary angioplasty
    t. coronary angioplasty
        guide wire
    t. coronary artery angioplasty
    t. endarterectomy catheter
    t. extraction atherectomy
    t. extraction catheter (TEC)

transluminal *(continued)*
    t. extraction-endarterectomy catheter
    t. lysing system

transmembrane
    t. potential
    t. pressure
    t. signaling
    t. voltage

transmitral
    t. Doppler E:A ratio
    t. E:A ratio
    t. E-wave deceleration time

transmitted murmur

transmural
    t. myocardial infarction
    t. pressure
    t. steal

transmyocardial
    t. laser revascularization
    t. pacing stylet
    t. perfusion pressure
    t. revascularization

transpericardial pacemaker

transplant
    allogeneic t.
    bone marrow t.
    cardiac t.
    t. coronary artery disease
    heart t.
    heart-lung t.
    heterologous cardiac t.
    heterotopic cardiac t.
    homologous cardiac t.
    Lower-Shumway cardiac t.
    mammary artery t.
    orthotopic cardiac t.
    rejection cardiomyopathy t.
    t. rejection classification
        system
    right pulmonary vein t.

transplantation

Transport
    T. dilatation balloon cathe-
      ter
    T. drug delivery catheter

transport
    active t.
    bulk t.
    exchange t.
    oxygen t.
    passive t.

transporter

transposition
    t. of arterial stems
    t. of great arteries
    t. of great vessels
    t. of pulmonary veins

transradial
    t. approach

transseptal
    t. angiocardiography
    t. cannula
    t. catheter
    t. left heart catheterization
    t. puncture

transthoracic
    t. approach
    t. catheter
    t. echocardiography (TTE)
    t. needle biopsy
    t. pacemaker
    t. pacing stylet

transvalvular
    t. aortic gradient
    t. flow

Transvene
    T. nonthoracotomy im-
      plantable cardioverter-de-
      fibrillator

transvenous
    t. approach
    t. aortovelography
    t. catheter pacemaker
    t. defibrillator lead

transvenous *(continued)*
    t. device
    t. digital subtraction angio-
      gram
    t. electrode
    t. implantation of pace-
      maker leads
    t. pacemaker
    t. pacer
    t. ventricular demand pace-
      maker

transventricular
    t. closed valvotomy
    t. dilator
    t. mitral valve commissur-
      otomy
    t. valvotomy

transverse
    t. arteriotomy
    t. artery of the face
    t. artery of neck
    t. artery of scapula
    t. cervical artery
    t. cervical veins
    t. circumflex vessels
    t. facial artery
    t. facial vein
    t. incision
    t. section of heart
    t. sinus
    t. sulcus of heart
    t. tomography
    t. tubule
    t. vein

transversus
    situs t.

trap-door approach

Traube
    T. bruit
    T. curve
    T. double tone
    T. heart
    T. murmur
    T. sign
    T. space
    T.-Hering waves

traumatic
    t. aortic aneurysm
    t. aortic disruption
    t. aortography
    t. heart disease
    t. hemopericardium
    t. hemorrhage
    t. hemothorax
    t. perforation
    t. pericarditis
    t. rupture
    t. tamponade
    t. thrombosis
    t. thrombus

treadmill
    t. echocardiography
    t. electrocardiogram
    exercise t.
    t. exercise stress test

treadmill-induced angina

treatment
    antianginal t.
    conservative medical t.
    empiric t.
    Fränkel t.
    Karell t.
    McPheeters t.
    Nauheim t.
    Oertel t.
    palliative t.
    prophylactic t.
    venous heart t.

trefoil balloon catheter

tremor
    flapping t.
    purring t.

Trendelenburg
    T. cannula
    T. position
    T. test
    T.-Crafoord clamp
    T.-Crafoord coarctation
        clamp

trendscriber

trendscription

trephocyte

trepidatio cordis

treppe
    t. phenomenon

triad
    acute compression t.
    adrenomedullary t.
    Beck t.
    hepatic t.
    t. of Herz
    Hull t.
    Kartagener t.
    Osler t.

triangle
    aortic t.
    axillary t.
    Burger's scalene t.
    cardiohepatic t.
    carotid t.
    clavipectoral t.
    Einthoven t.
    Farabeuf t.
    Gerhardt t.
    inferior carotid t.
    infraclavicular t.
    t. of Koch
    t. of safety
    sternocostal t.
    subclavian t.
    Todaro t.

triatrial heart

triatriatum
    cor t.

tricellular

trichinosis

trichocardia

tricrotic
    t. pulse
    t. wave

tricrotism

tricrotous

tricuspid
t. annuloplasty
t. aortic valve
t. atelectasis
t. atresia
t. commissurotomy
t. incompetence
t. insufficiency
t. murmur
t. opening snap
t. orifice
t. regurgitation (TR)
t. restenosis
t. stenosis
t. valve
t. valve annuloplasty
t. valve annulus
t. valve area
t. valve closure sound
t. valve disease
t. valve doming
t. valve flow
t. valve gradient
t. valve prolapse
t. valve strut
t. valve vegetation
t. valvular leaflet
t. valvuloplasty
t. valvotomy
t. valvulotomy

trifascicular block

trigeminal
t. pulse
t. rhythm

trigeminus
pulsus t.

trigeminy
ventricular t.

triggered
t. activity
atrial demand- t.
t. pacing

triggering mechanism

trigona
t. fibrosa cordis

trigone
fibrous t. of heart

trigonum
t. fibrosum dextrum cordis
t. fibrosum sinistrum cordis

Triguide catheter

trileaflet prosthesis

triloculare
cor t.

trilogy
t. of Fallot

Trimadeau sign

trinucleate

triolet
bruit de t.

Trios M pacemaker

trip-hammer pulse

"triple A" (abdominal aortic aneurysm)

triple-balloon valvuloplasty

triple bypass heart surgery

triple-lumen
t.-l. balloon flotation thermistor catheter
t.-l. central venous catheter
t.-l. perfused catheter system

triple-thermistor coronary sinus catheter

tripod
Haller's t.

tripolar
t. catheter
t. Damato curve catheter
t. defibrillation coil electrode

TriPort
  T. cannula
  T. hemostasis introducer
    sheath kit

trisection pulse

trisomy
  t. 13
  t. 18
  t. 21

trisomy-D syndrome

Triumph VR pacemaker

trocar
  Axiom thoracic t.
  Hunt angiographic t.
  Hurwitz thoracic t.
  Nelson thoracic t.
  Ochsner thoracic t.

trochocardia

trochorizocardia

Troisier sign

trophic changes

trophoblast

trophoblastic
  t. malignant teratoma
  t. tumor

trophospongium

tropical
  t. cardiospasm
  t. endomyocardial fibrosis

tropomyosin

troponin
  t. C
  t. I
  t. M
  t. T

trough
  t. concentration
  t. dosing
  t. level

trough *(continued)*
  peak and t.
  systolic t.

troughing
  venous t.

Trousseau syndrome

Tru-Arc blood vessel ring

true
  t. aneurysm
  t. restenosis

true-negative test result

true-positive test result

TrueTorque wire guide

truncal
  t. cushions
  t. septum

truncoaortic sac

truncoconal
  t. area
  t. septum

truncus
  t. arteriosus
  t. brachocephalicus
  t. fasciculi atrioventricula-
    ris

Trunecek symptom

trunk
  t. of atrioventricular bun-
    dle
  bifurcation of pulmonary t.
  brachiocephalic t.
  t. of bundle of His
  celiac t.
  jugular t.
  pulmonary t.
  t. valves

Trusler
  T. aortic valve technique
  T. rule for pulmonary ar-
    tery banding
  T. technique of aortic val-
    vuloplasty

trypanosomiasis

T system

TTE
transthoracic echocardiography

TTP
thrombotic thrombocytopenic purpura

T2 weighted image

TU
TU complex
TU wave

Tubbs
T. aortic dilator
T. mitral valve dilator
T. two-bladed dilator
T. valvulotome

tube
Baylor cardiovascular sump t.
chest t.
Cooley aortic sump t.
Cooley graft suction t.
Cooley intracardiac suction t.
Cooley vascular suction t.
DeBakey suction t.
DeBakey-Adson suction t.
endocardial t.
Humphrey coronary sinus-sucker suction t.
intracardiac suction t.
intracardiac sump t.
Methodist vascular suction t.
nasogastric t.
Sarns intracardiac suction t.
Southey-Leech t's

tubercle
intervenous t.
Lower's t.

tuberculoid myocarditis

tuberculous
t. arteritis
t. endocarditis
t. myocarditis
t. pericarditis

tuberculum
t. intervenosum

tubular
t. aneurysm
t. necrosis

tubulin

tucker
Cooley cardiac t.
Crafoord-Cooley t.

Tucker cardiospasm dilator

Tudor-Edwards
T.-E. costotome
T.-E. rib shears

Tuffier
T. arterial forceps
T. rib spreader
T. test

tumor
t. angiogensis factor
angiosarcoma t.
aortic t.
benign myocardial t.
bilateral atrial t.
t. of blood vessel
cardiac t.
t. embolism
endocardial t.
extrathoracic t.
myxoma t.
t. necrosis factor (TNF)
pericardiac t.
t. plop
primary malignant cardiac t.
pulmonary artery t.
Purkinje t.
teratoma t.
trophoblastic t.
vena caval t.

tunable
    t. dye laser
    t. pulsed dye laser

tunic
    Bichat t.

tunica
    t. adventitia vasorum
    t. externa vasorum
    t. intima vasorum
    t. media vasorum
    t. vasculosa

tunnel
    aortico-left ventricular t.
    Kawashima intraventricu-
        lar t.
    percutaneous t.
    saphenous t.
    vein t.
    t. view

tunneler
    Cooley t.
    CPI t.
    Crafoord-Cooley t.
    DeBakey t.
    DeBakey femoral bypass t.
    DeBakey vascular t.
    Diethrich-Jackson femoral
        graft t.
    Eidemiller t.
    Kelly-Wick vascular t.
    Noon AV fistular t.
    Noon modified vascular ac-
        cess t.
    Oregon t.
    Scanlan vascular t.
    vascular t.
    vascular access t.

tunnel graft

Tunturi EL400 bicycle ergome-
    ter

Tuohy
    T. aortography needle
    T. lumbar aortography nee-
        dle

Tuohy (continued)
    T.-Borst adapter
    T.-Borst introducer

turbulent
    t. diastolic mitral inflow
    t. jet

turgescent

turgid

turgor
    coronary vascular t.
    t. vitalis

Tuttle thoracic forceps

Tuttle-Singley thoracic forceps

twister
    Vital-Cooley wire t.
    Vital-Cooley-Baumgarten
        wire t.

two-block claudication

two-chamber view

two-dimensional (2D) echocar-
    diography

two-flight exertional dyspnea

two-patch technique

two-pillow orthopnea

two-step exercise test

two-turn epicardial lead

Tycos sphygmomanometer

Tygon tubing

tympanitic sound

tyramine

tyramine test

Tyshak
    T. balloon
    T. catheter

T-Y stent

U
  U loop
  U sutures
  U wave
  U wave alternans
  U wave inversion

UCG
  ultrasonic cardiography

UCI-Barnard
  UCI-B. aortic valve
  UCI-B. valve

Uhl
  U. anomaly
  U. disease
  U. malformation
  U. syndrome

ulcer
  atheromatous u.
  atherosclerotic u.
  decubitus u.
  hypertensive ischemic u.
  ischemic u.
  neurotrophic u.
  shaggy u.
  stasis u.
  varicose u.
  venous u.
  venous stasis u.

ulceration
  arteriolar ischemic u.
  ischemic u.

ulcerative
  u. endocarditis

ulcerosa
  angina u.

Uldall subclavian catheter

ulnar
  u. artery
  u. artery pulse
  compression test of u. artery
  occlusion of u. artery
  u. vein

ULP
  ultra low profile
  ULP catheter

ultimum moriens

Ultracor prosthetic valve

ultrafast
  u. computed tomographic scanner
  u. CT electron beam tomography

Ultraflex
  U. Microvasive stent
  U. self-expanding stent

ultra-low
  u. profile (ULP)
  u. profile fixed-wire balloon dilatation catheter

Ultramark
  U. 4 ultrasound
  U. 8 transducer

Ultra pacemaker

ultraphagocytosis

Ultra-Select nitinol PTCA guide wire

ultrasonic cardiography (UCG)

ultrasonography
  B-mode u.
  compression u.
  Doppler u.
  duplex B-mode u.
  duplex pulsed-Doppler u.
  intracaval endovascular u.
  intravascular u.
  pulsed wave Doppler u.

ultrasonoscope

ultrasound
  Acuson 128 Doppler u.
  Aloka u.
  u. angiography
  ATL u.
  B-mode u.

ultrasound *(continued)*
  cardiac u.
  u. cardiogram
  color vascular Doppler u.
  continuous-wave Dop-
    pler u.
  Doppler u.
  duplex u.
  echo-guided u.
  gray-scale u.
  Hewlett-Packard u.
  Interspec XL u.
  Intertherapy intravascu-
    lar u.
  intracoronary u.
  intraluminal u.
  intravascular u.
  Irex-Exemplar u.
  power Doppler u.
  real-time u.
  Shimadzu cardiac u.
  Siemens SI 400 u.
  transthoracic u.
  Ultramark 4 u.
  VingMed u.

Ultra-Thin balloon catheter

Ultravist contrast medium

umbilical
  u. arterial samples
  u. artery
  u. artery catheter
  u. artery catheterization
  u. artery velocimetry
  modified human u. vein
    graft
  u. tape
  u. vein catheter
  u. vein graft

umbilicalis
  arteritis u.

umbrella
  atrial septal defect u.
  Bard Clamshell septal u.
  Bard PDA u.
  Clamshell septal u.
  double u.
  u. filter

umbrella *(continued)*
  Mobin-Uddin u. filter
  patent ductus arteriosus u.
  Rashkind double u.
  transcatheter u.
  u. retractor

umbrella-type prosthesis

UMI transseptal Cath-Seal catheter introducer

underdrive
  u. pacing
  u. termination

underperfused myocardium

underloading
  ventricular u.

undersensing
  u. of pacemaker

undulating pulse

unequal pulse

unicommissural aortic valve

unidirectional block

unifocal
  u. PVCs
  u. ventricular ectopic beat

unilateral
  u. aortofemoral graft
  u. aortofemoral valve

Unilink anastomotic device

Unilith pacemaker

uninuclear

uninucleated

unipolar
  u. atrial pacemaker
  u. atrioventricular pace-
    maker
  u. defibrillation coil elec-
    trode
  u. limb lead
  u. pacemaker
  u. precordial lead

unipolar *(continued)*
    u. sequential pacemaker

UniPort hemostasis introducer
    sheath kit

unit
    acute coronary care u.
    BCD Plus cardioplegic u.
    Bipolar Circumactive Probe
        (BiCAP) u.
    coronary care u. (CCU)
    critical care u.
    digital fluoroscopic u.
    Multi Dopplex MDI vascular
        test u.
    peripheral resistance u.
    step-down u.
    Wood u.

Unity-C pacemaker

Unity VDDR pacemaker

univentricular
    u. atrioventricular connec-
        tion
    u. heart

universalis
    adiposis u.

University of Akron artificial
    heart

University of Illinois sternal
    puncture needle

University of Michigan Mixter
    thoracic forceps

University of Wisconsin solu-
    tion

Uniweave catheter

Unna boot

unoxygenated blood

Unschuld sign

unstable
    u. angina
    u. plaque

uPA
    u-type plasminogen activa-
        tor

upper
    u. lobe vein prominence on
        chest x-ray
    u. nodal extrasystole

upright
    u. tilt testing
    u. T wave
    u. U wave

upsloping ST segment depres-
    sion

upstairs-downstairs heart

upstream sampling method

upstroke
    brisk carotid u.
    diastolic u.
    u. pattern on apexcardi-
        ogram
    u. velocity

uptake
    C-11 palmitate u.
    diffuse myocardial u.
    fluorescein u.
    I-123 MIBG u.
    increased RV u.
    localized myocardial u.
    maximum oxygen u.
    myocardial oxygen u.
    oxygen u.
    u. studies
    venous u. cannula

uremia

uremic pericarditis

Uresil
    U. carotid shunt
    U. embolectomy thrombec-
        tomy catheter
    U. occlusion balloon cathe-
        ter
    U. radiopaque silicone
        band vessel loops

Uresil *(continued)*
   U. Vascu-Flo carotid shunt

Urografin-76 contrast medium

urokinase
   u.-type plasminogen activator (uPA)

USAFSAM treadmill exercise protocol

USCI
   United States Catheter & Instrument Company
      USCI angioplasty guiding sheath
      USCI angioplasty Y connector
      USCI arterial sheath
      USCI Bard catheter
      USCI bifurcated Vasculour II prosthesis
      USCI catheter
      USCI-DeBakey vascular prosthesis
      USCI Finesse guiding catheter
      USCI Goetz bipolar electrode

USCI *(continued)*
      USCI guide wire
      USCI guiding catheter
      USCI Hyperflex guide wire
      USCI introducer
      USCI Mini-Profile balloon dilation catheter
      USCI NBIH bipolar electrode
      USCI nonsteerable system
      USCI pacing electrode
      USCI Positrol coronary catheter
      USCI Probe balloon-on-a-wire catheter
      USCI Sauvage Bionit bifurcated vascular prosthesis
      USCI Sauvage EXS side-limb prosthesis
      USCI shunt
      USCI Vario permanent pacemaker

U-shaped catheter loop

Utah total artificial heart (TAH)

V
  V fib (ventricular fibrilla-
    tion)
  V lead
  V peak of jugular venous
    pulse
  V tach (ventricular tachy-
    cardia)
  V wave
  V wave of jugular venous
    pulse
  V wave of right atrial pres-
    sure
  V wave pressure on left or
    right atrial catheterization

v
  v wave on catheterization
  v wave on pulmonary capil-
    lary wedge tracing

VA
  ventriculoatrial
    VA block cycle length
    VA conduction
    VA interval

V_2A_2 curve

vacuus
  pulsus v.

VAD
  ventricular assist device
    Covaderm plus VAD
    Pierce-Donachy Thora-
      tec VAD
    Thoratec VAD

vagal
  v. attack
  v. block
  v. bradycardia
  v. escape
  v. response
  v. stimulation

vagolytic property

vagus
  v. arrhythmia
  v. nerve

vagus (continued)
  v. pulse
  v. reflex
  v. stimulation

Vairox high compression vascular stockings

Valsalva
  V. maneuver
  V. sinus
  V. test

valva
  v. aortae
  v. atrioventricularis dextra
  v. atrioventricularis sinistra
  v. mitralis
  v. pulmonaria
  v. tricuspidalis
  v. trunci pulmonalis

valve
  abnormal cleavage of car-
    diac v.
  Abrams-Lucas flap heart v.
  absent pulmonary v.
  Angell-Shiley bioprosthe-
    tic v.
  Angell-Shiley xenograph
    prosthetic v.
  Angiocor prosthetic v.
  annuloplasty v.
  aortic v.
  v. area
  artificial cardiac v.
  atrial v.
  atrioventricular v.
  ball-and-cage prosthetic v.
  ball-cage v.
  ball-occluder v.
  Baxter mechanical v.
  Beall mitral v.
  Beall-Surgitool 106 prosthe-
    tic v.
  Beall-Surgitool ball-cage
    prosthetic v.
  Beall-Surgitool disk prosth-
    etic v.
  Bianchi v.

valve *(continued)*
  Bicarbon Sorin v.
  Bicer-val prosthetic v.
  bicommissural aortic v.
  bicuspid aortic v.
  bicuspid v.
  bileaflet heart v.
  bileaflet tilting disk prosth-
    etic v.
  Biocor prosthetic v.
  bioprosthetic v.
  Bio-Vascular prosthetic v.
  Björk-Shiley v.
  Björk-Shiley convexocon-
    cave disk prosthetic v.
  Björk-Shiley mitral v.
  Björk-Shiley monostrut
    prosthetic v.
  Björk-Shiley prosthetic mi-
    tral v.
  Björk-Shiley prosthetic v.
  Blom-Singer v.
  bovine heart v.
  bovine pericardial v.
  Braunwald-Cutter ball
    prosthetic v.
  butterfly heart v.
  C-C (convexoconcave)
    heart v.
  caged-ball v.
  caged-ball occluder prosth-
    etic v.
  caged-disk occluder
    prosthetic v.
  calcified aortic v.
  calcified mitral v.
  calcified v.
  Capetown aortic prosthe-
    tic v.
  CarboMedics bileaflet pros-
    thetic heart v.
  CarboMedics top-hat su-
    pra-annular v.
  cardiac v.
  Carpentier-Edwards aor-
    tic v.
  Carpentier-Edwards bio-
    prosthetic v.

valve *(continued)*
  Carpentier-Edwards mitral
    annuloplasty v.
  Carpentier-Edwards peri-
    cardial v.
  Carpentier-Edwards por-
    cine prosthetic v.
  Carpentier-Edwards por-
    cine supra-annular v.
  caval v.
  cleft mitral v.
  commissural pulmonary v.
  competent v.
  congenital absence of pul-
    monary v.
  congenital anomaly of mi-
    tral v.
  congenital bicuspid aor-
    tic v.
  congenital unicuspid v.
  congenital quadricuspid
    aortic v.
  convexoconcave disk
    prosthetic v.
  Cooley-Bloodwell-Cutter v.
  Cooley-Cutter v.
  Cooley-Cutter disk prosthe-
    tic v.
  Coratomic prosthetic v.
  crisscross atrioventricu-
    lar v.
  Cross-Jones disk prosthe-
    tic v.
  Cross-Jones mitral v.
  cryopreserved allograft
    heart v.
  Cutter-Smeloff disk v.
  Cutter-Smeloff mitral v.
  DeBakey-Surgitool prosthe-
    tic v.
  v. debris
  v. dehiscence
  Delrin heart v.
  diastolic fluttering aortic v.
  disk-cage v.
  doming of v.
  Duostat rotating hemosta-
    tic v.
  Duraflow heart v.

valve *(continued)*
 Duromedics mitral v.
 dysplastic v.
 early opening of v.
 eccentric monocuspid tilting-disk prosthetic v.
 echo-dense v.
 Edmark mitral v.
 Edwards-Duromedics bileaflet v.
 Edwards-Duromedics
   prosthetic v.
 Elgiloy frame of prosthetic v.
 eustachian v.
 expiration of v.
 fenestrated v.
 fibrotic mitral v.
 flail mitral v.
 floating disk heart v.
 floppy mitral v.
 four-legged cage v.
 GateWay Y-adapter rotat-
   ing hemostatic v.
 glutaraldehyde-tanned bovine heart v.
 glutaraldehyde-tanned porcine heart v.
 Gott butterfly heart v.
 Guangzhou GD-1 prosthe-
   tic v.
 Hall-Kaster disk prosthetic v.
 Hall prosthetic heart v.
 hammocking of v.
 Hancock v.
 Hancock aortic 242 prosthetic v.
 Hancock bioprosthetic v.
 Hancock mitral prosthe-
   tic v.
 Hancock modified orifice v.
 Hancock pericardial
   prosthetic v.
 Hancock porcine hetero-
   graft v.
 Hancock prosthetic mi-
   tral v.
 Harken ball v.

valve *(continued)*
 Heimlich heart v.
 Hemex prosthetic v.
 hemostasis v.
 heterograft v.
 hockey-stick tricuspid v.
 Holter v.
 homograft v.
 Hufnagel disk heart v.
 Hufnagel caged-ball v.
 Hufnagel prosthetic v.
 hypoplastic v.
 incompetent v.
 Ionescu trileaflet v.
 Ionescu-Shiley bioprosthe-
   tic v.
 Ionescu-Shiley bovine peri-
   cardial v.
 Ionescu-Shiley heart v.
 Ionescu-Shiley low-profile
   prosthetic v.
 Ionescu-Shiley pericardial
   v. graft
 Ionescu-Shiley standard
   pericardial prosthetic v.
 Jatene-Macchi prosthetic v.
 Kay-Shiley caged- disk
   prosthetic v.
 Kay-Shiley mitral v.
 Kay-Suzuki disk prosthe-
   tic v.
 leaky v.
 Lillehei-Kaster pivoting
   disk prosthetic v.
 Lillehei-Kaster prosthetic
   mitral v.
 Liotta-Bioimplant LPB
   prosthetic v.
 low-profile prosthetic v.
 Magovern-Cromie ball-cage
   prosthetic v.
 mechanical v.
 Medtronic-Hall monocuspid
   tilting-disk v.
 Medtronic-Hall prosthetic
   heart v.
 Medtronic Hancock v.
 Medtronic Intact v.
 Medtronic prosthetic v.

valve *(continued)*
    midsystolic buckling of mi-
        tral v.
    midsystolic closure of aor-
        tic v.
    mitral v.
    Mitroflow pericardial
        prosthetic v.
    narrowed v.
    native v.
    noncalcified v.
    notching of pulmonic v.
    Omnicarbon v.
    Omnicarbon prosthetic v.
    Omniscience heart v.
    Omniscience prosthetic v.
    Omniscience tilting-disk v.
    v. orifice area
    v. outflow strut
    parachute mitral v.
    Pemco prosthetic v.
    porcine prosthetic v.
    premature closure of v.
    premature mid-diastolic
        closure of mitral v.
    prosthetic aortic v.
    prosthetic v.
    Puig Massana–Shiley annu-
        loplasty v.
    pulmonary autograft v.
    pulmonic v.
    quadricuspid pulmonary v.
    regurgitation of mitral v.
    v. replacement
    rheumatic mitral v.
    v. rupture
    St. Jude bileaflet prosthe-
        tic v.
    St. Jude Medical bileaflet
        tilting-disk aortic v.
    St. Jude Medical mitral v.
    St. Jude prosthetic aortic v.
    semilunar v.
    Shiley convexoconcave
        heart v.
    Silastic disk heart v.
    Smeloff prosthetic v.
    Smeloff-Cutter ball-cage
        prosthetic v.

valve *(continued)*
    Sorin cardiac prosthetic v.
    Starr-Edwards ball-and-
        cage v.
    Starr-Edwards mitral v.
    Starr-Edwards prosthetic v.
    Starr-Edwards Silastic v.
    Stellite ring material of
        prosthetic v.
    stenosis of mitral v.
    stenotic v.
    stentless porcine aortic v.
    stent-mounted allograft v.
    stent-mounted hetero-
        graft v.
    straddling atrioventricu-
        lar v.
    straddling tricuspid v.
    Surgitool 200 prosthetic v.
    v. of Sylvius
    systolic anterior motion of
        mitral v.
    Tascon prosthetic v.
    thebesian v.
    thickened mitral v.
    tilting-disk v.
    v. tip
    tissue v.
    top-hat supra-annular aor-
        tic v.
    Toronto SPV aortic v.
    track v.
    tricuspid v.
    tricuspid aortic v.
    trileaflet aortic v.
    Ultracor prosthetic v.
    unicommissural aortic v.
    Unistasis v.
    v. of veins
    Vascor porcine prosthe-
        tic v.
    v. vegetation
    venous v.
    v. of Vieussens
    Wada-Cutter disk prosthe-
        tic v.
    Wessex prosthetic v.
    Xenomedica prosthetic v.
    Xenotech prosthetic v.

valvotome

valvotomy
    aortic v.
    balloon aortic v.
    balloon mitral v.
    balloon pulmonary v.
    balloon tricuspid v.
    double-balloon v.
    Inoue balloon mitral v.
    v. knife
    Longmire v.
    mitral balloon v.
    mitral valve v.
    percutaneous mitral bal-
        loon v.
    pulmonary v.
    repeat balloon mitral v.
    single-balloon v.
    thimble v.
    transventricular closed v.

valvula
    v. coronaria dextra valvae
        aortae
    v. coronaria sinistra valvae
        aortae
    v. foraminis ovalis
    v. non coronaria valvae
        aortae
    v. semilunaris
    v. semilunaris anterior val-
        vae trunci pulmonalis
    v. semilunaris dextra val-
        vae aortae
    v. semilunaris dextra val-
        vae trunci pulmonalis
    v. semilunaris posterior
        valvae aortae
    v. semilunaris sinistra val-
        vae aortae
    v. semilunaris sinistra val-
        vae trunci pulmonalis
    v. sinus coronarii
    v. venae cavae inferioris

valvular
    v. aortic stenosis
    v. apparatus
    v. calcification

valvular *(continued)*
    v. dysfunction
    v. endocarditis
    v. heart disease
    v. incompetence
    v. opening
    v. orifice
    v. prolapse
    v. pulmonic stenosis
    v. regurgitation
    v. sclerosis
    v. thrombus

valvulitis
    aortic v.
    mitral v.
    rheumatic v.
    syphilitic aortic v.

valvuloplasty
    aortic v.
    bailout v.
    balloon v.
    balloon aortic v.
    balloon mitral v.
    balloon pulmonary v.
    Carpentier tricuspid v.
    catheter balloon v.
    double-balloon v.
    intracoronary thrombolysis
        balloon v.
    Kay tricuspid v.
    mitral v.
    multiple-balloon v.
    percutaneous balloon aor-
        tic v.
    percutaneous balloon mi-
        tral v.
    percutaneous balloon pul-
        monic v.
    percutaneous transluminal
        balloon v.
    pulmonary v.
    pulmonary balloon v.
    retrograde simultaneous
        double-balloon v.
    retrograde simultaneous
        single-balloon v.
    single-balloon v.
    triple-balloon v.

valvuloplasty *(continued)*
    Trusler technique of aortic v.

valvuloplasty balloon catheter

valvulotome
    angioscopic v.
    antegrade v.
    Bakst v.
    Brock v.
    Carmody v.
    Derra v.
    Dogliotti v.
    Dubost v.
    Gerbode mitral v.
    Gohrbrand v.
    Hall v.
    Harken v.
    Himmelstein v.
    Intramed angioscopic v.
    Leather antegrade v.
    Leather retrograde v.
    Leather venous v.
    Longmire v.
    Longmire-Mueller curved v.
    Mills v.
    Neider v.
    Potts expansile v.
    Potts-Riker v.
    retrograde v.
    Sellor v.
    Tubbs v.
    Universal malleable v.

valvulotomy
    open v.
    pulmonary v.

Van Tassel angled pigtail catheter

variability
    beat-to-beat v.
    cardiac v.
    heart rate v.

variable
    v. deceleration
    v. threshold angina

variant angina

variation
    circadian v.

variceal sclerotherapy

varicophlebitis

varicose
    v. vein
    v. vein stripping and ligation

varicosity
    saphenous vein v.

Variflex catheter

varix *pl.* varices
    anastomotic v.
    aneurysmal v.
    aneurysmoid v.
    arterial v.
    cirsoid v.

vas
    v. brevia
    v. vorticosa

vasalgia

vasa vasorum

Vas-Cath catheter

Vascor porcine prosthetic valve

Vascoray contrast medium

vascular
    v. access catheter
    v. bed
    v. bundle
    v. clamp
    v. clip
    v. compromise
    v. ectasia
    v. endothelial growth factor (VEGF)
    v. gene transfer
    v. graft prosthesis
    v. groove
    v. hemostatic device
    v. impedance
    v. injury
    v. murmur

vascular *(continued)*
   v. resistance index
   v. sclerosis
   v. sheath
   v. spasm
   v. spider
   v. stenosis
   v. stiffness
   v. tape

vascularity

vascularization

vascularize

vasculature
   pulmonary v.

vasculitic

vasculitis
   allergic v.
   Churg-Strauss v.
   consecutive v.
   hypersensitivity v.
   leukocytoclastic v.
   livedo v.
   necrotizing v.
   nodular v.
   overlap v.
   polyarteritis-like system-
     ic v.
   pulmonary v.
   segmented hyalinizing v.
   systemic necrotizing v.
   toxic v.
   urticarial v.

vasculogenesis

vasculogenic

vasculolymphatic

vasculomotor

vasculopathy
   allograft v.
   cardiac allograft v.
   cerebral v.
   graft v.
   hypertensive v.

vasculotoxic

Vascutek
   V. gelseal vascular graft
   V. knitted vascular graft
   V. vascular prosthesis
   V. woven vascular graft

vasoactive

vasoconstriction
   peripheral v.
   pulmonary v.

vasoconstrictive

vasoconstrictor

vasodepression

vasodepressor
   v. reaction

vasodepressor-cardioinhibitory
   syncope

vasodilatation
   coronary v.
   reflex v.

vasodilate

vasodilator
   v. agent
   peripheral v.

vasovenic

vasoinhibitor

vasomotion
   coronary v.

vasomotor
   v. angina

vasomotoria
   angina pectoris v.

vasoneuropathy

vasoneurosis

vasoparesis

vasopressor

vasoregulatory asthenia

vasorelaxation

vasoresponse

vasorum
    aortic vasa v.
    vasa v.

Vasoscope 3 Doppler probe

vasospasm
    coronary v.
    ergonovine-induced v.

vasospastic
    v. angina

vasotonic
    v. angina

vasovagal
    v. episode
    v. hypotension
    v. orthostatism
    v. phenomenon
    v. syncope

VAT
    ventricular activation time

Vaughn Williams classification
    of antiarrhythmic drugs

VCB
    ventricular capture beat

vector
    v. electrocardiogram
    v. loop
    mean QRS v.
    P v.
    QRS v.
    ST v.
    T v.
    T wave v.

vectorcardiogram
    frontal plane v.
    saggital plane v.
    transverse plane v.

vectorcardiography
    spatial v.

vegetation
    aortic valve v.
    bacterial v.

vegetation (continued)
    endocardial v.
    leaflet v.
    Libman-Sacks v.
    marantic v.
    prosthetic valve v.
    valvular v.
    ventricular septal defect v.
    verrucous v.

vegetative
    v. endocarditis

vein
    accompanying v. of hypo-
       glossal nerve
    afferent v's
    anastomotic v.
    angular v.
    anomalous pulmonary v.
    antebrachial v.
    anterior v's of heart
    anterior v's of right ventri-
       cle
    appendicular v.
    v. of aqueduct of cochlea
    v. of aqueduct of vestibule
    arterial v.
    articular v's
    atrial v's of heart,
    atrioventricular v's of heart
    auditory v's
    auricular v's
    autogenous v.
    axillary v.
    azygos v.
    basal v.
    basilic v.
    basivertebral v's
    Boyd perforating v.
    brachial v's
    brachiocephalic v.
    Breschet's v's
    bronchial v's
    Browning's v.
    v. of bulb of penis
    v. of bulb of vestibule
    Burow's v.
    v. of canaliculus of cochlea
    cardiac v.

vein *(continued)*

  v's of caudate nucleus
  cavernous v's of penis
  central v.
  central v's of hepatic lob-
    ules
  central v's of liver
  central v. of retina
  central v. of suprarenal
    gland
  cephalic v.
  cerebellar v's
  cerebral v's
  cervical v.
  choroid v., inferior
  choroid v., superior
  ciliary v's
  circumflex femoral v's
  circumflex iliac v.
  v. of cochlear canaliculus
  colic v.
  common femoral v.
  communicating v's
  conjunctival v's
  coronary v.
  v. of corpus callosum
  costoaxillary v's
  cubital v.
  cutaneous v.
  cystic v.
  deep v.
  deep v's of clitoris
  deep v's of lower limb
  deep v's of penis
  deep v. of thigh
  deep v. of tongue
  deep v's of upper limb
  digital v's, palmar
  digital v's, plantar
  digital v's of foot
  diploic v's
  Dodd perforating v.
  dorsal v. of clitoris
  dorsal v. of penis
  dorsal v's of tongue
  emissary v.
  emissary v., condylar
  emissary v., mastoid
  emissary v., occipital

vein *(continued)*

  emissary v., parietal
  v's of encephalic trunk
  epigastric v.
  epiploic v.
  episcleral v's
  esophageal v's
  ethmoidal v's
  facial v.
  femoral v.
  femoropopliteal v.
  fibular v's
  frontal v's
  Galen's v.
  gastric v.
  gastroepiploic v.
  gastroomental v.
  genicular v's
  gluteal v's
  gonadal v's
  hemiazygos v.
  hepatic v's
  ileal v's
  ileocolic v.
  iliac v., common
  iliac v., external
  iliac v., internal
  iliolumbar v.
  inferior v's of cerebellum
  infralobar v.
  infrasegmental v.
  innominate v.
  insular v's
  intercapitular v's of foot
  intercapitular v's of hand
  intercostal v's, anterior
  intercostal v., highest
  intercostal v., left superior
  intercostal v's, posterior
  intercostal v., right supe-
    rior
  interlobular v's of liver
  interosseous v's, anterior
  interosseous v's, posterior
  intersegmental v.
  interventricular v.
  intervertebral v.
  jejunal v's
  jugular v.

vein *(continued)*
    Kohlrausch v's
    Krukenberg's v's
    Kuhnt's postcentral v.
    Labbé's v.
    labial v's
    v's of labyrinth
    lacrimal v.
    laryngeal v.
    lateral direct v's
    v. of lateral recess of
        fourth ventricle
    v. of lateral ventricle, lat-
        eral
    v. of lateral ventricle, me-
        dial
    lingual v.
    lingual v., deep
    lingual v's, dorsal
    lobar v., middle
    v's of lower limb
    lumbar v's
    lumbar v., ascending
    labyrinthine v's
    colic v., intermediate
    mammary v's, external
    mammary v's, internal
    marginal v., lateral
    marginal v., left
    marginal v., medial
    marginal v., right
    v. of Marshall
    Marshall's oblique v.
    masseteric v's
    maxillary v's
    Mayo's v.
    median v. of elbow
    median v. of forearm
    median v. of neck
    mediastinal v's
    v's of medulla oblongata
    meningeal v's
    meningeal v's, middle
    mesencephalic v's
    mesenteric v., inferior
    mesenteric v., superior
    metacarpal v's, dorsal
    metacarpal v's, palmar
    metatarsal v's, dorsal

vein *(continued)*
    metatarsal v's, plantar
    musculophrenic v's
    nasal v's, external
    nasofrontal v.
    oblique v. of left atrium
    obturator v's
    obturator v., accessory
    occipital v.
    v. of olfactory gyrus
    ophthalmic v., inferior
    ophthalmic v., superior
    ophthalmomeningeal v.
    v's of orbit
    ovarian v., left
    ovarian v., right
    palatine v.
    palatine v., external
    palpebral v's
    palpebral v's, inferior
    palpebral v's, superior
    pancreatic v's
    pancreaticoduodenal v's
    paraumbilical v's
    parietal v's
    parietal v. of Santorini
    parotid v's
    parotid v's, anterior
    parotid v's, posterior
    parumbilical v's
    peduncular v's
    perforating v's
    pericardiac v's
    pericardiacophrenic v's
    peroneal v's
    petrosal v.
    pharyngeal v's
    phrenic v's, inferior
    phrenic v's, superior
    v's of pons
    pontomesencephalic v., an-
        terior
    popliteal v.
    portal v.
    posterior v. of left ventricle
    precentral v. of cerebellum
    prefrontal v's
    prepyloric v.
    v. of pterygoid canal

vein *(continued)*
 pudendal v's, external
 pudendal v., internal
 pulmonary v's
 pulmonary v., left inferior
 pulmonary v., left superior
 pulmonary v., right inferior
 pulmonary v., right superior
 pulp v's
 pyloric v.
 radial v's
 ranine v.
 rectal v's, inferior
 rectal v's, middle
 rectal v., superior
 retromandibular v.
 Retzius' v's
 Rosenthal's v.
 sacral v's, lateral
 sacral v., median
 sacral v., middle
 saphenous v., accessory
 saphenous v., great
 saphenous v., small
 v's of Sappey
 sausaging of v.
 scleral v's
 scrotal v's, anterior
 scrotal v's, posterior
 segmental v., apicoposter-
  ior
 segmental v., inferior lingular
 segmental v., superior lingular
 segmental v. of left lung,
  anterior
 segmental v. of left lung,
  superior
 segmental v. of right lung,
  anterior
 segmental v. of right lung,
  apical
 segmental v. of right lung,
  lateral
 segmental v. of right lung,
  medial

vein *(continued)*
 segmental v. of right lung,
  posterior
 segmental v. of right lung,
  superior
 v. of septum pellucidum,
  anterior
 v. of septum pellucidum,
  posterior
 sigmoid v's
 small v. of heart
 spermatic v.
 spinal v's, anterior
 spinal v's, posterior
 spiral v. of modiolus
 splenic v.
 Stensen's v's
 sternocleidomastoid v.
 striate v's
 stylomastoid v.
 subclavian v.
 subcostal v.
 subcutaneous v's of abdomen
 sublingual v.
 sublobular v's
 submental v.
 superficial v.
 superficial v's of lower limb
 superficial v's of upper
  limb
 superior v's of cerebellum
 supraorbital v.
 suprarenal v., left
 suprarenal v., right
 suprascapular v.
 supratrochlear v's
 sural v's
 sylvian v's
 v's of sylvian fossa
 temporal v's, deep
 temporal v., middle
 temporal v's, superficial
 temporomandibular articular v's
 terminal v.
 testicular v., left
 testicular v., right
 thalamostriate v's, inferior

vein *(continued)*
 thalamostriate v., superior
 thebesian v's
 v's of Thebesius
 thoracic v's, internal
 thoracic v., lateral
 thoracoacromial v.
 thoracoepigastric v's
 thymic v's
 thyroid v., inferior
 thyroid v's, middle
 thyroid v., superior
 tibial v's, anterior
 tibial v's, posterior
 trabecular v's
 tracheal v's
 transverse v. of face
 transverse v's of neck
 transverse v. of scapula
 Trolard's v.
 tympanic v's
 ulnar v's
 v. of uncus
 v's of upper limb
 uterine v's
 varicose v.
 ventricular v's of heart
 ventricular v., inferior
 v. of vermis, inferior
 v. of vermis, superior
 vertebral v.
 vertebral v., accessory
 vertebral v., anterior
 vertebral v's, superficial
 v's of vertebral column
 v's of vertebral column, external
 vesalian v.
 vesical v's
 vestibular v's
 vidian v.
 v's of Vieussens
 vorticose v's
 portal v., hepatic
 portal v. of liver
 basal v., anterior
 pericardial v's

vein harvesting

velocimetry
 Doppler v.
 laser-Doppler v.

velocity
 coronary blood flow v.
 diastolic regurgitant v.
 fiber-shortening (V_{CF}) v.
 maximal transaortic jet v.
 mean aortic flow v.
 mean posterior wall flow v.
 mean pulmonary flow v.
 meter per second (m/sec) v.
 peak aortic flow v.
 peak flow v.
 peak pulmonary flow v.
 peak transmitted v.
 regurgitant v.
 thrombotic threshold v.

vena *pl.* venae
 v. adrenalis dextra
 venae atriales dextrae
 venae atriales sinistrae
 venae atrioventriculares cordis
 venae auditivae internae
 venae bronchiales anteriores
 venae bronchiales posteriores
 v. canaliculi cochleae
 v. cardiaca magna
 v. cardiaca media
 venae cardiacae minimae
 v. cardiaca parva
 v. cava
 venae cavae
 v. cava inferior
 venae cerebri
 venae cerebri anteriores
 venae cerebri inferiores
 venae cerebri internae
 v. cerebri magna
 venae cerebri profundae
 venae cerebri superficiales
 venae cerebri superiores
 venae choroideae oculi

vena *(continued)*
- v. circumflexa iliaca profunda
- v. circumflexa iliaca superficialis
- venae circumflexae laterales femoris
- venae circumflexae mediales femoris
- venae cordis anteriores
- v. cordis magna
- v. cordis media
- venae cordis minimae
- v. cordis parva
- v. coronaria dextra
- v. coronaria sinistra
- venae costoaxillares
- venae digitales communes pedis
- venae digitales pedis dorsales
- v. dorsalis clitoridis profunda
- venae dorsales clitoridis superficiales
- v. dorsalis penis profunda
- venae dorsales penis superficiales
- v. epiploica dextra
- v. epiploica sinistra
- venae esophageae
- v. ethmoidalis anterior
- v. ethmoidalis posterior
- v. facialis anterior
- v. facialis communis
- v. facialis posterior
- v. faciei profunda
- v. femoropoplitea
- venae hepaticae mediae
- inferior v. cava (IVC)
- venae intercapitales
- venae intercapitales manus
- v. intermedia basilica
- v. intermedia cephalica
- v. interventricularis anterior
- v. interventricularis posterior
- v. lienalis

vena *(continued)*
- v. marginalis dextra
- venae massetericae
- v. intermedia antebrachii
- v. mediana basilica
- v. mediana cephalica
- v. mediana colli
- v. intermedia cubiti
- venae mesencephalicae
- venae metacarpeae dorsales
- venae metacarpeae palmares
- venae metatarseae dorsales
- venae metatarseae plantares
- v. ophthalmomeningea
- v. palatina
- venae pericardiales
- v. posterior ventriculi sinistri cordis
- v. pulmonalis inferior dextra
- v. pulmonalis inferior sinistra
- v. pulmonalis superior dextra
- v. pulmonalis superior sinistra
- v. sacralis media
- v. septi pellucidi anterior
- v. septi pellucidi posterior
- v. spiralis modioli
- venae striatae
- superior v. cava (SVC)
- superior v. cava, persistent left
- v. thoracalis lateralis
- v. thyroidea ima
- v. transversa scapulae
- venae vasorum
- venae ventriculares cordis
- venae ventriculi dextri anteriores
- v. ventriculi sinistri posterior
- v. vermis inferior
- v. vermis superior

vena *(continued)*
    venae cardiacae anteriores
    v. obliqua atrii sinistri
    venae esophageales

VenES II Medical Stockings

Venflon cannula

venipuncture

venoarterial admixture

venoatrial

venofibrosis

venogram
    isotope v.
    radionuclide v.
    technetium 99m v.

venography
    isotope v.
    radionuclide v.
    technetium 99m v.

venorrhaphy
    lateral v.

venosclerosis

venose

venosity

venostasis

venotomy

venous
    v. access
    v. cannula
    v. cutdown
    v. distention
    v. Doppler exam
    v. hum (nun's murmur)
    v. reservoir
    v. stasis
    v. ulcer

vent
    intracardiac v.
    pulmonary arterial v.
    slotted needle v.

Ventak automatic implantable
    cardioverter-defibrillator
    pacemaker

ventilation
    intermittent mandatory v.
    (IMV)
    mechanical v.
    pressure cycled v.
    synchronized intermittent
    mandatory v. (SIMV)
    time-cycled v.
    volume cycled v.

ventilator
    MA-1 v.
    pneuPAC v.

venting
    v. aortic Bengash-type nee-
    dle

vent the vein for air

ventricle
    akinetic left v.
    atrialized v.
    auxiliary v.
    common v.
    double-inlet v.
    double outlet v.
    double-outlet left v.
    double-outlet right v.
    dysfunctional left v.
    hypokinetic left v.
    hypoplastic v.
    left v. (LV)
    v. of heart
    left v. of heart
    Mary Allen Engle v.
    right v. (RV)
    right v. of heart
    rudimentary right v.
    single v.

Ventricor pacemaker

ventricular
    v. activation time (VAT)
    v. aneurysm
    v. apex
    v. capture beat

ventricular *(continued)*
  v. cavity
  v. contraction pattern
  v. dysfunction
  v. ectopy
  v. effective refractory period (VERP)
  v. enlargement
  v. extrastimulation
  v. fibrillation
  v. function curve
  v. hypertrophy
  v. lead
  maximum v. elastance (Emax)
  v. overdrive pacing
  v. paroxysmal tachycardia
  v. preexcitation
  v. premature contraction
  v. premature depolarization (VPD)
  v. rate
  recurrent intractable v. tachycardia
  v. refractoriness
  v. refractory period
  v. response
  v. rhythm disturbance
  right v. pressure
  v. segmental contraction
  v. septal defect (VSD)
  v. septal rupture
  v. septal summit
  v. single and double extrastimulation
  v. systole
  v. wall motion

ventricularization
  v. of left atrial pressure pulse

ventricularized
  v. morphology

ventriculoarterial conduit

ventriculoarterial discordance

ventriculoatrial
  v. effective refractory period

ventriculoatrial *(continued)*
  v. time-out

ventriculogram
  axial left anterior oblique v.
  biplane v.
  digital subtraction v.
  dipyridamole thallium v.
  exercise radionuclide v.
  LAO (left anterior oblique) projection v.
  left v. (LVG)
  radionuclide v. (RNV)
  RAO (right anterior oblique) projection v.
  retrograde left v.
  single plane left v.
  xenon v.

ventriculography
  first pass v.
  gated blood pool v.
  left v.
  radionuclide v.

ventriculorrhaphy
  linear v.
  Reed v.

ventriculotomy
  encircling endocardial v.
  endocardial v.
  partial encircling endocardial v.
  transmural v.

ventriculus
  v. cordis dexter/sinister
  v. dexter cordis
  v. sinister cordis

venula
  v. retinae medialis

venular

venule
  high endothelial v's
  macular v.
  nasal v. of retina
  postcapillary v.
  temporal v. of retina

venulitis
    cutaneous necrotizing v.

VeriFlex guide wire

VERP
    ventricular effective refractory period

verrucous carditis

VersaTrax
    V. pacemaker
    V. II pacemaker
    V. pulse generator

vertebrobasilar
    v. insufficiency
    v. occlusive disease

vertebrocarotid

vesicle
    intermediate v's

vessel
    anastomotic v.
    arterioluminal v's
    arteriosinusoidal v's
    atherectomized v.
    blood v.
    caliber of v.
    codominant v.
    collateral v's
    contralateral v.
    cross-pelvic collateral v.
    dominant v.
    great v's
    v. loop
    nondominant v.
    nutrient v's
    patent v.
    peripelvic collateral v.
    sinusoidal v.

Vesseloops rubber band

vestibule
    v. of aorta
    Sibson's v.

VF
    ventricular fibrillation

VH interval

viability
    tissue v.

Viagraph computerized exercise EKG system

Vicor pacemaker

Vicryl suture

videoangiography
    digital v.

Vieussens
    circle of V.
    valve of V.

view
    anterior v.
    apical four-chamber echocardiogram v.
    caudal v.
    four-chamber apical v.
    ice-pick M-mode echocardiogram v.
    LAO (left anterior oblique) v.
    LAO-cranial v.
    left anterior oblique (LAO) v.
    long-axis parasternal v.
    parasternal long-axis echocardiogram v.
    parasternal short-axis v.
    RAO (right anterior oblique) v.
    RAO-caudal v.
    right anterior oblique (RAO) v.
    short-axis parasternal v.
    sitting-up v.
    spider x-ray v.
    subcostal four-chamber echocardiogram v.
    subcostal long-axis echocardiogram v.
    subcostal short-axis echocardiogram v.
    subxiphoid echocardiography v.
    suprasternal notch echocardiogram v.

view *(continued)*
    weeping willow x-ray v.

Vigilon dressing

Vineburg cardiac revascularization procedure

VingMed ultrasound

visceral
    v. heterotaxy
    v. pericardium

viscosity
    blood v.
    plasma v.

Vista pacemaker

Vital
    V. Cooley microvascular
        needle holder
    V. Ryder microvascular
        needle holder

Vitalcor venous catheter

Vitatrax pacemaker

Vitatron
    V. catheter electrode
    V. pacemaker

VLDL
    very low density lipoprotein

VLDL-TG
    VLDL-triglyceride

V_1-like ambulatory lead system

V_5-like ambulatory lead system

Volkmann retractor

volt

voltage
    battery v.
    v. criteria
    increased v. (on EKG)
    low v.
    precordial v.

volume
    atrial emptying v.

volume *(continued)*
    blood v.
    cavity v.
    chamber v.
    circulation v.
    v. of circulation
    diastolic atrial v.
    Dodge area-length method
        for ventricular v.
    end-diastolic v.
    endocardial v.
    end-systolic v.
    epicardial v.
    forward stroke v.
    functional venous v.
    v. infusion
    intravascular v. depletion
    left ventricular chamber v.
    left ventricular end-diastolic v.
    left ventricular inflow v.
        (LVIV)
    left ventricular outflow v.
        (LVOF)
    left ventricular stroke v.
    LV (left ventricular) cavity v.
    mean corpuscular v.
    minute v.
    v. overload
    plasma v.
    prism method for ventricular v.
    pulmonary blood v.
    pyramid method for ventricular v.
    radionuclide stroke v.
    regurgitant stroke v. (RSV)
    right ventricular v.
    Simpson rule method for
        ventricular v.
    stroke v.
    systolic atrial v.
    thermodilution stroke v.
    total stroke v.
    ventricular end-diastolic v.
    von Recklinghausen test v.

von Willebrand blood coagulation factor

VOO pacemaker

Vorse-Webster clamp

vortex
v. cordis

VPB
ventricular premature beat

VPC
ventricular premature complex
ventricular premature contraction

VPT
ventricular paroxysmal tachycardia

VRT
venous return time

VSD
ventricular septal defect

VT
ventricular tachycardia

VT/VF
ventricular tachycardia/ventricular fibrillation

V_1–V_6 (precordial EKG leads)

V_1V_2 curve

VVI pacemaker

VVI/AAI pacemaker

VVT pacemaker

W
W pattern on right atrial
waveform
W wave on echocardi-
ogram

Waardenburg syndrome

Wada
W. hingeless heart valve
prosthesis
W. monocuspid tilting-disk
heart valve
W. prosthesis
W.-Cutter disk prosthetic
valve
W.-Cutter heart valve

waist
cardiac w.
w. of balloon catheter
w. of heart

Wakeling fetal heart monitor

Waldhausen subclavian flap
technique

walk-through angina

wall
akinetic w.
w. amplitude
aneurysm w.
anterior w.
anterior chest w.
anterior w. infarction
anterior left ventricle w.
anterobasal w.
anterolateral w.
anterolateral ventricular w.
aortic w.
apical w.
arterial w.
artery w.
atrial w.
basal w.
capillary w.
chest w.

wall *(continued)*
chest w. adhesions
diaphragmatic w.
dilation of ventricular w.
free w.
friable w.
inferior w.
inferior left ventricular w.
inferobasilar w.
inferoposterior w.
w. ischemia
lateral w.
left ventricular free w.
left ventricular posterior w.
left ventricular posterior w.
excursion
midventricular w.
w. motion
w. motion abnormality
w. motion analysis
w. motion score
w. motion score index
w. motion study
myocardial w.
posterior w.
posterior w. excursion
posterior w. infarct
posterior left ventricular w.
posterobasal w.
posterobasilar w.
posterolateral ventricu-
lar w.
posterolateral w.
posteroseptal w.
right ventricular free w.
w. sluggishness
septal w.
w. stress
w. structure
w. tension
w. thickening
thickening of ventricular w.
w. thickness
w. thinning
ventricular w.
vessel w.

Wall arterial stent

Wallace Flexihub central venous pressure cannula

Wallstent
W. flexible, self-expanding
wire-mesh stent
self-expanding W.
W. spring-loaded stent

Walter-Deaver retractor

wandering
w. atrial pacemaker (WAP)
w. baseline
w. heart

Wangensteen
W. anastomosis clamp
W. awl
W. patent ductus clamp

Ward-Romano syndrome

Wardrop method

warfarin
w. sodium
w. therapy

warmer
Bair Hugger w.
blood w.

WarmTouch patient warming
system

warm-up phenomenon

Warren shunt

washout
delayed w.
w. phase
w. rate
thallium w.

wasting
potassium w.

water
w. brash
w. wheel murmur

water-hammer pulse

watershed
w. infarction

watershed *(continued)*
w. region

Waterston
W. extrapericardial anasto-
mosis
W. groove
W. pacing wire
W. shunt
W.-Cooley procedure
W.-Cooley shunt

Watson heart valve holder

watt-seconds

wave
A w.
a w.
w. amplitude
anacrotic w.
anadicrotic w.
arterial w.
atrial pressure w.
atrial repolarization w.
bifid P w.
biphasic P w.
biphasic T w.
C w.
c w.
cannon a w.
catacrotic w.
catadicrotic w.
c-v systolic w.
D w.
deep S w.
delta w.
dicrotic w.
diphasic P w.
diphasic T w.
E w.
E w. to A w. (E:A)
enlarge T w.
F w.
f w. (jugular venous pulse)
fibrillary w.
flat P w.
flat T w.
flattening of T w.
flipped T w.

wave *(continued)*
    flutter w.
    flutter-fibrillation w's
    giant a w.
    giant a w.
    H w.
    h w.
    hyperacute T w.
    inverted P w.
    inverted Q w.
    inverted T w.
    inverted U w.
    w. inversion
    inversion of T w.
    J w.
    low-amplitude w.
    nonconducted w.
    nondiagnostic Q w.
    non-Q w.
    nonspecific T w.
    notched w.
    Mayer w.
    Osborne w.
    oscillation w.
    overflow w.
    P w.
    papillary w.
    pathologic Q w.
    peaked P w.
    percussion w.
    peridicrotic w.
    pointed P w.
    polymorphic slow w.
    post excitation w.
    postextrasystolic T w.
    precordial A w.
    predicrotic w.
    preexcitation w.
    propagation of R w.
    pseudonormalization of
     T w.
    pulse w.
    Q w.
    QRS w.
    QS w.
    R w.
    r w.
    R' w.
    R'R" w.

wave *(continued)*
    rapid filling w.
    recoil w.
    regurgitant w.
    respiratory w.
    retrograde P w.
    RF w.
    S w.
    sawtooth w.
    septal Q w.
    SF w.
    sharp w.
    sine w.
    slow filling w.
    ST w.
    ST-T w.
    T w.
    Ta w.
    tall P w.
    tall R w.
    terminal negativity of P w.
    tidal w.
    transverse w.
    Traube-Hering w's
    tricrotic w.
    TU w.
    T upright w.
    U w.
    upright R w.
    upright T w.
    upright U w.
    V w.
    v w.
    vasomotor w.
    ventricular w.
    W w.
    widened P w.
    x w.
    x' w. (right atrial catheteri-
     zation)
    x descent of the "a" w.
    X w. of Öhnell
    y w.
    y descent of the "a" w.

waveform
    w. analysis
    Edmark monophasic w.
    Gurvich biphasic w.
    pressure w.

waveform *(continued)*
    quasi-sinusoidal biphas-
        ic w.

wavelength

wax
    bone w.

waxing and waning
    w. a. w. chest pain
    w. a. w. in intensity

wean

weaned
    w. from respirator
    w. off cardiopulmonary by-
        pass

weaning
    ventilator w.

Weavenit
    W. patch graft
    W. prosthesis
    W. valve prosthesis
    W. vascular prosthesis

web
    inferior vena cava w.
    pulmonary arterial w.
    venous w.

Webb vein stripper

Weber aortic clamp

Weber-Christian disease

Weber-Osler-Rendu syndrome

Webster
    W. coronary sinus catheter
    W. infusion cannula
    W. orthogonal electrode
        catheter

Weck clip

wedge
    w. angiogram
    arterial w.
    w. arteriogram
    mediastinal w.
    w. position

wedge *(continued)*
    w. pressure
    w. pressure balloon
    pulmonary artery w.
    pulmonary capillary w.
    pulmonary w. pressure

weeping willow x-ray view

Wegener granulomatosis

Weinberg rib spreader

Weitlaner retractor

well
    pericardial w.

Wenckebach
    W. arterioventricular block
    W. cardioptosis
    W. cycle
    W. disease
    W. heart block
    W. pathway
    W. period
    W. phenomenon
    W. sign

Werlhof disease

Werner syndrome

Wesolowski
    W. bypass graft
    W. Teflon graft
    W. vascular prosthesis

Wessex prosthetic valve

Westergren
    W. method
    W. sedimentation rate

Westphal hemostatic forceps

wet reading of x-ray

Wexler catheter

whip
    catheter w.

whipping
    systolic w.

Whipple disease

white
  w. clot syndrome
  w. thrombus

white-coat hypertension

whole blood cardioplegia

Wholey
  W. Hi-Torque floppy guide
    wire
  W. Hi-Torque modified J-
    guide wire
  W. Hi-Torque standard
    guide wire
  W. wire

whoop
  systolic w.

whooping murmur

whorling of myocardial cells

wide
  w. complex rhythm
  w. QRS tachycardia

widely split second sound

widened cardiac silhouette

width
  atrial pulse w.
  pulse w.
  ventricular pulse w.

Wiener filter

Wigle scale for ventricular hypertrophy

Wilkie disease

Wiktor coronary stent

Willauer
  W. intrathoracic forceps
  W. thoracic scissors
  W.-Allis thoracic forceps
  W.-Allis thoracic tissue for-
    ceps

William
  W. Harvey arterial blood fil-
    ter

William (continued)
  W. Harvey cardiotomy res-
    ervoir

Williams
  W. cardiac device
  W. L-R guiding catheter
  W. syndrome
  W. vessel-holding forceps

Williamson sign

Willis
  circle of W.

Wilmer scissors

Wilms tumor

Wilson
  W. central terminal
  W. rib spreader
  W. vein stripper

Wilton-Webster coronary sinus
  thermodilution catheter

windkessel effect

windlass
  Spanish w.

window
  acoustic w.
  aortic w.
  aorticopulmonary w.
  aortic pulmonary w.
  aortopulmonary w.
  pericardial w.
  pleuropericardial w.
  tachycardia w.

windsock
  w. aneurysm
  w. sign

winged scapula

Winiwarter-Buerger disease

Wintrobe sedimentation rate

wire
  ACS microglide w.
  Amplatz torque w.
  angiographic guide w.

wire *(continued)*
    atrial pacing w.
    auger w.
    Babcock stainless steel suture w.
    Bentson w.
    central core w.
    coronary w.
    Cragg Convertible w.
    curved J-exchange w.
    w. cutter
    delivery w.
    dock w.
    docking w.
    Eder-Puestow w.
    epicardial pacing w.
    flexible steerable w.
    floppy-tipped guide w.
    guide w.
    Hancock test cardiac pacing w.
    high-torque w.
    J-tip guide w.
    J-tip w.
    Killip w.
    pacing w.
    steerable w.
    sternal w.
    Stertzer-Myler extension w.
    w. suture
    test pacing w.
    Waterston pacing w.
    Wholey w.

wiring
    sternal w.

wiry pulse

Wiskott-Aldrich syndrome

Wister vascular clamp

Wizard
    W. cardiac device
    W. disposable inflation device

Wolff-Parkinson-White (WPW)
    W.-P.-W. bypass tract
    W.-P.-W. reentrant tachycardia

Wolff-Parkinson-White *(continued)*
    W.-P.-W. syndrome

Wolf-Hirschorn syndrome

Wolman syndrome

Wolvek
    W. fixation device
    W. sternal approximation fixation instrument
    W. sternal approximator

Wood
    W. aortography needle
    W. units index for resistance

Woodbridge ligature

wooden-shoe heart

Woodward
    W. hemostat
    W. thoracic artery forceps

Woodworth phenomenon

woody
    w. edema
    w. thyroiditis

Wooler mitral annuloplasty

work
    w. capacity
    cardiac w. index
    left ventricular stroke w. (LVSW)
    right ventricular stroke w. (RVSW)
    stroke w. index

workload
    Bruce stage w.
    w. of heart
    increased w.
    5-MET w.
    7-MET w.

wound
    penetrating cardiac w.
    separate stab w.
    surgical w.
    thoracotomy w.

woven
  w. Dacron tube graft
  w. Teflon

woven-tube vascular graft prosthesis

WPW
  Wolff-Parkinson-White

wrap
  cardiac muscle w.

wrapping
  w. of abdominal aortic an-
    eurysm
  aneurysm w.

Wrisberg ganglion

Wylie
  W. carotid artery clamp
  W. endarterectomy set
  W. endarterectomy strip-
    per
  W. stripper

X
  x depression of jugular ve-
    nous pulse
  x descent of the "a" wave
  x descent of jugular venous
    pulse

xanthelasma

xanthogranuloma

xanthoma
  x. striatum palmare
  x. tendinosum
  tendinous x.

xenograft
  bovine pericardial heart
    valve x.
  Carpentier-Edwards porci-
    ne x.
  Hancock porcine x.
  Ionescu-Shiley pericar-
    dial x.
  stentless porcine x.

Xenomedica prosthetic valve

xenon
  x. 127
  x. 133
  x. chloride excimer laser
  x.-enhanced computed to-
    mography
  x. 133 scan
  x. 133 ventriculography

Xenotech prosthetic valve

xenotransplant

Xeroform
  X. gauze

Xeroform *(continued)*
  X. dressing

xiphisternum

xiphocostal

xiphodynia

xiphoid
  x. angle
  x. cartilage
  x. process

xiphoidectomy

xiphoiditis

X-linked dilated cardiomyopathy

XO syndrome

XT cardiac device

X wave of Öhnell

x wave
  venous pulse x w.

x′ wave
  x′ w. pressure on right
    atrial catheterization

XXXX syndrome

XXXY syndrome

xylol pulse indicator

Xyrel pacemaker

Xyticon 5950 bipolar demand
  pacemaker

XYZ lead system

Y
 Y axis
 Y connector
 Y-shaped graft
 Y stent

y
 y depression of jugular venous pulse
 y descent
 y descent of "a" wave
 y descent of jugular venous
  pulse
 y descent trough
 y descent wave
 y wave
 y wave pressure on right
  atrial catheterization

YAG
 yttrium-aluminium-garnet
 YAG laser

YAG/1064
 Laserscope Y.

Yankauer suction tube

Yasargil
 Y. aneurysm clip-applier
 Y. arachnoid knife
 Y. artery forceps
 Y. bayonet scissors
 Y. carotid clamp
 Y. microscissors

yeast

yttrium-aluminum-garnet (YAG)
 laser

Z
    Z line
    Z point
        Z point pressure on left atrial catheterization
        Z point pressure on right atrial catheterization
    Z stent

Zener diode

Zenotech graft material

zero-order kinetics

zigzag stent

Zimmer antiembolism support stockings

Zimmermann arch

zipper scar

Zipster rib guillotine

Zitron pacemaker

Z-Med catheter

Zoll
    Z. NTP noninvasive pacemaker
    Z. PD1200 external defibrillator

Zollinger
    Z.-Gilmore intraluminal vein stripper
    Z.-Gilmore vein stripper

zone
    ischemic z.
    subendocardial z.
    tendinous z's of heart
    transition z.
    vascular z.

Zucker
    Z. cardiac catheter
    Z. multipurpose bipolar catheter
    Z.-Myler cardiac device

Zuker bipolar pacing electrode

Zyrel pacemaker

Zytron pacemaker

APPENDIX A
Drugs Used in Cardiology

Below are the names of generic and ℞ brand name drugs used in cardiology, as shown in the *Saunders Pharmaceutical Xref Book*. The drugs are categorized by their "indications"—also called "designated use," "approved use," or "therapeutic action"—which group together drugs used for a similar purpose. The indications shown below are broad categories of therapeutic action. Individual drugs may be placed in subcategories or have specifically targeted diseases beyond the scope of this listing. For complete information about the drugs listed below, including each drug's availability, specific indications, forms of administration, and dosages, please consult the current edition of *Saunders Pharmaceutical Word Book*.

Anticoagulants
ancrod
anisindione
antithrombin III (AT-III)
ardeparin sodium
Arvin
ATnativ
bivalirudin
Calciparine
Carfin
Coumadin
coumarin
dalteparin sodium
danaparoid sodium
desirudin
dicumarol
enoxaparin sodium
Flocor
Fragmin
Fraxiparine ⓒⒶ⒩
Hep-Lock; Hep-Lock U/P
heparin calcium
heparin sodium
Heparin Lock Flush
Hirulog
Innohep
Kybernin
Liquaemin Sodium
Lovenox
Miradon
nadroparin calcium
Normiflo

Anticoagulants (cont.)
Orgaran
Revasc
Sofarin
Thrombate III
tinzaparin sodium
Vasoflux
Viprinex ⓒⒶ⒩
warfarin
warfarin sodium

Antihypertensives
[see also: Cardiac Agents]
Antihypertensives, α-Blockers
Apo-Terazosin ⓒⒶ⒩
Cardura
doxazosin mesylate
Hytrin
Hytrin ⓒⒶ⒩
labetalol HCl
Minipress
Minizide 1; Minizide 2; Minizide 5
Normodyne
Novo-Terazosin ⓒⒶ⒩
phentolamine mesylate
prazosin HCl
Regitine
terazosin HCl
Trandate
Antihypertensives, ACE Inhibitors
Accupril

Antihypertensives, ACE Inhibitors (cont.)
Accuretic ⓐ
Altace
benazepril HCl
Capoten
Capozide 25/15; Capozide 25/25;
    Capozide 50/15; Capozide 50/25
captopril
cilazapril
enalapril maleate
enalaprilat
fosinopril sodium
Inhibace
Lexxel
lisinopril
Lotensin
Lotensin HCT 5/6.25; Lotensin
    HCT 10/12.5; Lotensin HCT
    20/12.5; Lotensin HCT 20/25
Lotrel
Mavik
Mavik ⓐ
moexipril HCl
Monopril
Prinivil
Prinzide
Prinzide 12.5; Prinzide 25
quinapril HCl
ramipril
Renormax
spirapril HCl
Tarka
Teczem
trandolapril
Uniretic
Univasc
Vaseretic 5-12.5; Vaseretic 10-25
Vasotec
Vasotec I.V.
Zestoretic
Zestril

Antihypertensives, Angiotensin II Inhibitors
Atacand
Avalide
Avapro
candesartan cilexetil
Cozaar
Diovan

Antihypertensives, Angiotensin II Inhibitors (cont.)
Diovan HCT
Hyzaar
irbesartan
losartan potassium
Micardis
tasosartan
telmisartan
valsartan
Verdia

Antihypertensives, β-Blockers
acebutolol HCl
atenolol
Betachron E-R
betaxolol HCl
bisoprolol fumarate
Blocadren
celiprolol HCl
Corgard
Corzide 40/5; Corzide 80/5
Inderal
Inderal LA
Inderide 40/25; Inderide 80/25
Inderide LA 80/50; Inderide LA
    120/50; Inderide LA 160/50
Ipran
Kerlone
labetalol HCl
Levatol
Lopressor
Lopressor HCT 50/25; Lopressor
    HCT 100/25; Lopressor HCT
    100/50
metoprolol succinate
metoprolol tartrate
nadolol
Normodyne
penbutolol sulfate
pindolol
propranolol HCl
Sectral
Selecor
Tenoretic 50; Tenoretic 100
Tenormin
Timolide 10-25
timolol maleate
Toprol XL
Trandate
Visken

Antihypertensives, β-Blockers (cont.)
Zebeta
Ziac
Antihypertensives, Calcium Channel Blockers
Adalat
Adalat CC; Adalat Oros
amlodipine
amlodipine besylate
Baypress
Calan
Calan SR
Cardene
Cardene I.V.
Cardene SR
Cardizem
Cardizem SR; Cardizem CD
Chronovera ⓒ
Covera-HS
Dilacor XR
diltiazem HCl
diltiazem malate
DynaCirc
DynaCirc CR
felodipine
Isoptin
Isoptin SR
isradipine
lacidipine
Lacipil
Lexxel
Lotrel
mibefradil dihydrochloride
nicardipine HCl
nifedipine
nimodipine
Nimotop
nisoldipine
nitrendipine
Norvasc
Plendil
Posicor
Procardia
Procardia XL
Sular
Tarka
Teczem
Tiamate
Tiazac

Antihypertensives, Calcium Channel Blockers (cont.)
verapamil HCl
Verelan
Verelan PM
Antihypertensives, Diuretics
[see also: Diuretics]
Accuretic ⓒ
Aldactazide
Aldactone
Aldoclor-150; Aldoclor-250
Aldoril 15; Aldoril 25; Aldoril D30; Aldoril D50
Alodopa-15; Alodopa-25
amiloride HCl
Apresazide 25/25; Apresazide 50/50; Apresazide 100/50
Aprozide 25/25; Aprozide 50/50; Aprozide 100/50
Aquatensen
Avalide
bendroflumethiazide
benzthiazide
bumetanide
Bumex
Cam-Ap-Es
Capozide 25/15; Capozide 25/25; Capozide 50/15; Capozide 50/25
Chloroserpine
chlorothiazide
chlorthalidone
Combipres 0.1; Combipres 0.2; Combipres 0.3
Corzide 40/5; Corzide 80/5
Demadex
Demi-Regroton
Diovan HCT
Diucardin
Diupres-250; Diupres-500
Diurese
Diurigen
Diuril
Diutensen-R
Dyazide
Dyrenium
Edecrin
Edecrin Sodium
Enduron
Enduronyl; Enduronyl Forte
Esidrix

4   Antihypertensives, Diuretics

Antihypertensives, Diuretics (cont.)

Esimil
ethacrynate sodium
ethacrynic acid
Exna
Ezide
furosemide
Hydrap-ES
Hydrazide 25/25; Hydrazide 50/50
Hydro-Par
Hydro-Serp
hydrochlorothiazide (HCT; HCTZ)
HydroDIURIL
hydroflumethiazide
Hydromox
Hydropres-25
Hydropres-50
Hydroserpine #1; Hydroserpine #2
Hydrosine 25, Hydrosine 50
Hygroton
Hyzaar
indapamide
Inderide 40/25; Inderide 80/25
Inderide LA 80/50; Inderide LA
    120/50; Inderide LA 160/50
Lasix
Lopressor HCT 50/25; Lopressor
    HCT 100/25; Lopressor HCT
    100/50
Lotensin HCT 5/6.25; Lotensin
    HCT 10/12.5; Lotensin HCT
    20/12.5; Lotensin HCT 20/25
Lozol
mannitol (D-mannitol)
Marpres
Maxzide
Metahydrin
Metatensin #2; Metatensin #4
methyclothiazide
metolazone
Microzide
Midamor
Minizide 1; Minizide 2; Minizide 5
Moduretic
Mykrox
Naqua
Naturetin
Oretic
Osmitrol

Antihypertensives, Diuretics (cont.)

polythiazide
Prinzide
Prinzide 12.5; Prinzide 25
quinethazone
Rauzide
Regroton
Renese
Renese-R
Salazide; Salazide-Demi
Saluron
Salutensin; Salutensin-Demi
Ser-Ap-Es
Serpazide
Sodium Diuril
spironolactone
Tenoretic 50; Tenoretic 100
Thalitone
Timolide 10-25
torsemide
Tri-Hydroserpine
triamterene
trichlormethiazide
Unipres
Uniretic
Vaseretic 5-12.5; Vaseretic 10-25
Zaroxolyn
Zestoretic
Ziac

Antihypertensives, Vasodilators

Apresazide 25/25; Apresazide 50/50;
    Apresazide 100/50
Apresoline
Aprozide 25/25; Aprozide 50/50;
    Aprozide 100/50
Arfonad
Cam-Ap-Es
Corlopam
Cyclo-Prostin
diazoxide
epoprostenol
fenoldopam mesylate
Flolan
hydralazine HCl
Hydrap-ES
Hydrazide 25/25; Hydrazide 50/50
Hyperstat
Loniten
Marpres

Antihypertensives, Vasodilators (cont.)
minoxidil
Nitro-Bid IV
nitroglycerin
Nitropress
Proglycem
Ser-Ap-Es
Serpazide
sodium nitroprusside
Tri-Hydroserpine
Tridil
trimethaphan camsylate
Unipres
Antihypertensives, Other
Aldomet
Aldomet; Aldomet Ester HCl
Amodopa
Catapres
Catapres-TTS-1; Catapres-TTS-2; Catapres-TTS-3
clonidine HCl
Demser
deserpidine
Dibenzyline
guanabenz acetate
guanadrel sulfate
guanethidine monosulfate
guanfacine HCl
Hylorel
Inversine
Ismelin
mecamylamine HCl
methyldopa
methyldopate HCl
metyrosine
Moderil
phenoxybenzamine HCl
pinacidil
Pindac
Raudixin
Rauverid
rauwolfia serpentina
rescinnamine
reserpine
Serpalan
Tenex
Wytensin

Cardiac Agents
[see also: Antihypertensives; Diuretics]
Cardiac Agents, Antianginals
acebutolol HCl
Adalat
Adalat CC; Adalat Oros
amlodipine
amlodipine besylate
atenolol
bepridil HCl
Betachron E-R
Blocadren
Calan
Calan SR
Cardene
Cardilate
Cardizem
Cardizem SR; Cardizem CD
celiprolol HCl
Corgard
Covera-HS
Deponit
Dilacor XR
Dilatrate-SR
diltiazem HCl
diltiazem malate
Duotrate; Duotrate 45
erythrityl tetranitrate
Imdur
Inderal
Inderal LA
Ipran
Ismo
Iso-Bid
Isoptin
Isoptin SR
Isordil
isosorbide dinitrate
isosorbide mononitrate
Isotrate
Isotrate ER
Lopressor
metoprolol succinate
metoprolol tartrate
mibefradil dihydrochloride
Minitran
Monoket
nadolol
nicardipine HCl
nifedipine

Cardiac Agents, Antianginals (cont.)

Nitrek
Nitro-Bid
Nitro-Bid IV
Nitro-Derm
Nitro-Dur
Nitro-Time
Nitrocine
Nitrodisc
Nitrogard
nitroglycerin
Nitroglyn
Nitrol
Nitrolingual Pumpspray ⓒᴬ
Nitrong
NitroQuick
Nitrostat
Norvasc
NTS
pentaerythritol tetranitrate (PETN)
Pentylan
Peritrate
Peritrate SA
pindolol
Posicor
Procardia
Procardia XL
propranolol HCl
ranolazine HCl
Sectral
Selecor
Sorbitrate
Sorbitrate SA
Tenormin
Tiamate
Tiazac
timolol maleate
Toprol XL
Transderm-Nitro
Tridil
Trinipatch ⓒᴬ
Vascor
verapamil HCl
Verelan
Visken

Cardiac Agents, Antiarrhythmics

Adenocard
adenosine
Amio-Aqueous

Cardiac Agents, Antiarrhythmics (cont.)

amiodarone HCl
Betachron E-R
Betapace
bretylium tosylate
Bretylol
Brevibloc
Calan
Calan SR
Cardioquin
Cardizem
Cardizem SR; Cardizem CD
cifenline succinate
Cipralan
Cordarone
Corvert
Covera-HS
Crystodigin
digitoxin
digoxin
Dilacor XR
diltiazem HCl
diltiazem malate
disopyramide phosphate
esmolol HCl
Ethmozine
flecainide acetate
ibutilide fumarate
Inderal
Inderal LA
Ipran
Isoptin
Isoptin SR
Lanoxicaps
Lanoxin
lidocaine HCl
LidoPen
mexiletine HCl
Mexitil
moricizine HCl
Napamide
Norpace
Norpace CR
Pacerone
procainamide HCl
Procan SR
Procanbid
Promine
Pronestyl

Cardiac Agents, Antiarrhythmics (cont.)
Pronestyl-SR
propafenone HCl
propranolol HCl
Quin-Release
Quinaglute
Quinalan
Quinidex
quinidine gluconate
quinidine polygalacturonate
quinidine sulfate
Quinora
Rhythmin
RSD-921
Rythmol
sotalol HCl
Tambocor
Tiamate
Tiazac
tocainide HCl
Tonocard
verapamil HCl
Verelan
Xylocaine HCl IV for Cardiac Arrhythmias

Cardiac Agents, Congestive Heart Failure Agents
Accupril
Accuretic Ⓐ
Aldactazide
Aldactone
amiloride HCl
amrinone lactate
Aquatensen
Arkin Z
bumetanide
Bumex
Capoten
Capozide 25/15; Capozide 25/25; Capozide 50/15; Capozide 50/25
captopril
carvedilol
chlorthalidone
cilazapril
Combipres 0.1; Combipres 0.2; Combipres 0.3
Coreg
Crystodigin
Demadex

Cardiac Agents, Congestive Heart Failure Agents (cont.)
Demi-Regroton
digitoxin
digoxin
dobutamine HCl
Dobutrex
dopamine HCl
Dyazide
Dyrenium
Edecrin
Edecrin Sodium
enalapril maleate
enalaprilat
Enbrel
Enduron
Esidrix
etanercept
ethacrynate sodium
ethacrynic acid
Ezide
furosemide
Hydro-Par
hydrochlorothiazide (HCT; HCTZ)
HydroDIURIL
Hygroton
Inhibace
Inocor
Intropin
Lanoxicaps
Lanoxin
Lasix
levosimendan
lisinopril
Maxzide
methyclothiazide
metolazone
Microzide
Midamor
milrinone lactate
Moduretic
Mykrox
Natrecor
nesiritide
Oretic
Primacor
Primacor in 5% Dextrose
Prinivil
Prinzide
Prinzide 12.5; Prinzide 25

Cardiac Agents, Congestive Heart Failure Agents (cont.)
quinapril HCl
Simdax
spironolactone
Thalitone
torsemide
triamterene
Vaseretic 5-12.5; Vaseretic 10-25
Vasotec
Vasotec I.V.
vesnarinone
Zaroxolyn
Zestoretic
Zestril
Cardiac Agents, Vasopressors
Adrenalin Chloride
Ana-Guard
Aramine
dobutamine HCl
Dobutrex
dopamine HCl
dopamine HCl in 5% dextrose
ephedrine sulfate
epinephrine
epinephrine HCl
Epinephrine Pediatric
EpiPen; EpiPen Jr.
Intropin
isoproterenol HCl
Isuprel
Levophed
mephentermine sulfate
metaraminol bitartrate
methoxamine HCl
midodrine HCl
Neo-Synephrine
norepinephrine bitartrate
phenylephrine HCl
ProAmatine
Sus-Phrine
Vasoxyl
Wyamine Sulfate
Cardiac Agents, Other
5G1.1-SC
alprostadil
Berinert-P
C1-esterase-inhibitor, human
Indocin I.V.
indomethacin sodium trihydrate

Cardiac Agents, Other (cont.)
Pravachol
pravastatin sodium
Prostin VR Pediatric
simvastatin
TNK-tPA
Vasoprost
Zocor

Diuretics
[see also: Antihypertensives, Diuretics; Cardiac Agents, Congestive Heart Failure Agents]
acetazolamide
acetazolamide sodium
ammonium chloride
caffeine
caffeine, citrated
chlorothiazide
Daranide
Dazamide
Diamox
dichlorphenamide
Diurese
Diurigen
Diuril
Ismotic
isosorbide
Metahydrin
Naqua
Sodium Diuril
urea
Ureaphil

Enzymes
Enzymes, Thrombolytic
[see also: Thrombolytic Agents]
Abbokinase
Abbokinase Open-Cath
anistreplase
Eminase
Kabikinase
r-ProUK
Retavase
reteplase
saruplase
Streptase

Enzymes, Thrombolytic (cont.)
streptokinase (SK)
urokinase

Lipid-lowering Agents
Apo-Gemfibrozil 🇨🇦
atorvastatin calcium
Atromid-S
Baycol
cerivastatin sodium
CholestaGel
cholestyramine resin
Choloxin
clofibrate
colesevelam HCl
Colestid
colestipol HCl
dextrothyroxine sodium
fenofibrate
fluvastatin sodium
Gemcor
gemfibrozil
lecithin
Lescol
Lipitor
Lipo-Nicin/100
Lipo-Nicin/300
LoCholest; LoCholest Light
Lopid
Lorelco
lovastatin
Mevacor
niacin
Niacor
Niaspan
Nicolar
Novo-Gemfibrozil 🇨🇦
Pravachol
pravastatin sodium
Prevalite
probucol
Questran; Questran Light
simvastatin
Tricor
ZD 4522
Zocor

Peripheral Vasodilators
Cerespan
cilostazol
Cyclan
cyclandelate
Cyclo-Prostin
Cyclospasmol
Cyclospasmol 🇨🇦
epoprostenol
Ethaquin
Ethatab
ethaverine HCl
Ethavex-100
Flolan
flunarizine HCl
Genabid
Isovex
isoxsuprine HCl
Lipo-Nicin/100
Lipo-Nicin/300
niacin
Niacor
Niaspan
papaverine HCl
Pavabid
Pavabid HP
Pavagen TD
Pavarine
Pavased
Pavatine
Paverolan
pentoxifylline
Pletal
Priscoline HCl
Sibelium
tolazoline HCl
Trental
Vasodilan
Voxsuprine

Platelet Aggregation Inhibitors
[see also: Cardiac Agents]
abciximab
Aggrastat
Aggrenox
Apo-Ticlopidine 🇨🇦
aspirin
cilostazol
clopidogrel bisulfate

Platelet Aggregation Inhibitors
  (cont.)
  dipyridamole
  Easprin
  eptifibatide
  Integrilin
  Persantine
  Plavix
  Pletal
  ReoPro
  Ticlid
  ticlopidine HCl
  tirofiban HCl
  ZORprin

Thrombolytic Agents
  [*see also: Enzymes, Thrombolytic*]
  Abbokinase
  Abbokinase Open-Cath
  Activase
  Agrylin
  alteplase
  Eminase
  Kabikinase
  lanoteplase
  r-ProUK
  saruplase
  Streptase
  urokinase
  xemilofiban HCl